ADVANCES IN

Otolaryngology—Head and Neck Surgery®

VOLUME 14

ADVANCES IN

Otolaryngology—Head and Neck Surgery®

VOLUMES 1 THROUGH 11 (OUT OF PRINT)

VOLUME 12

Supracricoid Partial Laryngectomy, *by Jean-Louis Lefebvre and Dominique Chevalier*

Intratympanic Pharmacotherapy for Inner Ear Disorders, *by Lorne S. Parnes*

Guidelines for Inpatient Versus Outpatient Adenotonsillectomy in Children, *by Michael J. Cunningham*

Laser Surgery in the Management of Carcinoma of the Supraglottic Larynx and Hypopharynx, *by Heinrich H. Rudert*

The Special Child's Airway From Nose to Larynx, *by N. Wendell Todd*

What's New in the Management of Respiratory Papillomatosis? *by Frank L. Rimell*

Carcinoma of the Nasopharynx, *by William Ignace Wei*

The Use of Biological Therapy in Cancer of the Head and Neck, *by Jeffrey N. Myers*

Septoplasty and Rhinoplasty in the Pediatric Age Group, *by Stephen S. Park and Charles W. Gross*

Screening for Hearing Loss in Neonates: Where Do We Stand? *by Yvonne S. Sininger*

Management of the Abnormally Patulous Eustachian Tube, *by Charles D. Bluestone*

Contemporary Aspects of Nasal Reconstruction, *by Shan Baker*

Anesthesia for the Pediatric Otolaryngic Patient, *by Jimmy Scott Hill and Peter J. Davis*

VOLUME 13

Intrauterine Management of Congenital Anomalies, *by Marc H. Hedrick, Michael T. Longaker, and Michael R. Harrison*

Progressive Sensorineural Hearing Loss in Children: Diagnosis and Management, *by Margaret A. Kenna and Nancy Sculerati*

Communication Disorders in Children: Prevention, Identification, and Outcomes, *by Cheryl K. Messick*

Assistive Listening Devices, *by Noel L. Cohen and Susan B. Waltzman*

Habilitation of Hearing-Impaired Children, *by Annelle V. Hodges and Thomas J. Balkany*

Osseointegrated Implants in Otology, *by Lawrence R. Lustig and John Niparko*

Diagnosis and Management of Acute Facial Palsies, *by Brian P. Perry and Bruce J. Gantz*

Endoscopic Transnasal Hypophysectomy, *by Ricardo L. Carrau and Hae-Dong Jho*

Skull Base Cerebrospinal Fluid Leaks and Encephaloceles, *by Craig A. Buchman, Francisco J. Civantos, and Roy R. Casiano*

Nasal Obstruction in Infants and Children: Evaluation and Management, *by William S. Crysdale and Per G. Djupesland*

The Allergic Child: Chronic Sinusitis and Otitis, *by David S. Hurst*

Diagnosis and Treatment of Cervicofacial Masses in Children, *by David E. Tunkel and Steven M. Kelly*

Management of Cervical Metastasis in Head and Neck Cancer, *by Ehab Hanna and James Suen*

Cosmetic Laser Skin Resurfacing: A Practical Guide, *by Jeffrey N. Hausfeld*

Survival in the Era of Managed Care, *by K. J. Lee, Jill Cobert-Alvarez, and Mark E. Lee*

ADVANCES IN

Otolaryngology—Head and Neck Surgery®

VOLUME 14

Editor-in-Chief
Eugene N. Myers, MD
Professor and Chairman, Department of Otolaryngology, University of
Pittsburgh School of Medicine, Pittsburgh, Pa

Associate Editor
Charles D. Bluestone, MD
Professor of Otolaryngology, University of Pittsburgh School of
Medicine; Director, Department of Pediatric Otolaryngology, Children's
Hospital of Pittsburgh, Pittsburgh, Pa

Editorial Board
Derald E. Brackmann, MD
Clinical Professor of Otolaryngology and Neurosurgery, University of
Southern California School of Medicine; President, House Ear Clinic;
Board of Directors, House Ear Institute, Los Angeles

Charles J. Krause, MD
Professor, Department of Otolaryngology, Senior Associate Dean,
University of Michigan School of Medicine; Senior Associate Director,
University of Michigan Hospital, Ann Arbor

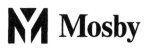 Mosby

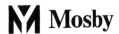

Publisher: Gretchen Murphy
Developmental Editor: Karen Moehlman
Manager, Periodical Editing: Kirk Swearingen
Production Editor: Pat Costigan
Project Supervisor, Production: Joy Moore
Composition Specialist, Production: Karie House
Manager, Literature Services: Idelle L. Winer

Printed in the United States of America
Printing/binding by The Maple-Vail Book Manufacturing Group

Editorial Office
Mosby, Inc.
11830 Westline Industrial Drive
St. Louis, Missouri 63146
Customer Service: periodical.service@mosby.com
            www.mosby.com/periodicals

International Standard Serial Number: 0887–6916
International Standard Book Number: 0–323-00937-9

Contributors

Eugene L. Alford, MD
Clinical Assistant Professor, Baylor College of Medicine; Director, Texas Center for Facial Plastic and Reconstructive Surgery, Houston

Thomas W. Braun, DMD, PhD
Interim Dean, School of Dental Medicine, University of Pittsburgh; Professor and Chairman, Department of Oral and Maxillofacial Surgery, University of Pittsburgh Medical Center, Pittsburgh, Pa

Ricardo L. Carrau, MD
Associate Professor, Department of Otolaryngology, University of Pittsburgh Medical Center, Pittsburgh, Pa

W. Gregory Chernoff, MD, BSc, FRCS(C)
Clinical Assistant Professor, Indiana University, Indianapolis

Rick A. Friedman, MD, PhD
Associate, House Ear Clinic; Section Chief, Hereditary Disorders of the Ear, House Ear Institute, University of Southern California, Los Angeles

Ann M. Gillenwater, MD
Assistant Professor of Medicine, University of Texas M. D. Anderson Cancer Center, Houston

Helmuth Goepfert, MD
Professor of Surgery and Chairman, Department of Head and Neck Surgery, University of Texas M. D. Anderson Cancer Center, Houston

Christian Guilleminault, MD, BiolD
Professor, Stanford University School of Medicine; Stanford Sleep Disorders Clinic, Stanford University Medical Center, Stanford, Calif

Daniel F. Jiannetto, MD
Fellow in Facial Plastic and Reconstructive Surgery, American Academy of Facial Plastic and Reconstructive Surgery, Baltimore, Md

Peter J. Koltai, MD
Head, Section of Pediatric Otolaryngology, Cleveland Clinic Foundation, Cleveland, Ohio

Jed A. Kwartler, MD
Clinical Associate Professor, Division of Otolaryngology–Head and Neck Surgery, UMDNJ–New Jersey Medical School, Newark, NJ; Ear Specialty Group, Springfield, NJ

Xiaoyan Cindy Li, MD
Senior Research Associate, House Ear Institute, Los Angeles

Anna H. Messner, MD
Assistant Professor of Surgery, Otolaryngology/Head & Neck Surgery, Stanford University, Palo Alto, Calif

Mary Lynn Moran, MD
Voluntary Clinical Faculty, Stanford University Hospital, Palo Alto, Calif

Michael J. O'Leary, MD
Clinical Assistant Professor, Uniformed Services University of the Health Sciences, and Chief of Neurotology/Skull Base Surgery, Naval Medical Center, San Diego, Calif

Ira D. Papel, MD
Associate Professor, Division of Facial Plastic and Reconstructive Surgery, Department of Otolaryngology–Head and Neck Surgery, The Johns Hopkins Medical Institutions, Baltimore, Md

Jonathan J. Park, DMD, MD
Chief Resident, Department of Oral and Maxillofacial Surgery, University of Pittsburgh Medical Center, Pittsburgh, Pa

Rafael Pelayo, MD
Assistant Clinical Professor, Stanford University School of Medicine; Stanford Sleep Disorders Clinic, Stanford University Medical Center, Stanford, Calif

Clough Shelton, MD
Professor, Division of Otolaryngology–Headn and Neck Surgery, University of Utah School of Medicine, Salt Lake City

Steven I. Sherman, MD
Associate Professor of Medicine and Associate Internist, University of Texas M. D. Anderson Cancer Center, Houston

Carl H. Snyderman, MD
Associate Professor, Department of Otolaryngology, University of Pittsburgh Medical Center, Pittsburgh, Pa

Robert F. Yellon, MD
Assistant Professor of Otolaryngology, University of Pittsburgh School of Medicine; Co-director, Department of Pediatric Otolaryngology; Director of Clinical Services, Children's Hospital of Pittsburgh, Pa

Preface

The Editorial Board of *Advances in Otolaryngology–Head and Neck Surgery* is quite proud of the content of Volume 14. We feel that this volume addresses all the subspecialty aspects of otolaryngology–head and neck surgery and consists of high-quality contributions.

"Advances in the Management of Sleep Disorders in Children" by Drs Christian Guilleminault and Rafael Pelayo is a special article written by an individual who is known as one of the world's foremost authorities on sleep disorders. Dr Guilleminault has contributed much to the literature, particularly with respect to adults, but this disorder in children is less well known. Following on in the pediatric section is an article by Dr Peter Koltai entitled "Powered Instrumentation in Pediatric Otolaryngology," which once again demonstrates the importance of technological advances in advancing our field to provide better care for patients. Dr Robert Yellon's chapter, "Update on Effects of Gastroesophageal Reflux Disease on Otolaryngologic Disorders in Infants and Children," and Drs Anna Messner and Mary Lynn Moran's chapter on "Management of Sinusitis in the Patient with Cystic Fibrosis," make this a strong and very informative section of *Advances*.

"Advances in the Management of Cancer of the Thyroid Gland," authored by Drs Helmuth Goepfert, Steven Sherman, and Ann Gillenwater of the M. D. Anderson Cancer Center, is an outstanding chapter that is comprehensive and yet reads very easily. Drs Thomas Braun and Jonathan Park give us the latest in "Diagnosis and Management of Temporomandibular Joint Syndrome." While otolaryngologists in general do not treat these disorders, we certainly diagnose them, and the Editorial Board felt that further information about the diagnosis and an overview of the management of temporomandibular joint disorders would be of interest to our readers.

Those interested in otology will find reading the chapter by Drs Clough Shelton and Jed Kwartler on "Office Treatment of the Draining Ear" a rewarding experience filled with "pearls" on this topic. Dr Michael O'Leary has given us yet another example of the power of technology in his chapter entitled "Stereotactic Advances in Otolaryngology–Head and Neck Surgery." Drs Rick Friedman and Cindy Li introduce us to the "Recent Advances in Molecular Genetics of Hereditary Hearing Loss" and leave us not only with the latest advances but a look into the future developments in this area.

Drs Carl Snyderman and Ricardo Carrau update a field common to most people in otolaryngology, and that is "The Treatment of Epistaxis." For those interested in facial plastic and cosmetic topics, we have Dr Eugene Alford's article on "Contemporary Management of Chronic Facial Parlaysis," Drs Daniel Jiannetto and Ira Papel's chapter on "Rhytidectomy in the Male Patient" and Dr Gregory Chernoff's article on "Laser Hair Modification."

I once again want to express my admiration for their creativity and my appreciation for their dedication to *Advances* to the hard-working members of our Editorial Board, Drs Charles Bluestone, Derald Brackmann and Charles Krause. Once again, I would like to thank Mary Jo Tutchko, our capable editorial assistant, and Sarah Zagarri and Terry Van Schaik from Mosby who have been attentive to our needs, and I welcome Karen Moehlman and Gretchen Murphy to the *Advances* team at Mosby.

Eugene N. Myers, MD
Editor-in-Chief

Contents

Contributors   vii
Preface   ix

1. Advances in the Management of Sleep Disorders in Children
By Rafael Pelayo and Christian Guilleminault   1
Normal Childhood Sleep   2
Sleep-Disordered Breathing   3
Narcolepsy   7
   Clinical Presentation   8
   Diagnosis   10
   HLA Class II Typing and Genetics   11
   Treatment Strategies   12
Other Causes of Excessive Daytime Sleepiness   14
   Idiopathic CNS Hypersomnia   15
   Delayed Sleep Phase Syndrome   16
   Periodic Limb Movements Disorder and Restless Leg Syndrome   17
Conclusion   18

2. Powered Instrumentation in Pediatric Otolaryngology
By Peter J. Koltai   25
Pediatric Endoscopic Sinus Surgery With Powered Instrumentation   26
Standard Pediatric FESS With Powered Instrumentation   27
Frontal Sinus Surgery for Children   29
Sphenoid Sinus Surgery for Children   30
Cystic Fibrosis   31
Mucoceles   31
Antrochoanal Polyps   31
Choanal Atresia   32
Adenoidectomy   33

Partial Adenoidectomy   36

Powered Instrumentation for Recurrent Respiratory Papillomatosis   36

Conclusion   37

3. Management of Sinusitis in the Patient With Cystic Fibrosis
By Anna H. Messner and Mary Lynn Moran   41

Diagnosis of CF   43

Sinonasal Symptoms   45

Medical Management   45

Surgical Management   45

ESS With Serial Antimicrobial Lavage   47

Lung Transplantation   48

New Treatments   49

Gene Therapy   50

Conclusion   51

4. Update on the Effects of Gastroesophageal Reflux Disease on Otolaryngologic Disorders in Infants and Children
By Robert F. Yellon   57

Diagnosis   57

Children's Hospital of Pittsburgh Study   58

Discussion and Review of the Literature   60

Sandifer's Syndrome   60

Reflux Rhinopharyngitis and Chronic Sinusitis   60

Chronic Cough   61

Reflux Laryngitis, Hoarseness, Vocal Cord Nodules, and Throat Clearing 61

Globus Pharyngeus   62

Oropharyngeal Dysphagia   62

Chronic Sore Throat   62

Otalgia and Otitis   63

Vocal Cord Granulomas and Ulcers   63

Airway Obstruction and GERD   63

Apnea   63

Asthma   64

Recurrent Croup/Spasmodic Croup   64

Laryngomalacia   65

Reflux-Induced Stridor and "Pseudolaryngomalacia"   66

Subglottic Stenosis   67

Treatment of GERD   68

Conclusion   69

5. Advances in the Management of Cancer of the Thyroid Gland
By Steven I. Sherman, Ann M. Gillenwater, and Helmuth Goepfert   75

Diagnostic Evaluation of the Solitary Thyroid Nodule   75

Thyroid Cancer Staging   77

Surgical Management   78

Management of Cervical Lymph Nodes   80

Management of the Recurrent Laryngeal Nerve   81

Management of Aerodigestive Tract Involvement   81

Outpatient Thyroidectomy   83

Management of Differentiated Thyroid Carcinoma in Children and Adolescents   83

Thyroid Carcinoma in Pregnant Women   84

Adjuvant Treatment   84

Radioiodine   85

Thyroid Hormone Suppression   87

External Beam Radiation Therapy   87

Long-term Follow-up   88

Radioiodine Scanning   89

Serum Thyroglobulin   89

Other Diagnostic Modalities   90

Medullary Thyroid Cancer   91

Initial Surgical Management   95

Adjuvant Radiation Therapy   95

Persistently Elevated Calcitonin   95

Prophylactic Surgery for Gene Carriers   96

6. Diagnosis and Management of Temporomandibular Joint Syndrome

By Jonathan J. Park and Thomas W. Braun   107

Embryology and Anatomy   108

Symptoms, Signs, and Pathogenesis of TMD   109

Evaluation and Differential Diagnosis   115

History   115

Physical Examination   116

Laboratory Studies   116

Imaging Studies   116

Treatment Approaches   117

Medical and Nonsurgical Treatments   118

Surgical Treatments   119

Conclusion   121

7. Stereotactic Advances in Otolaryngology–Head and Neck Surgery

By Michael J. O'Leary   127

Historical Developments   128

Stereotactic Principles   129

Technology   129

Cartesian Coordinates   130

Registration   132

Frame-Based Stereotactic Surgery   134

Gamma Knife Radiosurgery   135

Technology and Radiobiology   136

Technique   137

Case Reports   139

Discussion   144

Frameless Stereotactic Surgery   146

Technology   146

Technique   147

Case Reports   148

Discussion   155

Future Stereotactic Developments   156

Hardware 156

Software 157

Accessories 157

Conclusion 158

8. Office Treatment of the Draining Ear
By Jed A. Kwartler and Clough Shelton 165

Patient History 166

Examination and Cleaning 166

Bacteriology 168

Ototopical Therapy 169

Systemic Therapy 177

Summary 178

9. Recent Advances in Molecular Genetics of Hereditary Hearing Loss
By Xiaoyan Cindy Li and Rick A. Friedman 183

Human Chromosomes and Genetic Diseases 184

Methods of Identifying Hearing Loss Genes 189

Recent Progress in Hereditary Hearing Loss 194

Nonsyndromic Hearing Loss 194

Syndromic Hearing Loss 200

Mitochondrial Hearing Impairment 206

Conclusions 207

10. Advances in the Treatment of Epistaxis
By Carl H. Snyderman and Ricardo L. Carrau 213

Risk Factors 213

Nonsurgical Treatment 214

Surgical Treatment 214

Surgical Technique 215

Clinical Experience 221

Hereditary Hemorrhagic Telangiectasia 221

Summary 222

11. Contemporary Management of Chronic Facial Paralysis
By Eugene L. Alford   225

   Ancillary Procedures in the Treatment of Chronic Facial Paralysis   235

12. Rhytidectomy in the Male Patient
By Ira D. Papel and Daniel F. Jiannetto   239

   Historical Review   240

   Preoperative Considerations   241

   Intraoperative Considerations   244

   Postoperative Considerations   248

   Summary   250

13. Laser Hair Modification
By W. Gregory Chernoff   253

   Anatomy and Physiology   254

   Electrolysis and Electrothermolysis   255

   Lasers or Pulsed Light   256

     Wavelength   257

     Fluence   257

     Pulse Width   257

     Number of Treatments   258

     Dynamic Cooling   258

   Summary of Systems   258

     Nd:YAG Laser   258

     Ruby Laser   259

     Alexandrite Laser   261

     Laser Diode System   261

     Flash Lamp   261

     Microwave Technology   261

   Patient Selection   262

   Separating Fact from Fiction   268

Index   271

CHAPTER 1

Advances in the Management of Sleep Disorders in Children

Rafael Pelayo, MD
Assistant Clinical Professor, Stanford University School of Medicine;
Stanford Sleep Disorders Clinic, Stanford University Medical Center,
Stanford, Calif

Christian Guilleminault, MD, BiolD
Professor, Stanford University School of Medicine; Stanford Sleep
Disorders Clinic, Stanford University Medical Center, Stanford, Calif

The prevalence of sleep disorders in children is not well known. However, the overall impression of specialists in the field is that it is largely underestimated. This lack of recognition regarding this vulnerable population is unfortunate. Disturbances in such a fundamental part of life as sleep will affect the development of the child. Such disturbances may not only affect the child's immediate well-being but also carry over into adulthood. Unrecognized sleep disorders in children can lead to excessive daytime sleepiness, which is associated with learning difficulties and accidents. When the child's sleep disturbances carry over into adulthood, the young adult can occasionally be left with subtle but persistent problems. This effect can be seen with a wide variety of sleep disturbances that include parasomnias, sleep-disordered breathing, and disorders of initiating and maintaining sleep.

Typically, the same nosology is used to describe sleep disorders in adults and children. This is probably related to our meager knowledge of sleep disorders in the pediatric age group. Even if the sleep disorders of children may be phenomenologically the same as those of adults, the etiology, clinical presentation, complications, and treatment will often be very different. The child's age will affect the clinical situation. A teenager may have a different presentation than a younger child. Also, when a certain behavior is seen in a very large portion of the population at a given age but not at a later age, the distinction between normal and abnormal may be blurred. Klackenberg,[1] a pioneer in the study of sleep disorders in children, monitored 200 children born in Sweden from birth to age 20 years. He reported fundamental information on napping and parasomnias, the latter including night terrors, sleepwalking, nocturnal enuresis, and nightmares. This longitudinal study demonstrated that there are periods of development in a child's life when there is a greater chance to express certain behaviors associated with or linked to sleep. These behaviors normally disappear with maturity. Similar to the well-known neurologic concept, some persistent sleep behaviors that become increasingly out of the normal range and are at some point recognized as clearly pathological can be expressed as *developmental delay*. As the term *delay* implies, it is possible to see a return to normality within a short period, which would suggest an absence of pathology. This is why a clear cutoff age is not always attainable and clinical findings have to be adjusted for age and developmental stages. We review the sleep disorders associated with the syndromes leading to daytime somnolence, which can be devastating to a child.

NORMAL CHILDHOOD SLEEP

Before addressing the syndromes leading to daytime somnolence, it is necessary to review normal sleep in children. Daytime somnolence in a child may be obvious at first. The child identified as the "best napper" in kindergarten may be the same child who has difficulty staying alert in the first grade. Information about daytime sleep, such as naps and inadvertent sleep periods (eg, while a passenger in a car), has to be included when the history is obtained. The ontogeny of sleep has been extensively reviewed.[2] Sleep needs and patterns differ with age. A newborn child may typically sleep 17 hours, an amount that may gradually decrease until adolescence, when there may be an increased need for sleep.[3] It is important to be aware of daytime as well as nighttime sleep needs. Weissbluth[4] monitored a cohort of 172 children from 6 months to 7 years of age to determine how nap patterns change with age. Results showed that there were no differences in nap patterns based on gender, ordinal position, whether naps spontaneously disappeared or were stopped by the parents, and the number of naps at 6 months of age. Total daytime sleep remained a stable individual characteristic between 6 and 18 months of age. Age was associated with hours napping and number of naps. A pattern of 2 naps per day was well established by 9 to 12 months of age and 1 afternoon nap by 15 to 24 months. The modal duration of naps from 2 to 6 years was 2 hours. During the third and fourth year, the majority of children were napping but at decreasing rates. A minority of children were napping at 5 and 6 years, and naps usually disappeared by age 7.

SLEEP-DISORDERED BREATHING

Obstructive sleep apnea (OSA) can occur at any age. Charles Dickens[5] presented a classic Pickwickian description of a boy named Joe who had snoring with arousals and excessive daytime sleepiness. The first medical description of children with abnormal breathing in sleep is attributed to William Osler[6] in his 1892 textbook.

In the modern medical literature, Guilleminault et al[7] reported the first series of children with OSA in 1976. That report describes the essential clinical features of this condition. More recently, there has been a realization that patients may have symptoms in the absence of frank apneas.[8,9] This has led to the use of the terms *sleep-disordered breathing* and *sleep-related breathing disorders* to better describe the clinical spectrum that includes obstructive sleep apnea syndrome (OSAS), upper airway resistance syndrome (UARS), and obstructive hypopnea syndrome. Although sleep-disordered breathing in children has many important similarities to the adult version of this disease, there are also marked differences in presentation, diagnosis, and management.

The abnormal daytime sleepiness may be recognized more often by schoolteachers than by parents of young children. Parents may consider an increase in total sleep time or an extra long nap as normal. Most commonly, such nonspecific behavioral difficulties are mentioned to the pediatrician as abnormal shyness, hyperactivity, developmental delays, and rebellious or aggressive behavior. Other daytime symptoms may include speech defects, poor appetite, or swallowing difficulties.[7,8]

Many of these children are mouth breathers. Regular mouth breathing should always lead to suspicion of sleep-disordered breathing. Children with disordered breathing may avoid going to bed at night because of hypnagogic hallucinations. Upon awakening, these children may have morning headaches or dry mouth or they may be confused or irritable. As mentioned, daytime sleepiness may not be obvious depending on the age. It may be manifest only in a complaint of daytime tiredness. It may also be presented as a tendency to take naps easily anywhere. In schools, the tiredness and sleepiness may be labeled "inattentive in class," "daydreaming," or "not being there." An abrupt and persistent deterioration in grades must also raise suspicion of abnormal sleep and sleep-disordered breathing.[7,8]

The most obvious nocturnal symptom is snoring. Our opinion is that "chronic" snoring should be investigated and never be considered normal. Although it may be caused by allergies, it is commonly associated with some degree of sleep-disordered breathing.

Clinical signs include increased respiratory efforts with nasal flaring, suprasternal or intercostal retractions, abnormal paradoxical inward motion of the chest that may occur during inspiration, and sweating during sleep. The sweating may be limited to the nuchal region, particularly for infants, but it may be severe enough to necessitate changing clothes during the night. The parents may mention that the child feels warm at night or prefers to sleep without a blanket. Parents may also observe the child stop breathing, then gasping for breath. It is surprising how often parents have observed abnormal breathing patterns during sleep but were never questioned about it by pediatricians during regular visits. Information regarding the sleep position is helpful. Typically, the neck is hyperextended and the mouth is open. Another typical sleeping position is prone with the knee tucked under the chest with head turned to the side and hyperextended. The child with sleep-disordered breathing rarely prefers to sleep propped up on several pillows.[8]

Ohayon et al[10] have found that individuals identified with sleep-disordered breathing have a much higher incidence of nightmares, with reports of drowning, being buried alive, choking, and so on. These reports must be related to the known association of night terrors and sleepwalking with sleep-disordered breathing. Night terrors probably have similar content as nightmares. Night terrors may lead to escape behavior and sleepwalking. If sleep fragmentation induced by the breathing events occurs during slow wave sleep, night terrors and sleepwalking may undoubtedly be triggered.[7,8]

A physical finding that may be overlooked in a child with sleep-disordered breathing is a narrow and high-arched palate.[8] Interestingly, the Diagnostic and Statistical Manual of Mental Disorders (DSM-IV) description of attention deficit disorder mentions that minor physical anomalies such as high-arched palates may be present.[11] Because both conditions may include similar daytime behavior in the same age group, a child with sleep-disordered breathing could be misidentified as having attention deficit disorder. The possibility of a sleep disorder being present should be considered in any child being evaluated for attention deficit disorder. This is particularly important because treatment of sleep-disordered breathing may improve behavior and academic performance.[12,13]

The diagnostic criteria used for adults with OSAS cannot be used reliably in children.[14,15] The diagnosis of sleep-disordered breathing is based on the history, physical findings, and supportive data. Laboratory testing should ideally be tailored to the clinical question. For example, if there are concerns about excessive daytime sleepiness, a multiple sleep latency test (MSLT) may be indicated.[16] The MSLT is ideally performed in subjects who are at least 8 years old.

The polysomnogram for a child uses the same technology, and the same type of information is recorded as for adults. Airflow, respiratory effort, and pulse oximetry make up the breathing measurements that are usually monitored. The respiratory effort is measured most accurately in a clinical sleep study using esophageal pressure measurements with a water-filled catheter.[8,17] Esophageal pressure measurements are not yet part of the routine polysomnogram in most sleep laboratories. An alternative measurement can be obtained using end-tidal CO_2 monitoring, which can detect important transient episodes of hypercarbia.[17] More recently, a technique to measure airflow with the use of a nasal cannula has been introduced. This promising technique may replace nasal thermistors and may be less invasive than esophageal manometry.[18,19]

Along with the absence of controlled studies, another problem in the attempt to understand pediatric sleep-disordered breathing is that definitions for key terms vary. OSAs are defined as lasting at least 10 seconds in adults. However, because children have faster respiratory rates, clinically significant apneas can occur in less time. Apneas as brief as 3 or 4 seconds may have oxygen desaturations. There are no uniform measures of hypopneas in children. The clinician needs to know how apneas and hypopneas are defined and scored when interpreting a polysomnogram report.[20]

The UARS is present in individuals with symptoms of sleep-disordered breathing who on the polysomnogram have evidence of sleep disruption associated with increased work of breathing without a significant degree of apneas or hypopneas.[9] For children, the work of breathing can be measured by using esophageal pressure. During the calibration of the recording, the awake esophageal pressure is measured. This value is usually between −3 and −5 cm of water. A repetitive breathing pattern can be identified, with increasing negative esophageal pressure culminating in a brief arousal.[8]

Controversy exists over whether a diagnosis of OSA, or the larger spectrum of sleep-disordered breathing, can be made without a formal polysomnogram. Although some have suggested that this diagnosis can be made in patients with the use of either the history and physical, or the history, physical, and an audio or videotape, others have found an inability of clinical history alone to distinguish primary snoring from OSAS in children.[21-24] The situation is further complicated by the recent description of UARS in children, which may have been missed in the studies cited above. The sleep study is the most definitive test for sleep-disordered breathing.[17] Currently, some otolaryngologists who treat children with sleep-disordered breathing may make the surgical recommendation based on clinical findings of airway obstruction, sometimes after reviewing an audiotape or videotape.[25-28] The clinicians must be aware of the potential pitfalls to this practice. Certainly there are individual cases in which a diagnostic sleep study is not available, but ideally this should be the exception. The challenge we face in sleep medicine is providing easily accessible and cost-effective care while working within a multidisciplinary model. We do not know with certainty how accurate a clinical diagnosis is without appropriate testing. Until we have a better answer, the gold standard of diagnosis should not be disregarded, particularly in a tertiary care setting. Both the American Thoracic Society[17] and the American Academy of Sleep Medicine[29] support the use of sleep studies in the pediatric age group.

Sleep-disordered breathing is not the only sleep disorder a child may have. Clinical impression may have both false-negatives and false-positives, resulting in a possible misdiagnosis or unnecessary surgery. For example, without confirmatory testing, a child with only "simple" snoring and symptomatic periodic limb movements may inevitably be misdiagnosed with sleep-disordered breathing and undergo unnecessary surgery. Periodic limb movements of sleep and restless leg syndrome (RLS) are not uncommon in children.[30] These syndromes can have a vague or difficult history to elicit.

Adenotonsillectomy is the most common initial treatment for sleep-disordered breathing in children; however, it does not always cure the sleep disorder. The true cure rate by surgery for sleep-disordered breathing is unknown.

Some may argue that clear-cut cases of sleep-disordered breathing may skip the sleep study.[26-28] However, experience with adults teaches us that it is precisely these obviously more severe or "clearcut" cases that will have residual disease. Adenotonsillectomy will not change the relationship of tongue size and shape to the palate. The parents may report that the child is 100% better, yet the child may have residual disease. If the child still has trouble paying attention in school, a sleep problem may no longer be considered a possible explanation. The child may end up labeled as having attention deficit disorder because no sleep test was done in the postoperative period.[31]

What is the role of the polysomnogram for children? It is a tool that the treating physician can use as needed to objectively evaluate the patient's condition. In adult sleep medicine, our surgical colleagues are a component of the multidisciplinary treatment options offered to the patient. Advances in the surgical management of OSA would not have occurred without a strong relationship between the surgeon and the sleep specialist.[32,33]

NARCOLEPSY

Narcolepsy is a chronic neurological disorder in which the boundaries between the awake, sleeping, and dreaming brain are blurred. The awake narcoleptic will feel sleepy. The sleeping narcoleptic will have disturbed sleep due to arousals. Historically, the word *narcolepsy* was coined by Gélineau in 1880 to designate a pathological condition characterized by irresistible episodes of sleep of short duration recurring at close intervals. In the same article, he wrote that attacks were sometimes accompanied by falls or "astasias." The cardinal features of narcolepsy are daytime somnolence, cataplexy, sleep paralysis, and hypnagogic hallucinations.[15] These symptoms were called the "tetrad" of narcolepsy by Yoss and Daly.[34] Rechtschaffen et al[35] and Hishikawa[36] reported the presence of abnormal sleep onset rapid eye movement (REM) sleep periods in narcolepsy.

Narcolepsy is not a rare condition. The prevalence of narcolepsy has been calculated at about 0.04% of the general population.[37] The age at onset varies from early childhood to the fifth decade, with a peak in the second decade. It is important to consider narcolepsy, especially in young patients, because it can take up to 20 years between the initial onset of the first symptom, commonly sleepiness, and development of the full clinical syndrome. During this lapse of time, the patient may be mislabeled with a wide variety of diagnoses. The patient may be considered lazy or depressed.

Before being correctly diagnosed, the patient may turn to illegal drugs such as "crank" amphetamine to combat the sleepiness.

CLINICAL PRESENTATION

Narcolepsy is characterized by abnormal sleep, including excessive daytime sleepiness with often-disturbed nocturnal sleep later in life and pathological manifestations related to REM sleep. The REM sleep–related abnormalities include early REM sleep onset and cataplexy.

Cataplexy is an abrupt and reversible decrease or loss of muscle tone that is most frequently provoked by emotion, particularly laughter. Consciousness typically remains intact. It may involve only certain muscles or the entire voluntary musculature. Most typically, the jaw sags, the head falls forward, the arms drop to the side, and the knees buckle. The severity and extent of cataplectic attacks can range from a state of absolute powerlessness, which seems to involve the entire body, to no more than a fleeting sensation of weakness. Although the extraocular muscles are supposedly not involved, the patient may complain of blurred vision. Speech may be impaired. Respiration may become irregular during an attack, which may be related to weakness of the abdominal muscles. Complete loss of muscle tone, which results in a fall with risk of serious injuries including skull and other bone fractures, may be noted during a cataplectic attack. The attacks may also be subtle and not noticed by nearby individuals. An attack may consist only of a slight buckling of the knees. Patients may perceive this abrupt and short-lasting weakness and may simply sit or stand against a wall. Speech may be slurred because of intermittent weakness affecting the arytenoid muscles. As seen during nocturnal REM sleep, the abrupt muscle inhibition is interrupted by sudden bursts of returning muscle tone, which at times even seems enhanced. If the weakness involves only the jaw or speech, the subject may have wide masticatory movement or odd attacks of stuttering. If it involves the upper limbs, the patient will complain of clumsiness, reporting activity such as dropping cups or plates or spilling liquids when surprised or laughing. These attacks are short and do not resemble the "classic" full-blown attack of cataplexy (ie, with a complete fall).

In early childhood, cataplexy attacks are more often the complete fall type. The child may be initially seen for repetitive falls that cannot be easily explained. Atonic seizures or drop attacks are the most common initial misdiagnoses for children younger than 5 years old.[38] The duration of each cataplectic attack, partial or total, is highly variable. The attacks usually range from a few seconds to 2 minutes and, on rare occasions, up to 30 minutes. Attacks can be elicited by emotion, stress, fatigue, or heavy meals. Laughter and anger seem to be the most common triggers, but the attacks can also be induced by a feeling of elation while listening to music, reading a book, or watching a movie. Cataplexy may be induced merely by remembering a funny situation, and it may also occur without obvious precipitating acts or emotions. It often occurs in children who are playing with others.

A pathway similar to the one leading to REM atonia is used in cataplexy.[39] Cataplexy is associated with an inhibition of monosynaptic H-reflexes and of the multisynaptic tendon reflexes.[40] H-reflex activity is fully suppressed physiologically during REM sleep, which emphasizes the relationship between the motor inhibition of REM sleep and the sudden atonia and areflexia seen during a cataplectic attack.[41]

Apart from overwhelming sleepiness, patients may feel abnormally drowsy. They may spend the day at a low level of alertness that is responsible for poor performance at school, memory lapses, and even gestural, or speech automatisms. This low alertness may persist despite the use of stimulant medication.[42]

Daytime sleepiness may not be obvious to parents of very young children, and it may easily be missed before a child attends kindergarten.[38] Sleepy behavior is more often recognized by teachers, who may complain of apathy in the child. The parents may misjudge the behavior as normal napping. Prolonged nocturnal sleep, difficulty waking up in the morning, and aggressiveness before being awakened are commonly seen. However, sleepiness can be hidden behind other abnormal behavior such as hyperactivity or social withdrawal and shyness.

Sleep paralysis can be a terrifying experience that occurs in narcolepsy when a child falls asleep or during awakenings. Children find themselves suddenly unable to move the limbs, to speak, or even to breathe deeply. This state is frequently accompanied by hallucinations. During episodes of sleep paralysis, particularly the first occurrence, the patient may have extreme anxiety associated with fear of dying. This anxiety is often greatly intensified by the hallucinations, sometimes terrifying, that may accompany the sleep paralysis. Children are often reluctant to talk about these events. These experiences are so frightful that the child may resist going to bed.

Visual hypnagogic hallucinations usually consist of simple forms (eg, colored circles, parts of objects) that are constant or changing in size. The image of an animal or a person may present itself abruptly, sometimes in black and white but more often in color. Auditory hallucinations are also common. The auditory hallucinations can range from simple sounds to an elaborate melody. The patient may also be menaced by threatening sentences or harsh invectives.

Hypnagogic hallucinations and sleep paralysis do not affect all subjects and can be transitory. Disturbed nocturnal sleep seldom occurs initially and generally worsens during adulthood.

DIAGNOSIS

Unless cataplexy is unequivocally witnessed by the examiner, an objective sleep study will be necessary to obtain an accurate diagnosis of narcolepsy.[15] Unfortunately, no objective test has been developed to confirm the diagnosis for the child younger than 8 years. For these younger children, the diagnosis is made as a process of elimination when there is an otherwise clear history. Clinical electroencephalogram and MRI findings are normal. A key finding in this age group is the absence of another sleep disorder such as periodic limb movement disorder, as demonstrated on a complete overnight polysomnogram. The polysomnogram should be normal with the possible exception of a short REM sleep latency. The polysomnogram monitoring should include either a nasal cannula or esophageal pressure to not miss a more subtle condition, such as UARS.[8]

For children 8 years or older, objective testing is available to aid in the diagnosis of narcolepsy. After a full nocturnal polysomnogram is completed the following morning, an MSLT is necessary.[16] The MSLT was designed to measure physiologic sleep tendencies in the absence of alerting factors. The time or latency between lights-out and sleep onset is calculated for each nap. The type of sleep, REM or non-REM, is also noted. After each nap, patients must stay awake until the following scheduled nap. The MSLT records the sleep latency for each nap, the mean sleep latency, and the presence or absence of REM sleep in any of the naps. REM sleep that occurs within 15 minutes of sleep onset is considered a sleep-onset REM period.

In normal populations, MSLT scores vary with age—puberty being the critical landmark—with prepubertal children between the ages of 8 and 11 years appearing relatively hyperalert. The maximum mean MSLT score obtainable is 20 minutes, which corresponds to a subject staying awake during all naps. Mean MSLT scores under 8 minutes are generally considered to be in the pathological sleepiness range; those over 10 minutes are considered normal in adults. Before puberty, as mentioned above, children are very alert in the daytime and the normal adult MSLT cutoff value of 10 minutes may be too low. Even scores of 12 minutes for a prepubertal child may be abnormal. For children undergoing an MSLT, the presence of 2 or more sleep onset REM periods is always abnormal and consistent with narcolepsy.

HLA CLASS II TYPING AND GENETICS

HLA typing had been recommended as an adjuvant test for narcolepsy when it was found in Japan to have an association with the DR2 marker.[43] A more specific HLA marker, DQB1*0602, was later found be associated with narcolepsy.[44] However, this marker is neither sufficient nor necessary for the diagnosis because it is present in 10% to 15% of the general population.[45] Determination of HLA haplotypes in children suspected of having narcolepsy is usually not helpful in making the diagnosis.[46,47] The results are, of course, valuable in understanding the genetics underlying narcolepsy. Recently, narcolepsy has been shown to be a neurological disorder known to be tightly associated with 2 HLA markers, DQA1*0102 and DQB1*0602.[48] Clinical research has shown that the relative risk for narcolepsy was 2 to 4 times higher in DQB1*0602 homozygotes versus heterozygotes. In contrast, symptom severity does not differ between DQB1*0602 homozygous and heterozygous subjects. These results indicate that HLA-DQB1*0602 homozygosity increases susceptibility to narcolepsy but does not appear to influence disease severity.[49]

Normal subjects with positive DQB1*0602 marker have been studied.[50] Results indicated shorter REM sleep latency, increased sleep efficiency, and decreased time percentage spent in stage 1 sleep during nocturnal polysomnography in DQB1*0602 subjects. However, there was no difference in the degree of daytime sleepiness based on the results gathered using the MSLT or the Epworth and Stanford sleepiness scales. The authors concluded that these results support the hypothesis that polymorphisms at the level of HLA-DQ modulate sleep tendencies in humans.[50]

An animal model that used dogs has been studied for narcolepsy. With the use of positional cloning, an autosomal recessive mutation responsible for narcolepsy was recently discovered in this canine model. Canine narcolepsy is caused by disruption of the hypocretin (orexin) receptor 2 gene (Hcrtr2). Hypocretins appear to be major sleep-modulating neurotransmitters.[51] Abnormally low hypocretin levels have been found in the cerebrospinal fluid of human narcoleptics.

TREATMENT STRATEGIES

Succesful management of narcolepsy must include both behavioral and pharmacologic treatments. The situation is analogous to that of juvenile diabetes mellitus, in which a combination of diet and medication can control the condition. With the recent discovery of a gene responsible for narcolepsy, potentially novel therapeutic approaches may be discovered.[51]

Behavioral Treatment

Treatment strategies must include conservative behavioral treatment such as the use of short naps, emotional support to parents and child, and education of school authorities. Repetitive 15- to 20-minute naps at 3-hour intervals are helpful in restoring alertness. Behavioral and emotional disturbances are reported in adolescents with narcolepsy.[52] Subjects and families should be referred to narcolepsy support groups led by therapists who can address issues created by this chronic condition.

Pharmacologic Approaches

Drug therapy must take into account possible side effects, with the fact kept in mind that narcolepsy is a lifelong illness and patients will have to receive medication for years. Tolerance or addiction may occur with some of these compounds. Treatment of narcolepsy must try to balance avoidance of side effects, including tolerance, with maintenance of an active life. Physicians need to be alert to the development of hypertension, abnormal liver function, depression, irritability, anorexia, insomnia, or psychosis associated with medications.

There are no double-blind placebo-controlled trials of medication specifically for children with narcolepsy. The drugs most widely used to treat excessive daytime sleepiness are the central nervous system (CNS) stimulants.[53] Amphetamines were first proposed in 1935.[34] The alerting effect of a single oral dose of amphetamine is at its maximum 2 to 4 hours after administration, and many patients require a single or twice-daily dose. However, a number of side effects including irritability, anxiety, nervousness, headache, psychosis, tachycardia, hypertension, nocturnal sleep disturbances, tolerance, and drug dependence may arise. The use of methylphenidate was later encouraged because of a shorter half-life and lower incidence of similar side effects.[54] Pemoline, an oxazolidine derivative with a longer half-life and a slower onset of action, is less efficient but is well tolerated.[54] It had previously been the first stimulant used in children, but pemoline should now be discouraged because of the possibility of severe liver damage. The manufacturer, Abbot, has recommended that baseline liver function tests be obtained before starting pemoline and every 2 weeks thereafter. It should be avoided. Mazindol, an imidazoline derivative, has been shown to reduce the number of daytime sleep episodes in narcoleptics in a dose range of 0.5 to 4 mg.[55]

There are 2 drugs with different modes of action that have been recently considered for narcolepsy. The first, modafinil, is considered more a somnolytic than a nonspecific stimulant.[56-58] The drug, which has been recently approved in the United States, has been reported in adults to bring substantial improvement.[59,60] The mechanism of action of modafinil is not entirely clear, but it is not dopamine-mediated.[61,62] The neuronal targets for modafinil in the brain include nuclei of the hypothalamus and amygdala.[63,64] The initial dose should be relatively low, 100 mg, to avoid headaches. The dosage can later be increased to 200 to 400 mg per day divided twice daily. The second dose should be given before 2 PM because of the long half-life of the medication. Modafinil does not have the typical side effects of amphetamine.[65] The most common side effect is headache, and this negative effect may be eliminated if there is a progressive dose increase over time. Unlike amphetamines, dependency signs have never been observed.[57]

The second drug is γ-hydroxybutyrate, which has been banned in the United States outside of clinical trials approved by the US Food and Drug Administration (FDA). This substance is known to have powerful CNS depressant effects.[66] γ-Hydroxybutyrate can increase slow wave sleep.[67,68] This medication, when given at bedtime, may be of value to reduce cataplexy and perhaps daytime sleepiness.[69,70] The future role of γ-hydroxybutyrate in the treatment of narcolepsy is uncertain. It may be more useful for cataplexy than for excessive daytime sleepiness, particularly if insomnia is also present. However, this medication has been known to be used recreationally and may be abused.[71,72]

The other symptoms of narcolepsy, such as cataplexy, are typically treated with different medications than those used for excessive daytime sleepiness. Cataplexy seems to respond best to medications with noradrenergic reuptake blocking properties.[73] Again, there are no systematic trials of anticataplexy drugs on children. Postpubertal teenagers are usually treated as young adults. In this group, 2 medications, clomipramine and fluoxetine, have been used. Both have active noradrenergic reuptake blocking metabolites (desmethylclomipramine and norfluoxetine). It is through these metabolites that the therapeutic effect may be mediated.[74]

Other compounds have been found to be effective in children with cataplexy, particularly imipramine and desipramine, and in Europe, viloxazine hydrochloride. Clomipramine and imipramine have atropinic side effects that undoubtedly also have a beneficial impact on the auxiliary symptoms of narcolepsy. These side effects, however, may be problematic and lead to treatment with fluoxetine or viloxazine instead. Fluoxetine can help cataplexy with somewhat less efficacy than the other medications.[75]

OTHER CAUSES OF EXCESSIVE DAYTIME SLEEPINESS

There are more than 100 different sleep disorders described in *The International Classification of Sleep Disorders.*[15] Of these conditions, more than 30 are categorized by excessive sleepiness. Further complicating this situation, conditions that are primarily considered under the category of insomnia can be initially seen clinically as excessive daytime sleepiness. This highlights the emergence of sleep disorders medicine as a medical specialty and the importance of formal training to provide appropriate care. Among the conditions that may be associated with excessive daytime sleepiness in children are the following:

- Delayed sleep phase syndrome
- Non–24-hour sleep-wake syndrome
- Irregular sleep-wake pattern
- Recurrent hypersomnia (Kleine-Levin syndrome)
- Inadequate sleep hygiene
- Inadequate sleep syndrome
- Limit-setting sleep disorder
- Environmental sleep disorder
- Central alveolar hypoventilation syndrome
- Central sleep apnea syndrome
- Posttraumatic hypersomnia
- Periodic limb movement disorder
- Mood disorders
- Idiopathic hypersomnia

All of the above conditions should be considered under the appropriate clinical situation because they may improve with correct management. Of the above conditions, the most challenging may be idiopathic hypersomnia, also referred to as idiopathic CNS hypersomnia.

IDIOPATHIC CNS HYPERSOMNIA

Idiopathic CNS hypersomnia is a condition that is characterized by chronic sleepiness without cataplexy; it is presumed to be of neurologic origin. The daytime sleepiness is isolated. Historically, this syndrome has had a number of labels, including essential narcolepsy, independent narcolepsy, non-REM sleep narcolepsy, functional hypersomnia, and harmonious hypersomnia.[76-80] It is important to clearly differentiate idiopathic hypersomnia from the narcolepsy syndrome, with its auxiliary symptoms, and from the daytime sleepiness related to nocturnal sleep disturbances such as sleep apnea or periodic leg movement syndrome.[15] The distinction from narcolepsy can be difficult, however, because the 2 disorders have many similarities, including age at onset of symptoms, duration, and a familial or genetic predisposition. UARS adds to create a difficult differential diagnosis.[81] Idiopathic CNS hypersomnia syndrome is a disorder of exclusion that renders diagnosis and treatment more difficult. A strong genetic component has been suggested by the high proportion of familial cases. No association with HLA has been evidenced to date.[82]

Polygraphic monitoring and MSLT are needed to confirm the presence of the syndrome. Classically, no sleep onset REM sleep periods are seen in a 5-nap MSLT. When a large group of patients with narcolepsy and those with CNS hypersomnia are compared, the mean sleep latency score is usually higher in the CNS hypersomnia group. Guilleminault et al,[83] reviewing polygraphic results of 50 patients with CNS hypersomnia, found a mean MSLT of 6.3 + 3.5 minutes and only 10% of the population had a score of 3.7 minutes or less. Van den Hoed et al[84] found a mean MSLT of 6.5 + 3.2 minutes for patients with CNS hypersomnia versus 3.3 + 3.3 minutes for patients with narcolepsy. The diagnostic criteria in *The International Classification of Sleep Disorders* requires a mean sleep latency on the MSLT of less than 10 minutes and fewer than 2 sleep onset REM periods.[15]

For lack of a better treatment, management of idiopathic hypersomnia is symptom-based. Behavioral approaches and sleep hygiene techniques must be recommended, but they have little positive impact alone. Daytime naps are long and, unlike narcolepsy, most commonly are nonrefreshing. The most commonly used medications that have brought a partial, and often intermittent, relief have been the same stimulant drugs used in narcolepsy. Modafinil has been used successfully in idiopathic hypersomnia, and it has not been associated with tolerance or drug dependence after 3 years of use.[85] Given the minimal side effects reported, modafinil should be considered the initial drug of choice for idiopathic hypersomnia.

DELAYED SLEEP PHASE SYNDROME

The circadian rhythm sleep disorder, delayed sleep phase syndrome, is characterized by chronic sleep onset difficulty and an inability to arise at an appropriate time in the morning. Once the major sleep episode has been initiated, there is the ability to sleep soundly and for a normal duration.[86] When not required to maintain a strict sleep schedule (eg, weekends, vacations, and holiday periods) patients will awaken spontaneously, albeit at a late morning or early afternoon hour. They will have a normal nocturnal total sleep time.[15] This may be the most common sleep disorder of adolescence and may be associated with depression.[87,88]

The original treatment for delayed sleep phase syndrome was called chronotherapy by Weitzman.[86] Chronotherapy resets the patient's sleep cycle by a series of consecutive delayed adjustments of the bedtime that are made over several days. To maintain the readjusted sleep pattern, the patient is encouraged to adhere strictly to the new sleep onset and wake times. This treatment can be impractical because the progressive forward bedtime shifts will have the child at one point temporally sleeping in the daytime. While awake, the child must be constantly supervised to avoid falling asleep at the wrong time.

Another treatment technique resets the sleep-wake rhythm by using bright morning light, combined with evening light restriction, to phase-shift the patient's sleep time.[89] The term *phototherapy* is used for this treatment. The essential principles of phototherapy are that bright light in the morning can phase advance sleep onset and bright light in the evening can phase delay sleep onset. Different phototherapy protocols have been used with various success rates.[89-91] Our practice is to use light intensity of 10,000 lux for 45 minutes within a few minutes of the subject's awakening at a predetermined time for several weeks. The subject is typically 3 feet away from the light source, depending on the rating of the device. Phototherapy may be contraindicated in the presence of retinal-ocular disease.

Treatment with melatonin has been described.[92-94] Melatonin is a hormone secreted by the pineal gland, and its primary function seems to be to convey information about the changing length of the night in the course of the year. This information is used by photoperiodic animals to ensure the correct timing of seasonally variable functions such as reproduction, coat growth, and probably the duration and organization of sleep.[94] The clinical use of melatonin may be difficult and probably should be discouraged by nonspecialists. Melatonin is not regulated as a pharmaceutical in the United States but rather is classified as a food additive. This lack of regulation may make the quality of over-the-counter melatonin highly variable. The timing of the dose must be individually determined based on the core body temperature rhythm of the subjects.[92] The patients' motivation to modify their lifestyle is essential for successful treatment. Adolescents may have to vary social and academic pressures to avoid going to bed at an earlier time. A large difference between the bedtimes and wake-up times from school nights compared with weekends can reinforce the delayed sleep phase.

PERIODIC LIMB MOVEMENTS DISORDER AND RESTLESS LEG SYNDROME

Periodic limb movements disorder and RLS are distinct sleep disorders that are usually associated with older adults. However, recent reports suggest that it may be more common in children than had previously been considered, and it may affect children at a very young age.[95,96] RLS is a movement disorder characterized by unusual sensations that occur typically in the legs, occasionally in the arms, and infrequently in other body parts. The patients feel a need to move the affected extremity to achieve relief. RLS is worse during the evening and at night, and it can lead to insomnia and excessive daytime sleepiness.[15,97] Periodic limb movements disorder is characterized by recurrent episodes of repetitive and highly stereotyped limb movements that occur during sleep. The movement in the leg is the extension of the big toe, while at the same time the ankle, knee, and sometimes the hip are partly flexed. These repetitive episodes of muscle contraction last from a half second to 5 seconds with an interval of about 20 to 40 seconds. They tend to occur in the first third of the night.[15,98]

These conditions can be treated with different medications. Medications working through dopamine receptors seem to be the most effective.[99] Recently, specific dopamine agonists pramipexole and pergolide tested in double-blind placebo-controlled studies have been shown to be effective.[100,101] Before starting the child on medication, behavioral treatments include avoidance of caffeine, including chocolate, and giving the child a warm bath before going to bed.

Children with either periodic limb movements disorder or RLS can mimic the daytime symptoms of attention deficit disorder. These symptoms resolve or improve when the movement disorder is treated.[28,95,96] RLS has been reported to have an autosomal dominant pattern of inheritance.[102] Therefore, it is very important to suspect this condition in any child with behavioral problems who has a first-degree relative with RLS. At the same time, the parents of any child who is diagnosed with RLS should also be questioned about possibly having this disorder.

CONCLUSION

The evaluation of excessive daytime sleepiness in children requires a broader differential diagnosis beyond OSAS. The polysomnogram can assist not only for the diagnosis but also to monitor the clinical course of the child. The development of new therapies for these conditions should allow better treatment options for these children.

ACKNOWLEDGEMENT

The work of Dr Guilleminault was supported by an Academic Award from the Sleep Center of the National Heart, Lung, and Blood Institute, NIH.

REFERENCES

1. Klackenberg G: Sleep behaviour studied longitudinally: Data from 4-16 years on duration, night-awakening and bed-sharing. *Acta Paediatr Scand* 71:501-506, 1982.
2. Anders TF, Sadeh A, Appareddy V: Normal Sleep in Neonates and Children, in *Principles and Practice of Sleep Medicine in the Child.* Philadelphia, WB Saunders, 1995, pp 7-19.
3. Carskadon MA, Wolfson AR, Acebo C, et al: Adolescent sleep patterns, circadian timing, and sleepiness at a transition to early school days. *Sleep* 21:871-881, 1998.
4. Weissbluth M: Naps in children: 6 months-7 years. *Sleep* 18:82-87, 1995.
5. Dickens C: *The Posthumous Papers of the Pickwick Club,* London, Chapman & Hall, published in serial form 1836-1837.
6. Osler W: Chronic tonsillitis, in *The Principles and Practice of Medicine.* New York, Appleton and Co., 1892, pp 335-339.
7. Guilleminault C, Eldridge F, Simmons F, et al: Sleep apnea in eight children. *Pediatrics* 58:23-30, 1976.
8. Guilleminault C, Pelayo R, Clerk A, et al: Recognition of sleep-disordered breathing in children. *Pediatrics* 98:871-882, 1996.
9. Downey R III, Perkin RM, MacQuarrie J: Upper airway resistance syndrome: Sick, symptomatic but underrecognized. *Sleep* 16:620-623, 1993.
10. Ohayon MM, Guilleminault C, Priest RG: Night terrors, sleepwalking, and confusional arousals in the general population: Their frequency and relationship to other sleep and mental disorders. *J Clin Psychiatry* 60:268-276, 1999.

11. American Psychiatric Association: *Diagnostic and Statistical Manual of Mental Disorders: DSM-IV.* Washington: Amer Psychiatric Pr, 1994.
12. Gozal D: Sleep-disordered breathing and school performance in children. *Pediatrics* 102:616-620, 1998.
13. Guilleminault C, Korobkin R, Winkle R: A review of 50 children with obstructive sleep apnea syndrome. *Lung* 59:275-287, 1981.
14. Carroll JL, Loughlin GM: Diagnostic criteria for obstructive sleep apnea syndrome in children. *Pediatr Pulmonol* 14:71-74, 1992.
15. Diagnostic Classification Steering Committee, Thorpy MJ (Chairman). *International Classification of Sleep Disorders Diagnostic and Coding Manual.* Rochester, Mich, American Association of Sleep Disorders, 1990.
16. Carskadon MA, Dement WC, Mitler M, et al: Guidelines for the multiple sleep latency test (MSLT): A standard measure of sleepiness. *Sleep* 9:519-524, 1986.
17. Standards and indications for cardiopulmonary sleep studies in children. American Thoracic Society. *Am J Respir Crit Care Med* 153:866-878, 1996.
18. Norman RG, Ahmed MM, Walsleben JA, et al: Detection of respiratory events during NPSG: Nasal cannula/pressure sensor versus thermistor. *Sleep* 20:1175-1184, 1997.
19 Hosselet JJ, Norman RG, Ayappa I, et al: Detection of flow limitation with a nasal cannula/pressure transducer system. *Am J Respir Crit Care Med* 157:1461-1467, 1998.
20. Marcus CL, Omlin KJ, Basinki DJ, et al: Normal polysomnographic values for children and adolescents. *Am Rev Respir Dis* 146:1235-1239, 1992.
21. Thach BT: Pediatric aspects of the sleep apnea syndrome. *Ear Nose Throat J* 63:214-221, 1984.
22. Carroll JL, McColley SA, Marcus CL, et al: Inability of clinical history to distinguish primary snoring from obstructive sleep apnea syndrome in children. *Chest* 108:610-618, 1995.
23. Goldstein NA, Sculerati N, Walsleben JA, et al: Clinical diagnosis of pediatric obstructive sleep apnea validated by polysomnography. *Otolaryngol Head Neck Surg* 111:611-617, 1994.
24. Nieminen P, Tolonen U, Lopponen H, et al: Snoring children: Factors predicting sleep apnea. *Acta Otolaryngol Supp* 529:190-194, 1994.
25. Guilleminault C, Pelayo R: ... And if the polysomnogram was faulty? [editorial; comment]. *Pediatr Pulmonol* 26:1-3, 1998.
26. Messner AH: Evaluation of obstructive sleep apnea by polysomnography prior to pediatric adenotonsillectomy. *Arch Otolaryngol Head Neck Surg* 125:353-356, 1999.
27. Coleman J: Sleep studies: Current techniques and future trends. *Otolaryngol Clin North Am* 32:195-210, 1999.
28. Sculerati N: Clinical opinion: Preoperative sleep studies. *Arch Otolaryngol Head Neck Surg* 125:357, 1999.

29. Practice parameters for the indications for polysomnography and related procedures. Polysomnography Task Force, American Sleep Disorders Association Standards of Practice Committee. *Sleep* 20:406-422, 1997.

30. Picchietti DL, England SJ, Walters AS, et al: Periodic limb movement disorder and restless legs syndrome in children with attention-deficit hyperactivity disorder. *J Child Neurol* 13:88-94, 1998.

31. Chervin RD, Dillon JE, Bassetti C, et al: Symptoms of sleep disorders, inattention, and hyperactivity in children. *Sleep* 20:1185-1192, 1997.

32. Riley RW, Powell NB, Guilleminault C: Obstructive sleep apnea syndrome: a review of 306 consecutively treated surgical patients. *Otolaryngol Head Neck Surg* 108:117-125, 1993.

33. Powell NB, Riley RW, Troell RJ, et al: Radiofrequency volumetric tissue reduction of the palate in subjects with sleep-disordered breathing. *Chest* 113:1163-1174, 1998.

34. Yoss RE, Daly DD: On the treatment of narcolepsy. *Med Clin North Am* 52:781-877, 1968.

35. Rechtschaffen A, Dement W: Studies on the relation of narcolepsy, cataplexy, and sleep with low voltage random EEG activity. *Res Publ Assoc Res Nerv Ment Dis* 45:488-505, 1967.

36. Hishikawa Y: [Neurophysiological characteristics of narcoleptic symptoms]. *Rev Neurol (Paris)* 116:675-676, 1967.

37. Hublin C, Kaprio J, Partinen M, et al: The prevalence of narcolepsy: An epidemiological study of the Finnish Twin Cohort. *Ann Neurol* 35:709-716, 1994.

38. Guilleminault C, Pelayo R: Narcolepsy in prepubertal children. *Ann Neurol* 43:135-142, 1998.

39. Wu MF, Gulyani SA, Yau E, et al: Locus coeruleus neurons: Cessation of activity during cataplexy [In Process Citation]. *Neuroscience* 91:1389-1399, 1999.

40. Guilleminault C, Heinzer R, Mignot E, et al: Investigations into the neurologic basis of narcolepsy. *Neurology* 50:S8-15, 1998.

41. Hishikawa Y, Shimizu T: Physiology of REM sleep, cataplexy, and sleep paralysis. *Adv Neurol* 67: 245-271, 1995.

42. Randomized trial of modafinil for the treatment of pathological somnolence in narcolepsy. US Modafinil in Narcolepsy Multicenter Study Group. *Ann Neurol* 43:88-97, 1998.

43. Juji T, Satake M, Honda Y, et al: HLA antigens in Japanese patients with narcolepsy: All the patients were DR2 positive. *Tissue Antigens* 24:316-319, 1984.

44. Mignot E, Hayduck R, Black J, et al: HLA class II studies in 509 narcoleptic patients. *Sleep Research* 1997.

45. Matsuki K, Grumet FC, Lin X, et al: DQ (rather than DR) gene marks susceptibility to narcolepsy. *Lancet* 339:1052, 1992.

46. Guilleminault C: Narcolepsy and its differential diagnosis, in Guilleminault C (ed): *Sleep and Its Disorders in Children*. New York, Raven Press 1987, pp 181-194.

47. Mignot E, Won C, Grument FC, et al: DQB1-0602 negative narcolepsy a different trigger for cataplexy? *Sleep Research* 1997.
48. Faraco J, Lin X, Li R, et al: Genetic studies in narcolepsy, a disorder affecting REM sleep. *J Hered* 90:129-132, 1999.
49. Pelin Z, Guilleminault C, Risch N, et al: HLA-DQB1*0602 homozygosity increases relative risk for narcolepsy but not disease severity in two ethnic groups: US Modafinil in Narcolepsy Multicenter Study Group. *Tissue Antigens* 51:96-100, 1998.
50. Mignot E, Young T, Lin L, et al: Nocturnal sleep and daytime sleepiness in normal subjects with HLA-DQB1*0602. *Sleep* 22:347-352, 1999.
51. Lin L, Faraco J, Li R, et al: The sleep disorder canine narcolepsy is caused by a mutation in the hypocretin (orexin) receptor 2 gene. *Cell* 98:365-376, 1999.
52. Dahl RE, Holttum J, Trubnick L: A clinical picture of child and adolescent narcolepsy. *J Am Acad Child Adolesc Psychiatry* 33:34-41, 1994.
53. Mitler MM: Evaluation of treatment with stimulants in narcolepsy. *Sleep* 17:103-106, 1994.
54. Mitler MM, Shafor R, Hajdukovich R, et al: Treatment of narcolepsy: Objective studies on methylphenidate, pemoline, and protriptyline. *Sleep* 9:260-264, 1986.
55. Iijima S, Sugita Y, Teshima Y, et al: Therapeutic effects of mazindol on narcolepsy. *Sleep* 9:265-268, 1986.
56. Bastuji H, Jouvet M: Successful treatment of idiopathic hypersomnia and narcolepsy with modafinil. *Prog Neuropsychopharmacol Biol Psychiatry* 12:695-700, 1988.
57. Besset A, Chetrit M, Carlander B, et al: Use of modafinil in the treatment of narcolepsy: A long term follow-up study. *Neurophysiol Clin* 26:60-66, 1996.
58. Mitler M: Modafinil for the treatment of pathological somnolence in patients with narcolepsy. *Sleep Research* 26:527, 1997.
59. Broughton RJ, Fleming JA, George CF, et al: Randomized, double-blind, placebo-controlled crossover trial of modafinil in the treatment of excessive daytime sleepiness in narcolepsy. *Neurology* 49:444-451, 1997.
60. Randomized trial of modafinil for the treatment of pathological somnolence in narcolepsy. US Modafinil in Narcolepsy Multicenter Study Group. *Ann Neurol* 43:88-97, 1998.
61. Lyons TJ, French J: Modafinil: Unique properties of a new stimulant. *Aviat Space Environ Med* 62:432-435, 1991.
62. Edgar DM, Seidel WF: Modafinil induces wakefulness without intensifying motor activity or subsequent rebound hypersomnolence in the rat. *J Pharmacol Exp Ther* 283:757-769, 1997.
63. Ferraro L, Antonelli T, O'Connor WT, et al: The effects of modafinil on striatal, pallidal and nigral GABA and glutamate release in the conscious rat: Evidence for a preferential inhibition of striato-pallidal GABA transmission [In Process Citation]. *Neurosci Lett* 253:135-138, 1998.

64. Engber TM, Dennis SA, Jones BE, et al: Brain regional substrates for the actions of the novel wake-promoting agent modafinil in the rat: Comparison with amphetamine. *Neuroscience* 87:905-911, 1998.

65. Laffont F, Mayer G, Minz M: Modafinil in diurnal sleepiness. A study of 123 patients. *Sleep* 17:S113-S115, 1994.

66. Tunnicliff G: Sites of action of gamma-hydroxybutyrate (GHB): A neuroactive drug with abuse potential. *J Toxicol Clin Toxicol* 35:81-90, 1997.

67. Scharf MB, Hauck M, Stover R, et al: Effect of gamma-hydroxybutyrate on pain, fatigue, and the alpha sleep anomaly in patients with fibromyalgia: Preliminary report. *J Rheumatol* 25:986-990, 1998.

68. Van Cauter E, Plat L, Scharf MB, et al: Simultaneous stimulation of slow-wave sleep and growth hormone secretion by gamma-hydroxybutyrate in normal young men. *J Clin Invest* 100:45-53, 1997.

69. Scharf MB, Lai AA, Branigan B, et al: Pharmacokinetics of gammahydroxybutyrate (GHB) in narcoleptic patients. *Sleep* 21:507-514, 1998.

70. Lammers GJ, Arends J, Declerck AC, et al: Gammahydroxybutyrate and narcolepsy: A double-blind placebo-controlled study. *Sleep* 16:216-220, 1993.

71. Adverse events associated with ingestion of gamma-butyrolactone: Minnesota, New Mexico, and Texas, 1998-1999. *MMWR Morb Mortal Wkly Rep* 48:137-140, 1999.

72. Galloway GP, Frederick SL, Staggers FE Jr, et al: Gamma-hydroxybutyrate: An emerging drug of abuse that causes physical dependence. *Addiction* 92:89-96, 1997.

73. Mignot E, Renaud A, Nishino S, et al: Canine cataplexy is preferentially controlled by adrenergic mechanisms: evidence using monoamine selective uptake inhibitors and release enhancers. *Psychopharmacology* 113:76-82, 1993.

74. Nishino S, Arrigoni J, Shelton J, et al: Desmethyl metabolites of serotonergic uptake inhibitors are more potent for suppressing canine cataplexy than their parent compounds. *Sleep* 16:706-712, 1993.

75. Frey J, Darbonne C: Fluoxetine suppresses human cataplexy: A pilot study. *Neurology* 44:707-709, 1994.

76. Berti-Ceroni G, Coccagna G, Gambi D, et al: Considerazioni clinico poligrafiche sulla narcolessia essenziola "a son nolento." *Sist Nerv* 19:81-89, 1967.

77. Mouret J, Renaud B, Quenin P, et al: Monoamines et regulation de la vigilance: Apport et interprétation biochimique des données polygraphiques, in Girard P, Couteaux R (eds): *Les Mediateurs Chimiques.* Paris, Masson, 1972, pp 139-155.

78. Roth B: Functional hypersomnia, in Guilleminault C, Dement WC, Passouant P (eds): *Narcolepsy. Advances in Sleep Research.* Vol 3. New York, Spectrum Publications, 1976, pp 333-350.

79. Guilleminault C, Faull KF: Sleepiness in non-narcoleptic, nonsleep apneic EDS patients: The idiopathic CNS hypersomnolence. *Sleep* 5:S175-S181, 1982.
80. Aldrich M: The clinical spectrum of narcolepsy and idiopathic hypersomnia. *Neurology* 46:393-401, 1996.
81. Guilleminault C, Stoohs R, Clerk A, et al: A cause of excessive daytime sleepiness: The upper airway resistance syndrome. *Chest* 104:781-787, 1993.
82. Billiard M, Merle C, Carlander B, et al: Idiopathic hypersomnia. *Psychiatry Clin Neurosci* 52:125-129, 1998.
83. Guilleminault C, Partinen M, Quera-Salva MA: Daytime sleepiness in non-narcoleptic subjects: Central nervous system hypersomnia and obstructive sleep apneic patients, in Smirne S, Franceschi M, Ferini-Strambi L (eds): *Sleep in Medical and Neuropsychiatric Disorders.* Milan, Masson, 1988, pp 111-124.
84. Van den Hoed J, Kraemer H, Guilleminault C, et al: Disorders of excessive daytime somnolence: Polygraphic and clinical data for 100 patients. *Sleep* 4:23-38, 1981.
85. Bastuji H, Jouvet M: Successful treatment of idiopathic hypersomnia and narcolepsy with modafinil. *Prog Neuropsychopharmacol Biol Psychiatry* 12:695-700, 1988.
86. Weitzman ED, Czeisler CA, Coleman RM, et al: Delayed sleep phase syndrome. A chronobiological disorder with sleep-onset insomnia. *Arch Gen Psychiatry* 38:737-746, 1981.
87. Thorpy MJ, Korman E, Spielman AJ, et al: Delayed sleep phase syndrome in adolescents. *J Adolesc Health Care* 9:22-27, 1988.
88. Dagan Y, Stein D, Steinbock M, et al: Frequency of delayed sleep phase syndrome among hospitalized adolescent psychiatric patients. *J Psychosom Res* 45:15-20, 1998.
89. Rosenthal NE, Joseph-Vanderpool JR, Levendosky Alytia A, et al: Phase-shifting effects of bright morning light as treatment for delayed sleep phase syndrome. *Sleep* 13:354-361, 1990.
90. Watanabe T, Kajimura N, Kato M, et al: Effects of phototherapy in patients with delayed sleep phase syndrome. *Psychiatry Clin Neurosci* 53:231-233, 1999.
91. Chesson AL Jr, Littner M, Davila D, et al: Practice parameters for the use of light therapy in the treatment of sleep disorders. *Sleep* 22:641-660, 1999.
92. Nagtegaal JE, Kerkhof GA, Smits MG, et al: Delayed sleep phase syndrome: A placebo-controlled cross-over study on the effects of melatonin administered five hours before the individual dim light melatonin onset. *J Sleep Res* 7:135-143, 1998.
93. Dagan Y, Yovel I, Hallis D, et al: Evaluating the role of melatonin in the long-term treatment of delayed sleep phase syndrome (DSPS). *Chronobiol Int* 15:181-190, 1998.
94. Arendt J, Middleton B, Stone B, et al: Complex effects of melatonin: Evidence for photoperiodic responses in humans? *Sleep* 22:625-635, 1999.

95. Picchietti DL, England SJ, Walters AS, et al: Periodic limb movement disorder and restless legs syndrome in children with attention-deficit hyperactivity disorder. *J Child Neurol* 13:588-594, 1998.
96. Picchietti DL, Walters AS: Moderate to severe periodic limb movement disorder in childhood and adolescence. *Sleep* 22:297-300, 1999.
97. Walters AS: Toward a better definition of the restless legs syndrome. The International Restless Legs Syndrome Study Group. *Mov Disord* 10:634-642, 1995.
98. Recording and scoring leg movements: The Atlas Task Force. *Sleep* 16:748-759, 1993.
99. Kaplan PW, Allen RP, Buchholz DW, et al: A double-blind, placebo-controlled study of the treatment of periodic limb movements in sleep using carbidopa/levodopa and propoxyphene. *Sleep* 16:717-723, 1993.
100. Montplaisir J, Nicolas A, Denesle R, et al: Restless legs syndrome improved by pramipexole: A double-blind randomized trial. *Neurology* 52:938-943, 1999.
101. Wetter TC, Stiasny K, Winkelmann J, et al: A randomized controlled study of pergolide in patients with restless legs syndrome. *Neurology* 52:944-950, 1999.
102. Lazzarini A, Walters AS, Hickey K, et al: Studies of penetrance and anticipation in five autosomal-dominant restless legs syndrome pedigrees. *Mov Disord* 14:111-116, 1999.

CHAPTER 2

Powered Instrumentation in Pediatric Otolaryngology

Peter J. Koltai, MD*

Head, Section of Pediatric Otolaryngology, Cleveland Clinic Foundation, Cleveland, Ohio

* Dr Koltai is a consultant for Linvatec Corporation.

Introduced in 1993 by Setliff and Parsons,[1] powered instrumentation for sinonasal surgery has rapidly become an important tool for the pediatric otolaryngologist. The relevance of powered instrumentation is underscored by the conceptual similarities between the ears and the sinuses. Both the ears and the sinuses are air-containing, mucosal-lined structures that communicate with the nose through small holes. Both organ systems are prone to infection with identical risk factors. Their infections can be acute, subacute, or chronic and can result from identical pathogens. Finally, both require medical and sometimes surgical management.

Ear surgery and sinus surgery are also conceptually similar. Both are done in small cavities that have complex configurations, and those cavities are in close proximity to important structures, such as the brain and the eyes. Otolaryngologists routinely use powered instrumentation for ear surgery. The hammer and gouge were long ago replaced by the otologic drill; with its high speed, sharp burs, and continuous irrigation, it is a tool of precision and accuracy. The power microdébrider system, which was initially used for sinonasal surgery, has some common features with contemporary otologic drills. Originally developed for orthopedic arthroscopic surgery, it has been modified for endoscopic sinus surgery and, more recently, for laryngeal surgery as well. It consists of a control console, a foot switch, and a handle that houses the motor. A coaxial disposable blade fits into the handpiece. The external shaft is static while the hollow inner shaft oscillates at various speeds. Suction draws soft tissue into the superimposed windows, where it is cut off by the rotating inner blade. Some of the blades can also be bent, since the inner shaft is made of a flexible material. Several companies produce prebent blades for use around corners. New blade designs for use on thick bone include covered drill burs, which are hooded on one side to protect the surrounding soft tissues.

In an important article in 1996, Parsons[2] described the use of powered instrumentation for a variety of procedures other than sinus surgery, including transnasal resection of sinonasal tumors, management of choanal atresia and recurrent papillomatosis, and dacryocystorhinostomy. This chapter reviews the contemporary uses of powered instrumentation for pediatric otolaryngology.

PEDIATRIC ENDOSCOPIC SINUS SURGERY WITH POWERED INSTRUMENTATION

Setliff and Parsons[1] were the first to describe the use of an endoscopic shaver for pediatric endoscopic sinus surgery. They reported on 345 patients, 90 of whom were children. Other authors[3-6] have described their anecdotal experiences with functional endoscopic sinus surgery (FESS) using powered instrumentation, but there are no controlled studies comparing it with standard techniques and there are certainly no reports specific to children. Krouse and Christmas[5] described a nonblinded, nonrandomized study comparing 250 patients who had FESS with powered instrumentation with 225 previous patients who had "traditional" FESS. No difference in operating time was noted. The power instrument group averaged 20 mL of blood loss, whereas the traditional group averaged 45 mL of blood loss. There were no synechiae in the power instrument group and 4 in the traditional group. One had reocclusion of the ostia in the powered instrument group compared with 7 in the traditional group. The success rate, defined as being symptom-free 6 months after surgery, was the same for both, at 85%. The authors felt that the patients in the powered instrument group healed faster.

Our own experience is with 62 children with a variety of sinus pathologies (chronic sinusitis, cystic fibrosis with chronic polyposis, ethmoid and sphenoid mucoceles, and antrochoanal and sphenoethmoidal polyps) for whom powered instrumentation was used as part of the surgical procedure. We agree with the anecdotal experience of most surgeons that powered instruments provide a precise tool for the removal of diseased mucosa and the intervening bone from pediatric paranasal sinuses. However, powered instrumentation is not a panacea that renders surgical technique easy and risk-free, and it is not entirely devoid of technical problems, some of which can compromise its utility. Our technique for a variety of sinus procedures is outlined below.

STANDARD PEDIATRIC FESS WITH POWERED INSTRUMENTATION

We begin the procedure by having the child start with 2 squirts of .05% oxymetazoline hydrochloride nasal spray in each nostril, repeated every 5 minutes before the actual surgery begins. Once the child is anesthetized, the nose is further packed with cottonoid pledgets soaked in the same vasoconstrictor. These are then removed, and on both sides the leading edge of the uncinate and the medial edge of the middle turbinate are injected with 1% xylocaine with 1:20,000 units of epinephrine. No more than 2 mL (1 mL per side) of this solution is used in total. A 4 mm 0° endoscope with a slip-on telescope irrigator (Endoscrub; Xomed, Jacksonville, Fla) is introduced into the nose and used to visualize the uncinate and middle turbinate. A Freer elevator is used to medialize the middle turbinate, and it is used to incise the uncinate. In the circumstance where the middle turbinate cannot be sufficiently medialized, the microdébrider can remove the anterior leading edge of it to provide a larger opening into the middle meatus. This maneuver can also be done with a "true cut" forceps. The endoscopic microdébrider is then introduced, with the cutting edge facing laterally to protect the lateral middle turbinate mucosa, and the uncinate is removed. Occasionally, uncinate bone will clog the microdébrider, so larger pieces of bone should be removed with conventional instruments. The removal of the uncinate allows endoscopic inspection of the lower lateral nasal wall and identification of the natural ostia of the maxillary sinus and the bulla ethmoidalis. Identification of the maxillary ostium provides an opportunity to enlarge this structure with a backbiting forceps. If the natural ostium cannot be seen, a ball tip seeker can usually be safely passed into the maxillary sinus by riding laterally over the bony insertion of the inferior turbinate at a point posterior to the posterior wall of the bulla ethmoidalis. The opening can be further enlarged, and surrounding disease can then be removed with the microdébrider. Bendable or precurved blades will facilitate this procedure, especially along the posterior and inferior edges of the antrostomy. Parsons et al[7] advocate a retrograde dissection of the uncinate process, starting in the hiatus semilunaris along the mid portion of the uncinate. Setliff[8] suggests that a powered removal of the inferior uncinate to the anterior limit of the infundibulum and exposure of the natural maxillary ostium is sufficient to return health to the maxillary sinus. Once the uncinate has been removed, the ethmoidectomy is begun with the opening of the bulla ethmoidalis. Tapping on the thin bone of the bulla ethmoidalis with the tip of the microdébrider will crack it like an eggshell, allowing a precise medial to lateral dissection. Again, larger pieces of bone can be removed with small Blakesly forceps to prevent clogging of the microdébrider. In this fashion, the inferior, medial, and posterior walls of the bulla are removed, exposing the sinus lateralis and the vertical portion of the basal lamella.

Access to the posterior ethmoids can be obtained by once again eggshelling the basal lamella with the tip of the microdébrider and then enlarging the opening by routering its edges. The posterior ethmoid complex is variably pneumatized in children, and additional air cells may need to be opened. It is imperative to visualize and maintain an accurate perspective on the roof of the ethmoid after entry into the posterior ethmoid complex. Dissection is then directed medially and inferiorly to avoid the fovea ethmoidalis and the posterior portion of the lamina papyracea.

With the opening of the posterior ethmoid air cells, one of the methods of accessing the sphenoid sinus becomes feasible. Removing the floor and medial wall of the large posterior ethmoid air cell with the microdébrider results in exposure of the anterior surgical wall of the sphenoid sinus. The sphenoid ostium is inferomedial to the opening. Parsons et al[9] have described a "ridge" of bone just lateral to the ostium and the superior turbinate as a landmark. The blunt tip of the microdébrider blade can eggshell the anterior face of the sphenoid and, once the sinus is opened, the blade can be used like a router to enlarge the opening. It is important to stay low and medial to avoid injury to vital structures.

After completion of the dissection, the ethmoid cavity can be further touched up with the microdébrider used like a polishing tool to remove or shave down irregular bony edges, débride diseased mucosa, and enlarge and smooth the openings that have been created. A gelatin film roll is generally placed between the lateral nasal wall and the middle turbinate and is left in place for 2 weeks to prevent synechiae formation. Postoperative care is the same as with traditional technique. We encourage hypertonic saline irrigations and prescribe oral amoxicillin for 4 weeks after surgery. Children are seen 2 weeks postoperatively and if they are cooperative, they are endoscopically examined and their cavities are cleaned. This is repeated every 2 weeks until their sinuses have re-mucosalized and healed.

Several points are worth mentioning. The microdébrider is only as precise as the surgeon using it, and the powerful and rapid oscillations of the instrument pose specific threats to the orbital contents. Violating the lamina papyracea with traditional instruments, while best avoided, is generally not a major problem. However, getting into the orbital fat with the microdébrider can result in a rapid and significant fat loss with a potential for orbital hemorrhage. The medial rectus muscle, especially toward the posterior orbit where it is closely approximated to the lamina papyracea, is also particularly vulnerable to injury from the microdébrider.

A major inconvenience of the microdébrider during sinus surgery is its propensity to become clogged with bits of bone that enter the cutting window and become caught within the shaft of the blade. This problem can be addressed with the use of an irrigating blade, now available from most of the blade vendors. Clogging can also be reduced by maintaining suction above 150 mm Hg and flushing saline through it whenever the blade is removed from the nose.

FRONTAL SINUS SURGERY FOR CHILDREN

The frontal sinus is not commonly involved with disease in children; however, after 11 years of age, it is usually developed sufficiently to be susceptible to disease. In most cases, adequate opening of the frontal recess is sufficient to maintain drainage. This can be accomplished by using the microdébrider in the angle between the lateral nasal wall and the middle turbinate, directing it superiorly and laterally. The bone gets thick laterally and may require a hand rongeur. After opening the junction between the lateral nasal wall and middle turbinate, and after removing the superior uncinate, the floor of the agger nasi cell becomes accessible for opening. Once opened, a ball tipped seeker is passed posteromedial to the posterior wall of the agger nasi, which is the anterior wall of the nasofrontal duct. The seeker is gently pulled anteriorly and inferiorly, creating a widened frontal sinus opening. After the down fracture, the mucosa and bone can then be removed with the microdébrider, with a 30° telescope used to visualize the site.

For more refractory frontal sinus disease in older children, Gross et al[10] have described a modified transnasal endoscopic Lothrop procedure or "frontal drill out" that results in one common opening that combines both the natural frontal ostia. The opening starts with endoscopic exposure of the frontal recess on both sides. The anatomically more favorable frontal recess is canulated for anatomical orientation. With a 30° and a 70° telescope to visualize and the use of a soft tissue microdébrider blade, the mucosa is removed from the perpendicular plate of the ethmoid on both sides of the nasal septum anterior to the frontal recess; mucosa is also taken (or sacrificed) from the anterior face of the frontal recess, bounded by the anterior-superior insertion of the middle turbinate. A cannula is then passed into the nasofrontal duct once again for anatomic guidance. The blade in the microdébrider is changed to a covered bone cutting drill (available from the various blade vendors) and is used to bur away bone from the anterior face of the frontal recess on one side, carefully staying in front of the cannula in the nasofrontal duct. The bone being drilled away on the anterior face of the frontal recess is what is known as the "nasofrontal beak." The perpendicular plate of the ethmoid, which has been denuded of mucosa is burred away from the floor of the frontal sinus, staying anterior to the reference cannula. The anterior floor of the frontal sinus is drilled away, going from lateral to medial and then crossing over to the contralateral nasofrontal duct and recess. Gross et al[10] recommend as much bone removal anteriorly between the nasofrontal ducts as possible, leaving a thin shell of bone under the glabellar region.

SPHENOID SINUS SURGERY FOR CHILDREN

The transethmoid access to the sphenoid sinuses has already been described. However, for some children with isolated sphenoid sinus disease, the small diameter and 8 cm length of the shaver blades facilitate direct access. This is not to suggest that sphenoidotomy is simple; there are many vital surrounding structures and tolerances for error are measured in millimeters. The complex anatomy is further complicated by the changing size and distance to the sphenoid sinuses in a growing child. Smith et al[11] described the variations of distance to the sphenoid sinus from the nasal spine in children between 4.7 cm to 8.2 cm.

The anterior face of the sphenoid sinus is best approached by placing the shaver between the septum and the posterior end of the middle turbinate, utilizing a 0° telescope for visualization. The middle turbinate attaches to the lateral posterior wall of the nose, just in front of the anterior wall of the sphenoid. The microdébrider is used to remove the mucosa around the posterior septum as it flares out onto the anterior sphenoid sinus wall. The anterior wall is eggshelled as close to the midline as technically feasible. The sinus is entered with the microdébrider, which is then used to further enlarge the opening. In some children, the close proximity of the middle turbinate to the septum precludes easy access to the anterior sphenoid wall and requires its removal, a maneuver that is controversial among pediatric sinus surgeons.

CYSTIC FIBROSIS

Nasal polyposis in children with cystic fibrosis is particularly well managed with the endoscopic shaver. The uncinate and the bony sinus partitions are frequently demineralized and thinned, facilitating resection with the microdébrider. The polyps themselves are rapidly evacuated without tearing the more normal surrounding mucosa. The microdébrider's sharp cutting of the polypoid tissue subjectively appears to result in less bleeding than encountered with traditional techniques. By shaving out the polyps rapidly and with less bleeding, the important landmarks amid the distorted anatomy are more readily defined, enhancing safety in primary procedures. With revision cystic fibrosis sinus surgery, the boundaries of the existing sinus spaces are readily established with the resection of the recurrent polyps.

MUCOCELES

As with cystic fibrosis, expansile mucoceles of the ethmoid sinus tend to thin and demineralize the bony septae that contain them. This renders the cyst amenable to exenteration with the microdébrider. The blunt tip of the shaver can be used to gently eggshell the bone of the cyst wall. Upon entry into the mucocele, the continuous suction of the blade evacuates the mucinous contents. The remainder of the cyst wall can be shaved away, although larger or thicker pieces of bone are often best removed by conventional instruments.

ANTROCHOANAL POLYPS

As with any polypoid sinus disease in any age group, the microdébrider is ideal for resecting antrochoanal polyps in children. The anterior component of the polyp is resected toward the middle meatus, which is generally widened by the polyp. Once the middle meatus is entered, the stalk of the polyp is followed to the hiatus semilunaris from which the posterior portion of the polyp can usually be pulled out en bloc. An uncinectomy is then performed and the unnaturally enlarged maxillary ostium, from the lower edge of which the polyps usually arise, is readily identified. The remaining lateral stalk of the polyp is shaved away from the enlarged ostium. This opening can then be further widened if the polyp arises from within the sinus and from where the diseased polyp-generative mucosa needs to be removed. A curved shaver blade may be of some help; however, the more lateral antral cleanout is often best accomplished with conventional instruments. A transbuccal puncture, through the anterior maxillary sinus wall, may be necessary in some children for better visualization and control of resection.

CHOANAL ATRESIA

Parsons[2] was the first to suggest the use of powered instrumentation for choanal atresia repair. April and Ward[12] have also described their experience with 5 unilateral cases and 2 bilateral cases. They reported that all their unilateral cases remain patent while both bilateral cases showed stenosis. Their technique is to vasoconstrict the nasal mucosa both topically and with injection. A spinal needle is passed through the atresia plate under nasopharyngeal telescopic (120°) control. Under telescopic guidance, a sickle knife is used to create mucosal flaps on the atresia plate in primary cases. A covered bone cutting drill is then used to resect the atresia plate by widening the opening created by the spinal needle. They emphasized the importance of removing the remaining lateral pterygoid lamina. Their final step is to remove the posterior vomer with a backbiting forceps. No stent is used on the unilateral cases, instead a Merocel sponge (Xomed, Jacksonville, Fla) is left in place for 24 to 48 hours. For bilateral cases, they use a 3.5 endotracheal tube as a stent for 4 to 6 weeks.

Our own technique with unilateral choanal atresia is similar, although with some minor variations. We prefer to operate after the children are over 1 year of age. Experience suggests that posterior mucosal flaps are ephemeral and of questionable value in preserving the neochoana. Instead, the mucosa of the posterior nose is resected with the microdébrider under telescopic control and the bony atresia plate is exposed. The atresia plate is pierced by a No. 6 curved urethral sound, which can be visualized or palpated in the nasopharynx. The opening is then enlarged as described by April and Ward.[12]

With bilateral choanal atresia, the small size of a neonate's nose presents an unresolved challenge in getting both a telescope and the microdébrider blade inside. For 2 infants, we've overcome this limitation by using a technique suggested by Kazanjian[13] more than 50 years ago. An incision is made through the base of the columella and extended deep into the posterior nose along the junction of the floor and the septum to the atresia plate on both sides. The cartilage of the septum, which in the neonate extends back into the atresia plate, is then dislocated along its entire length from the maxillary crest. This mobilization of the septum allows it to be freely pushed to either side of the nose to provide sufficient room for the telescope and the shaver blade. The resection of the atresia plate and the creation of the neochoana are then performed as previously described, but on both sides. Prior to closure, mitomycin is topically applied to the neochoana. The collumellar incisions are closed with 5-0 fast-absorbing cat gut (Ethicon, Somerville, NJ). The septum is allowed to swing back into the midline and is stabilized with small Merocel packs in either side of the nose for 48 hours while the infants are kept intubated. In follow-up, both of our children have maintained a patent posterior nose with no sign of choanal stenosis. Some will question the wisdom of detaching the nasal septum of a neonate in light of concerns about nasal and midfacial growth.

ADENOIDECTOMY

Koltai et al[14] introduced power-assisted adenoidectomy (PAA) in 1997. We developed the idea for this procedure during a demonstration of a bendable shaver blade for endoscopic sinus surgery. The bent cannula had a similar curve as the bend we had been shaping for our disposable suction cautery units for control of bleeding after adenoidectomy. We found that if we overbent the cannula, it comfortably fit into the nasopharynx and that the action of the shaver resecting the adenoids was easily controlled through visualization with a mirror. The rapid oscillations of the blade removes small, discrete quantities of adenoid tissue exactly at the point where the instrument is placed. In most children, the blade can reach into the choanal sill and posterior nose to remove adenoid vegetations around the vomer and choana. The cannula can also be passed through the nose while tissue resection is observed in the mirror. This specificity in the roof of the nasopharynx is ideal for children needing partial adenoidectomy.

As with any new technique, there's a learning curve to PAA. Initially, there appears to be more bleeding with the shaver than with the curet. This is because of the way the shaver removes small pieces of tissue with each oscillation, leaving a raw surface that bleeds as the remainder of the adenoidectomy is performed. However, with the hand piece on continuous suction, the blood is evacuated along with the tissue, leaving an unobstructed view of the operative field. We have found that the most efficient way to perform the procedure is to start high in the nasopharynx with the resection of the superiormost layer of adenoid and working down to the base in an orderly fashion, with the cutting edge of the shaver in continuous view.

Our initial study tried to quantify our perception that PAA was an improvement over traditional curet adenoidectomy.[14] We retrospectively reviewed the first 40 consecutive children to have PAA and compared them with the last 40 consecutive children who underwent adenoidectomy performed with conventional technique and compared operative time, blood loss, and length of hospitalization after the procedure.

With PAA, the mean operative time was significantly faster (11 minutes vs 19 minutes for the conventional method), mean blood loss was not significantly different (22 ml vs 32 ml for the conventional method), mean length of hospitalization after the procedure was not significantly different (2.95 hours vs 2.8 hours for the conventional method), and there were no surgical complications with either technique.

After establishing the utility of PAA, we sought to demonstrate the safety of this new procedure in a large cohort of patients. A retrospective review of 329 patients who had an adenoidectomy by powered instrumentation was performed.[15] Postoperative complications were documented and compared with a similar group that had curet adenoidectomy. Complications watched for included prolonged recovery, postoperative hemorrhage, readmission for dehydration, velopharyngeal insufficiency, and nasopharyngeal stenosis. No postoperative complications were seen in the PAA group. Our review confirmed the safety of PAA.

Despite demonstrating the elegance and safety of PAA, these retrospective studies had several limitations. The operative time for adenoidectomies was recorded by the anesthesiologists. The estimated blood loss was recorded in the chart by the operating room nurses. Issues that were not addressed include a comparison of the quality of the adenoid resection and the recovery periods between the 2 groups. For these reasons, a controlled, randomized, prospective study was performed to accurately assess the merits of PAA.[16] The parameters evaluated were operative time, blood loss, completeness and depth of resection, injuries to the surrounding structures, short- and long-term complications, the surgeon's satisfaction with the operation, and the parent's assessment of the child's postoperative recovery.

There were 90 children (ages 1 to 13 years) in the PAA group and 87 children (ages 1 to 12 years) in the curet adenoidectomy group. We found that PAA was 20% faster ($P < .001$) and had 27% less blood loss ($P < .001$) than curet adenoidectomy. It provided a more complete resection ($P < .001$) and better control of the depth of resection ($P < .05$). Surgeon satisfaction was greater with PAA ($P < .001$).

There were no differences in the recovery period or parent satisfaction. One patient in the PAA group returned to the operating room for postoperative bleeding and 1 child in the curet adenoidectomy group returned to the hospital for postoperative dehydration. We concluded that PAA provided a faster, dryer, more complete, and more surgically satisfying resection than curet adenoidectomy. The principal drawback of the PAA remains the $65 cost of each shaver blade.

Our technique begins the same way as traditional adenoidectomy with orotracheal intubation. The child is placed into the Rose's position with a roll under the shoulder, the head extended, and the body covered with sterile drapes. A left curved Crow-Davis mouth gag, which provides higher nasopharyngeal access than a right curved retractor, is used to retract the jaw. The soft palate is palpated for occult clefting, and if none is found, 2 red rubber catheters are passed through the nose, past the adenoids into the oropharynx, and retrieved through the mouth. The distal and proximal ends of the catheters are crossed and clamped so that they retract the soft palate providing access to the nasopharynx. The adenoids are examined with a No. 5 laryngeal mirror.

The disposable cannula of the endoscopic shaver is bent to the curvature required for the adenoidectomy with the use of the bending tool that comes with the instrument. This bendable cannula was originally developed for endoscopic sinus surgery, and the manufacturer recommends that the blade be placed 1 cm into the bending tool and given a single full bend, which yields an arch of 15°. We have found that this is an inadequate curve for oral access to the nasopharynx, and we have developed a way of overbending the cannula. We begin the bend with the window of the cannula facing upward underneath the fulcrum of the bending tool, and a full bend is given to the cannula. The cannula is then pushed 1 cm into the bending tool and then another full bend is given to the cannula. The cannula is then pushed in as far as it goes and given a final full bend. This technique yields a suitable curvature of approximately 45° for the adenoidectomy.

The cannula is then seated in the handpiece, the suction tubing is attached, and continuous suction is turned on. The adenoid tissue is collected in a sock seated in the vacuum bottle. The overbent cannula is introduced into the nasopharynx under direct mirror visualization, and the foot pedal control switch is depressed to activate the oscillating blade. The adenoidectomy is begun high in the nasopharynx near the choanal sill and the resection is performed side to side, progressing on an even level until the inferior edge of the adenoid pad is reached. The depth of adenoid resection is precisely controlled, the dissection around the torus tubarius is accurately circumspect, and resection of intranasal adenoid tissue can be performed by directly extending the cannula up toward the posterior choana or by passing it transnasally and resecting the intranasal adenoids through the nose. Transnasal use of the shaver benefits from vasoconstriction of the nasal mucosa with .05% oxymetasoline hydrochloride solution. It is imperative that the tip of the oscillating cannula be always under visual control with the use of the laryngeal mirror. Blind use of the endoscopic shaver is contraindicated.

After adenoidectomy is completed, a sponge is placed in the nasopharynx for several minutes. The sponge is removed and the bleeding is controlled with suction cautery. When hemostasis has been achieved, the hardware is removed and the child is turned back to the anesthetist for awakening and extubation.

Subsequent to our development of PAA using the bendable shaver blade (Rhinotec Blade System, Linvatec Corp, Largo, Fla), other companies have developed precurved adenoidectomy blades that are equally useful for this procedure (RADnoidectomy Blade, Xomed, Jacksonville, Fla).

PARTIAL ADENOIDECTOMY

In our original description of PAA, we noted the specificity of the microdébrider for performing partial adenoidectomy for children at risk for velopharyngeal insufficiency due to palatal abnormalities. We have performed 26 partial adenoidectomies using powered instrumentation on children with such vulnerability without subsequent problems with hypernasality. Recently, Murray et al[17] described a nonrandom series of 100 children undergoing partial adenoidectomy with powered instrumentation compared with 40 children undergoing conventional partial adenoidectomy with curets. They found that operative time was 58% shorter with the microdébrider group while blood loss was comparable for both groups. There were no complications with either group and surgical satisfaction with the microdébrider group was high. They concluded that the degree of control afforded by the microdébrider technique was of high value and consider it a preferred technique for partial adenoidectomy. Their conclusions are consistent with our own experience.

POWERED INSTRUMENTATION FOR RECURRENT RESPIRATORY PAPILLOMATOSIS

The first reference to the use of powered instrumentation for recurrent respiratory papillomatosis is by Parsons[2] in 1996. Myer et al[18] presented their experience with laryngeal powered instrumentation on 2 patients with massive recurrent respiratory papillomatosis at the 1998 annual meeting of the American Bronchoesophogologic Association. Several companies (eg, Xomed, Linvatec) have developed specialized laryngeal blades for their microdébrider systems. The initial blades were simply longer versions of the blades used for sinus surgery, typically with a proximal bend that allowed them to be used in the larynx by way of a suspended laryngoscope. These early blades, with their large-toothed cutting windows, were not precise enough for the delicate tissues of the vocal fold after the initial bulky lesions had been shaved away. Moreover, the straight distal shaft of the blade made visualization of the tissue being resected difficult. Subsequent blade refinements have included downsizing of the shaft of the blade from 4 mm to 3.5 mm, adding a slight bend to the distal tip for better visualization, reducing the distal aperture size, and replacing the aggressive toothed cutting windows with a sharp toothless cutting edge. A large 4 mm blade with a 2.0 mm toothed aperture can still be used for resecting the bulk of the papilloma, while the smaller 3.5 mm blade with a 1.4 mm toothless biting window is used for the final tissue shaving near the vocal folds.

We have had experience with 5 children with recurrent respiratory papillomatosis using the new laryngeal blades. Typically, standard laryngoscopic jet ventilation is used, although spontaneous ventilation or an endotracheal tube can also be used for anesthesia. The shaver is maintained in an oscillating mode, but the speed of the oscillations is kept well below the 1500 oscillations per minute used for sinus surgery and adenoidectomy. Bleeding can be a problem for some patients, and this can usually be controlled with topically applied epinephrine on small cottonoid pledgets. There may be a theoretical risk of distal papilloma spread from the bleeding, although we do not believe this to be a real issue.

The laryngeal blades can be used for subglottic and proximal tracheal papilloma, utilizing a 0° 4 mm Hopkins rod telescope for visualization. We have also used the shaver blades to successfully resect a child's thin subglottic web, as well as several suprastomal granulomas using the telescope for visualization. There may be further airway applications for this novel technology.

CONCLUSION

Powered instrumentation is an important tool in the surgical armamentarium of the pediatric otolaryngologist. It is applicable for sinonasal surgery, for adenoidectomy, and for the resection of laryngeal lesions such as recurrent respiratory papillomatosis and granulations. As with any tool, its utility depends on the skill and care of the surgeon. The rapid oscillations of the shaver and the high speed of the covered burs are a greater potential risk to the surrounding tissues than are conventional instruments. On the other hand, the speed and the power of these tools, when appropriately applied, broaden the scope of minimally invasive procedures for our specialty in a variety of anatomical sites. The problems encountered with the early powered instruments—such as bulky hand units, easy clogging, and insufficient power—have been sufficiently ameliorated with the refinements of the second generation of microdébriders. Unfortunately, the problem of their excessive costs has yet to be resolved.

ACKNOWLEDGEMENTS

We gratefully acknowledge the help of Dr Paul Stanislaw in performing the literature search for this chapter, and the assistance of Mr Grant Van Ulbrich in the preparation of the manuscript.

REFERENCES

1. Setliff RC, Parsons DS: The hummer: New instrumentation for endoscopic sinus surgery. *Am J Rhinol* 8:275-278, 1994.
2. Parsons DS: Rhinologic uses of powered instrumentation in children beyond sinus surgery. *Otolaryngol Clin North Am* 29:105-114, 1996.
3. Hawke WM, McCombe AW: How I do it: Nasal polypectomy with an arthroscopic bone shaver: The Stryker "Hummer." *J Otolaryngol* 24:57-59, 1995.
4. Christmas DA, Krouse JH: Powered instrumentation in functional endoscopic sinus surgery I: Surgical technique. *Ear Nose Throat J* 75:33-38, 1996.
5. Krouse JH, Christmas DA: Powered instrumentation in functional endoscopic sinus surgery II: A comparative study. *Ear Nose Throat J* 75:42-44, 1996.
6. Gross CW, Becker DG: Powered instrumentation in endoscopic sinus surgery. *Operative Techniques Otolaryngol Head Neck Surg* 7:236-241, 1996.
7. Parsons DS, Stivers FE, Talbot AR: The missed ostium sequence and the surgical approach to revision functional endoscopic sinus surgery. *Otolaryngol Clin North Am* 29:169-183, 1996.
8. Setliff RC: Minimally invasive sinus surgery: The rationale and the technique. *Otolaryngol Clin North Am* 29:115-129, 1996.
9. Parsons DS, Bulger W, Boyd E: The "Ridge" – a safer entry to the sphenoid sinus during functional endoscopic surgery in children. *Operative Techniques Otolaryngol Head Neck Surg* 5:43-44, 1994.

10. Gross CW, Gross WE, Becker DG: Modified transnasal endoscopic Lothrop procedure: Frontal drillout. *Operative Techniques Otolaryngol Head Neck Surg* 6:193-200, 1995.
11. Smith WC, Boyd EM, Parsons DS: Pediatric Sphenoidotomy. *Otolaryngol Clin North Am* 29:159-167, 1996.
12. April MM, Ward RF: Cholanal atresia repair: Use of powered instrumentation. *Operative Techniques Otolaryngol Head Neck Surg* 7:248-251, 1996.
13. Kazanjian DMD: The treatment of congenital atresia of the choana. *Ann Otol Rhinol Laryngol* 51:704-711, 1942.
14. Koltai PJ, Kalathia AS, Stanislaw P, et al: Power-assisted adenoidectomy. *Arch Otolaryngol Head Neck Surg* 123:685-688, 1997.
15. Heras HA, Koltai PJ, Stanislaw P: The safety of power-assisted adenoidectomy. *Int J Peds Otolaryngol* 44:149-153, 1998.
16. Stanislaw P, Koltai PJ, Fustel PJ: Comparison of power-assisted adenoidectomy versus adenoid curette adenoidectomy. *Arch Otolaryngol Head Neck Surg*, submitted for publication.
17. Murray NL, Fitzpatrick P, Guarisco JL: Powered partial adenoidectomy: A clinical trial. Presented at the Annual Meeting of the American Society of Pediatric Otolaryngology, Palm Desert, Calif, May 1999.
18. Myer CM, Willging JP, McMurray S, et al: The use of a laryngeal micro resector system for treatment of recurrent respiratory papillomatosis. Presented at the Annual Meeting of the American Broncho Esophalogical Association, Palm Beach, Fla, May 1998.

CHAPTER 3

Management of Sinusitis in the Patient With Cystic Fibrosis

Anna H. Messner, MD
Assistant Professor of Surgery, Otolaryngology/Head & Neck Surgery, Stanford University, Palo Alto, Calif

Mary Lynn Moran, MD
Voluntary Clinical Faculty, Stanford University Hospital, Palo Alto, Calif

Ten years have passed since the discovery of the cystic fibrosis (CF) gene on the long arm of chromosome 7.[1] Since then, great strides have been made in understanding the pathogenesis of CF and improving its treatment. At present, the average lifespan for a patient with CF is 29 years—a vast improvement over the 14-year life span predicted in 1969.[2] In addition, it is estimated that a patient born today will live approximately 40 years, even with no further advances in CF treatment.[3] The mainstay of CF treatment is intravenous antibiotic therapy. Despite this, pulmonary function for patients with CF declines approximately 2% per year; eventually, 90% of patients die of lung disease.[2]

The CF protein, called the cystic fibrosis transmembrane conductance regulator (CFTR), is a cyclic adenosine monophosphate–dependent ion channel whose activation is defective in CF cells. This defect causes the cells lining the exocrine glands of patients with CF to have reduced chloride permeability, impairing fluid and electrolyte secretion into the lumen and resulting in abnormally viscous mucus of the upper and lower airways and the pancreas. The mucostasis results in obstruction of sinus ostia, leading to sinus disease for patients with CF.

Radiographic sinus disease is nearly universal among patients with CF.[4] Coronal computed tomography is considered the most useful radiographic test to evaluate the sinuses; sinus plain films have little diagnostic value.[5] A triad of findings are typical on the coronal CTs of patients with CF (in contrast to chronic sinusitis patients without CF). These include (1) a higher prevalence of maxillary and ethmoid sinus opacification, (2) medial bulging of the lateral nasal wall, and (3) a higher prevalence of frontal sinus agenesis (Fig 1).[6,7] Demineralization of the uncinate process also has been described.[8] Some authors believe, however, that the uncinate process is not reabsorbed but is displaced against the septum or rolled 180 degrees so that the free edge points anteriorly.[9] Mucoceles are not uncommon in patients with CF and have been seen in a child as young as 13 months of age.[10-12]

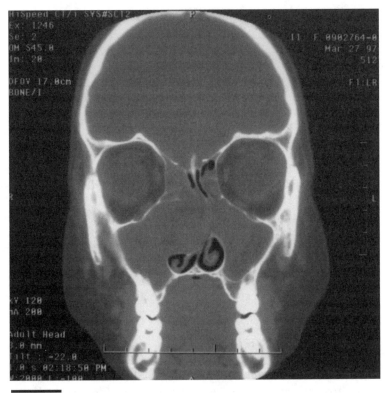

FIGURE 1.
Coronal CT scan of the sinuses from an 11-year-old girl with CF and extensive sinonasal polyposis. Scan demonstrates typical features of sinusitis in patients with CF including opacification of the maxillary and ethmoid sinuses and medialization of the lateral nasal wall.

DIAGNOSIS OF CF

Occasionally, a child will have chronic sinusitis and no other systemic symptoms that would lead to a diagnosis of CF.[8,13] For this reason, it is important for the practicing otolaryngologist to have a basic understanding of the fundamentals of CF diagnosis. The incidence of CF among whites is 1 in 3200 newborns in the United States, 1 in 15,000 blacks, and 1 in 31,000 Asian Americans.[14] Approximately 3.3% of whites in the United States are asymptomatic carriers of the CF gene.[2] The most common mutation causing malfunction of the CFTR is a deletion of a phenylalanine at position 508 (ΔF508). This deletion is found on approximately 70% of CF chromosomes. The ΔF508 mutation is most commonly found among whites and is responsible for only 30% of the mutations in black CF populations. Another 600 abnormalities of the CF gene have been described.[15] Genotype analysis of patients with CF who have undergone sinus surgery for polyposis showed a higher prevalence of the ΔF508/ΔF508 and ΔF508/G551D genotypes.[16,17]

The CF foundation consensus panel has stated that a diagnosis of CF should be based on the presence of one or more characteristic phenotypic features (Table 1) and an increased sweat chloride concentration.[14] Alternative criteria for diagnosing CF are delineated in Table 2. The only acceptable sweat test is the quantitative pilocarpine iontophoresis sweat test.[14] A sweat chloride concentration of more than 60 mmol/L is consistent with a diagnosis of CF. Testing should be carried out by experienced personnel at facilities that perform adequate numbers of tests to maintain laboratory quality control.

Commercial mutation screening panels that detect the most common CF DNA mutations are now available. For individuals with clinical features consistent with CF, identification of two known CF mutations by a Clinical Laboratory Improvement Amendment-accredited DNA diagnostic laboratory confirms the diagnosis. Many hospitals do not offer sweat tests, and it is tempting to rely on the DNA analysis to make the diagnosis of CF. The inability to detect CF mutations does not rule out a diagnosis of CF because the current commercially available mutation screening panels only detect 80% to 85% of CF mutations.[14] Conversely, the diagnosis of CF should not be made based on the presence of two mutations alone because there can be additional mutations that mitigate the abnormal mutations, leading to erroneous identification of CF.[18]

Nasal potential difference measurements also can help confirm the diagnosis of CF in the 2% of patients with an "atypical" phenotype consisting of chronic sinopulmonary disease, normal pan-

TABLE 1.

Phenotypic Features Consistent with a Diagnosis of CF

1. Chronic sinopulmonary disease manifested by
    a. Persistent colonization/infection with typical CF pathogens including *Staphylococcus aureus*, nontypeable *Haemophilus influenzae*, mucoid and nonmucoid *Pseudomonas aeruginosa*, and *Burkholderia cepacia*
    b. Chronic cough and sputum production
    c. Persistent chest radiograph abnormalities (e.g., bronchiectasis, atelectasis, infiltrates, hyperinflation)
    d. Airway obstruction manifested by wheezing and air trapping
    e. Nasal polyps; radiographic or CT abnormalities of the paranasal sinuses
    f. Digital clubbing
2. Gastrointestinal and nutritional abnormalities including
    a. Intestinal: meconium ileus, distal intestinal obstruction syndrome, rectal prolapse
    b. Pancreatic: pancreatic insufficiency, recurrent pancreatitis
    c. Hepatic: chronic hepatic disease manifested by clinical or histologic evidence of focal biliary cirrhosis or multilobular cirrhosis.
    d. Nutritional: failure to thrive (protein-calorie malnutrition), hypoproteinemia and edema, complications secondary to fat-soluble vitamin deficiency
3. Salt loss syndromes: acute salt depletion, chronic metabolic alkalosis
4. Male urogenital abnormalities resulting in obstructive azoospermia (congenital bilateral absence of vas deferens.)

(Courtesy of Rosenstein BJ, Cutting GR: The diagnosis of cystic fibrosis: A consensus statement. *J Pediatr* 132:590, 1998.)

TABLE 2.

Criteria for the Diagnosis of CF

One or more characteristic phenotypic features
    —or a history of CF in a sibling
    —or a positive newborn screening test
AND an increased sweat chloride concentration by pilocarpine iontophoresis on two or more occasions
    —or identification of two CF mutations
    —or demonstration of abnormal nasal epithelial ion transport.

(Courtesy of Rosenstein BJ, Cutting GR: The diagnosis of cystic fibrosis: A consensus statement. *J Pediatr* 132:594, 1998.)

creatic function, and either borderline (40 to 60 mmol/L) or normal (<40 mmol/L) sweat chloride concentrations.

SINONASAL SYMPTOMS

Sinonasal symptoms are a frequent but not universal complaint of patients with CF, despite the nearly universal severe disease seen radiographically. Some believe that because of the long-standing, congenital nature of the sinusitis, patients with CF psychologically adapt and do not recognize that anything is amiss in their nose or sinuses, even though typical CF radiographic findings in a patient without CF would likely elicit significant complaints.[9] Theoretically, patients with CF would benefit from treatment of their "asymptomatic" sinus disease by the establishment of a new baseline for comparison that allows them to recognize their symptoms.

When present, the most common symptoms include nasal obstruction, nasal drainage, headaches, anosmia, facial pain, postnasal drip, and recurrent sinusitis.[19-21] Gentile and Isaacson[22] reported that if polyps were present, the major complaint was nasal obstruction; if chronic sinusitis without polyps was present, the major complaint was headaches. Polyps were present in approximately 43% of patients with CF when nasal endoscopy was used in the examination.[23]

MEDICAL MANAGEMENT

Medical management of chronic CF paranasal sinus disease is largely ineffective.[24,25] Oral or intravenous antibiotics may decrease the inflammatory response that contributes to chronic sinusitis, but they do not alter the underlying problem—the increased viscosity of the mucus. Topical nasal steroids are often used to decrease nasal inflammation and polyposis, but no controlled trials have been performed on the efficacy of nasal steroids in this population. Some anecdotal evidence suggests that topical steroids have little effect on massive nasal polyposis, although they may have some effect on small polyps.[7,26]

SURGICAL MANAGEMENT

Indications for surgical management in CF sinus disease are controversial.[27,28] Some authors[25,26,29] believe that only actively symptomatic patients should consider surgery. Specifically, these authors recommend surgery when persistent nasal obstruction is present with nasal polyposis or medial bulging of the lateral nasal wall or chronic facial pain or headaches with associated sinus disease. Nishioka et al[9] have recommended the following additional indications: (1) medialization of the lateral nasal wall, without subjective nasal airway obstruction, because of the high prevalence of mucocelelike formation; (2) pulmonary exacerbations that appear to correlate with sinonasal disease exacerbations (particularly with a reactive airway component and the presence of purulent postnasal drainage) or worsening of the patient's pulmonary status or activity level despite appropriate medical management; and more generally, (3) "a desire for improvement in symptom profile beyond what medical management has achieved in a patient with significant nasal cavity and paranasal sinus symptoms."

This last recommendation is based on two theories. First, the physical comfort and sense of well-being of patients with CF may be improved after sinus surgery, even though they did not have active symptoms because of "symptom adaptation." Second, sinusitis may adversely affect the lower respiratory tract, as is commonly believed to be the case in asthma.[30] If the sinusitis improves, the lower respiratory tract symptoms may improve. In support of this second theory, Umetsu et al[31] found an improvement in respiratory symptoms and a decrease in hospital admissions among a small number of patients with CF who had undergone sinus surgery. The question of whether objective measures of pulmonary function improve after surgery is controversial, with authors presenting data both pro and con.[31-33] In addition to the above, we consider potential lung transplantation to be a valid indication for sinus surgery, as discussed below.

The success of sinus surgery depends somewhat on the type of surgery performed. Polypectomy with or without nasal antral irrigation generally results in short-term benefit only.[34,35] Polypectomy with additional sinus surgery, specifically ethmoidectomy and maxillary antrostomy, appears to reduce the rate of recurrence or prolong the time between recurrences.[34,36] During the last decade, endoscopic sinus surgery (ESS) has been shown to be safe and has become the standard surgical method for patients with chronic CF sinusitis who decide to undergo surgery.[37]

Several series have reported successful initial resolution of sinus symptoms, particularly nasal obstruction, after endoscopic sinus surgery.[22,26,32,38-40] Additionally, Nishioka et al.[20] reported significant improvements in olfactory function, purulent nasal discharge, activity level, facial pain, and snoring after surgery in the only prospective study evaluating this subject. Most series have reported no significant postoperative improvement in headaches,[20,25,38] although this finding is not universal.[22] It is likely that headaches persist because of other etiologies, such as the chronic hypoxia that patients with CF experience as a result of their lung disease. ESS has been shown to be safe, with none of the above series reporting any serious complications. Over time, clinically undetectable unilateral or bilateral reduced maxillary sinus volume may develop in the patient with CF who undergoes ESS.[41] The incidence of this anatomic abnormality is not known.

Although improvement in patients' sinus symptoms is significant, their paranasal sinus disease may recur because surgery does not affect the underlying mucosal defect. Rowe-Jones and Mackay[40] reported that 50% of their 46 patients with CF who underwent ESS returned to their preoperative symptom state or required a second operation within 18 and 24 months. Not surprisingly, those whose main complaint was nasal obstruction and who had larger intranasal polyps were more likely to suffer a deterioration in symptoms or require further surgery, compared with the group who underwent ESS for a main complaint of pain or mucopurulent rhinorrhea. Similarly, Nishioka et al[20] reported that polyps recurred in 6 of the 13 patients with preoperative polyps, but none was symptomatically obstructive. No patient in this series of 29 patients had recurrence of medial bulging of the lateral nasal wall.

ESS WITH SERIAL ANTIMICROBIAL LAVAGE

The persistence or recurrence of paranasal sinus disease among patients with CF after ESS is a difficult problem. At our institution, Moss and King[42] developed a program of repeated antimicrobial lavage of the maxillary sinuses during the first postoperative week, followed by monthly lavage treatments, to combat the recurrence of signs and symptoms after ESS. Typically, their patients were colonized with aminoglycoside-sensitive *Pseudomonas aeruginosa* and were treated with topical tobramycin. Moss and King compared the results of 19 patients who underwent ESS alone with 32 patients who underwent ESS and antimicrobial lavage. The group that underwent lavage had fewer operations per patient and a decrease in repeated surgery at 1-year (10% vs 47%) and 2-year (22% vs 72%) follow-ups. Other practitioners have adopted this protocol during the postoperative period[32] and after.[43]

The rationale for the use of topical antimicrobial lavage is supported by the studies on inhaled tobramycin for pulmonary care of patients with CF. Intravenous antibiotics have long been the mainstay of therapy for pulmonary infections in this patient population. Inhaled tobramycin, however, is being used increasingly for those patients whose lungs are colonized with *P aeruginosa*. In two multicenter, double-blind, placebo-controlled trials involving

520 patients, long-term intermittent inhaled tobramycin was compared with a placebo group.[44] The treatment group was found to have an average improvement of 10% of forced expiratory volume in 1 second (FEV_1), compared with the control group, which had a 2% decline in FEV_1 ($P < .001$). The patients in the tobramycin group were 26% less likely to be hospitalized than those in the placebo group. Although not statistically significant, the trend in this study was toward increased minimal inhibitory concentration of tobramycin for the treatment group.

ESS with repeated long-term antimicrobial lavage has become the standard at our institution. Although it is not necessary for all patients with CF (we have a few patients who have had no recurrence of their sinus disease since ESS), we have found that the sinus disease is reasonably well controlled with monthly (on average) instillation of tobramycin. Not surprisingly, sinusitis among patients with a history of extensive nasal polyposis is harder to control. A butterfly catheter, with the needle and a portion of the tubing removed, attached to a 3-cc syringe is used to apply the antibiotic to the maxillary sinuses. Those patients who are not colonized with *P aeruginosa* or who are resistant to tobramycin are lavaged with other antibiotics, most commonly piperacillin. Sulfite-free tobramycin is available to patients who are allergic to sulfa. The primary disadvantage of this program is that repeated visits to the otolaryngology office are required. We have tried to teach some of our patients to lavage their sinuses at home. We have found, however, that they have difficulty cannulating the maxillary sinus, and that an aerosolized spray bottle does not provide an optimum concentration of tobramycin into the sinuses. A similar approach used by practitioners in San Diego involves a dental irrigator (eg, Water-pik) attachment to irrigate the sinuses on a daily basis.[43]

ESS with repeated antibiotic lavage theoretically could lead to an increase in resistant organisms among patients with CF who follow this protocol. Data from our institution[45] of sinus and sputum cultures of 35 patients who underwent sinus surgery with subsequent antimicrobial lavage were compared with a control group (n = 92) who did not undergo sinus surgery. Monthly application of tobramycin to the maxillary sinuses did not contribute significantly to the development of resistance in the sputum or sinus secretions of patients with CF.

LUNG TRANSPLANTATION

More than 700 patients with CF have undergone lung transplantation.[46] Patients with CF are transplant candidates when they have progressive respiratory insufficiency that will probably cause death shortly after the expected waiting period for donor lungs. (The waiting period is currently 6 to >24 months.) The 3-year survival rate for CF transplants performed since 1992 is 56%, and the current 5-year survival rate for patients with CF is 48%.[46] Survival rates of CF lung transplant recipients are comparable to those of lung transplant patients with other underlying diagnoses.

Physicians in some transplant centers believe that the paranasal sinuses are an important reservoir of posttransplant lung infection for patients with CF.[46] Although survival does not appear to be affected, lung transplant patients with CF have an increased rate of allograft *Pseudomonas* infection after transplant, compared with non-CF lung transplant patients, and the infections occur earlier after the transplant.[47] Walter et al[48] examined the *P aeruginosa* species infecting the airways before and after lung transplantation. They found that each of 11 lung transplant recipients harbored one identical *P aeruginosa* clone before and after transplantation. They concluded that "the chronic drainage of *P. aeruginosa* into the lung allografts is caused by the bacterial reservoir in the paranasal sinuses and the trachea." For this reason, some centers require that transplant candidates undergo endoscopic sinus surgery with serial antimicrobial lavage or inhaled antimicrobials.[43,49] Others recommend that the sinuses be evaluated pretransplant, but they only advise surgery if severe polyp disease or significant symptoms are present.[50] At our institution, patients with CF and radiographic paranasal sinus disease who are transplant candidates undergo ESS with monthly postoperative lavage, even if they have no sinus-related symptoms.

NEW TREATMENTS

Anti-inflammatory medicines, including ibuprofen, oral corticosteroids, and inhaled corticosteroids have been used by patients with CF to decrease airway inflammation and preserve pulmonary function. In a double-blind trial, 85 patients with mild lung disease received either high-dose ibuprofen or placebo twice daily for 4 years.[51] The group that received the ibuprofen had a significantly slower rate of decline in their FEV_1 and forced vital capacity (FVC) compared with the placebo group; also, patients in the ibuprofen group better maintained their weight.

Oral steroids also have been used by patients with CF. In a 4-year multicenter trial of alternate-day prednisone therapy involving 285 patients, prednisone in a dose of 1 mg/kg resulted in improved pulmonary function compared with placebo in those patients colonized with *P aeruginosa.*[52] This trial also included a group receiving 2 mg/kg on alternate days, but that therapy was terminated early because of a high incidence of side effects (glucose abnormalities, growth retardation.) Growth retardation also developed in the 1 mg/kg group after 2 years of alternate-day therapy.

Approximately 12% of patients with CF use inhaled corticosteroids.[53] Three short-term trials of inhaled corticosteroids demonstrated inconclusive effects on the pulmonary status of patients with CF.[54-56]

Distal airway obstruction among patients with CF is caused by the accumulation of thick, purulent secretions. Two components of the thick secretions are mucus glycoproteins and DNA. Extracellular DNA is released by leukocytes into the airway in response to the chronic bacterial infection present in CF, making the secretions particularly viscous. Deoxyribonuclease I (DNase I) is an enzyme, normally present in blood, saliva, urine, and pancreatic secretions, that digests extracellular DNA. Aerosolized recombinant human DNase I (rhDNase, dornase alfa [Pulmozyme]) is currently being used by patients with CF to decrease the viscosity of their pulmonary secretions. Used twice a day, rhDNase has been shown to decrease respiratory exacerbations by 37% and to improve FEV_1 by a mean of approximately 5%.[57] Laryngitis with hoarseness is more common in rhDNase-treated patients. Thus far, aerosolized rhDNase has not been used in the paranasal sinuses of patients with CF. Theoretically, because rhDNase has been effective in decreasing the viscosity of pulmonary secretions, it also may be effective in decreasing the secretions that accumulate in the paranasal sinuses, even after sinus surgery. Chronic sinusitis and its acute exacerbations could potentially be decreased with this new therapy. Further investigation is needed.

GENE THERAPY

Cloning of the CFTR gene in 1989 enabled the development of gene therapy. Theoretically, if the normal gene can be introduced into the abnormal cells lining the respiratory tract, then chloride transport can be restored, leading to improved viscosity of luminal secretions. In vitro studies suggest that correction of 10% of airway epithelial cells should be sufficient for clinical benefit.[58] Various vectors to introduce the CF gene into respiratory cells are currently being investigated. Adenovirus vectors have been found to result in only transient expression of the gene and to cause a rapid inflammatory response from patients with CF, thus far limiting the viability of these vectors.[59,60] Adeno-associated virus vectors are currently under investigation. In a recent phase I study using the maxillary sinus as the test site, CFTR cDNA was transferred to the mucosal cells and found to persist for up to 10 weeks.[61] Two nonviral systems being studied to provide for CFTR gene transfer are liposome-DNA complexes and molecular conjugates.[62]

The nose and maxillary sinuses have been used in several gene therapy trials to test the safety and efficacy of CF gene therapy.[62] The nasal and sinus epithelia contain the same defects as the lung epithelium, and they allow for the administration of a low volume of vectors to accessible areas of epithelium.[63] In addition, the maxillary sinuses are attractive for evaluating new CF treatments because they have similar microbiology as the lower respiratory tract; theoretically, clinical efficacy can be measured by the recurrence of sinusitis.[64] Nasal endoscopy can be used in conjunction with patient symptoms to assess the recurrence of sinusitis in the patient undergoing CF gene therapy. Recurrent sinusitis can be used as a surrogate model for infectious exacerbations of CF lung disease.

The primary focus of gene therapy is to correct the genetic defect in the lungs of patients with CF because the most significant morbidity of this disease is found in the lungs. If gene therapy becomes widespread, however, sinusitis may also be treated with aerosolized gene therapy.

CONCLUSION

During the past 10 years, the discovery of the genetic basis of CF has led to major advances in CF diagnosis and treatment. ESS is currently the standard therapy for patients with CF and chronic sinusitis, although the indications for ESS among patients with CF are somewhat controversial. Patients with CF who undergo ESS can expect significant symptom improvement after their surgery, although they must be informed that their symptoms are likely to return. Serial antimicrobial lavage after ESS can lead to prolonged symptom resolution and is the standard of care for potential recipients at some lung transplant centers. RhDNase and gene therapy are potential treatments for patients with CF to improve both their pulmonary and nasal function.

REFERENCES

1. Kerem B, Rommens JM, Buchanan JA, et al: Identification of the cystic fibrosis gene: Genetic analysis. *Science* 245:1073-1080, 1989.
2. FitzSimmons SC: The changing epidemiology of cystic fibrosis. *J Pediatr* 122:1-9, 1993.

3. Collins FS: Cystic fibrosis: Molecular biology and therapeutic implications. *Science* 256:774-779, 1992.
4. Ledesma-Medina J, Osman MZ, Girdany BR: Abnormal paranasal sinuses in patients with cystic fibrosis of the pancreas. *Pediatr Radiol* 9:61-64, 1980.
5. Kerrebijn JDF, Poublon RML, Overbeek SE: Nasal and paranasal disease in adult cystic fibrosis patients. *Eur Respir J* 5:1239-1242, 1992.
6. Nishioka GJ, Cook PR, McKinsey JP, et al: Paranasal sinus computed tomography scan findings in patients with cystic fibrosis. *Otolaryngol Head Neck Surg* 114:394-399, 1996.
7. Brihaye P, Jorrissen M, Clement R: Chronic rhinosinusitis in cystic fibrosis (mucoviscidosis). *Acta Otorhinolaryngol Belg* 51:323-337, 1997.
8. April MM, Zinreich SJ, Baroody FM, et al: Coronal CT scan abnormalities in children with chronic sinusitis. *Laryngoscope* 103:985-990, 1993.
9. Nishioka GJ, Cook PR: Paranasal sinus disease in patients with cystic fibrosis. *Otolaryngol Clin North Am* 29:193-205, 1996.
10. Tunkel DE, Naclerio RM, Baroody FM, et al: Bilateral maxillary sinus mucoceles in an infant with cystic fibrosis. *Otolaryngol Head Neck Surg* 111:116-120, 1994.
11. Alvarez RJ, Liu NJ, Isaacson G: Pediatric ethmoid mucoceles in cystic fibrosis: Long-term follow-up of reported cases. *Ear Nose Throat J* 76:538-546, 1997.
12. Davis WE, Barbero GJ, LaMear, et al: Paranasal sinus mucoceles in cystic fibrosis. *Am J Rhinol* 7:31-35, 1993.
13. Wiatrak BJ, Myer CM, Cotton RT: Cystic fibrosis presenting with sinus disease in children. *Am J Dis Child* 147:258-260, 1993.
14. Rosenstein BJ, Cutting GR: The diagnosis of cystic fibrosis: A consensus statement. *J Pediatr* 132:589-595, 1998.
15. Rubin BK: Emerging therapies for cystic fibrosis lung disease. *Chest* 115:1120-1126, 1999.
16. Kingdom TT, Lee KC, FitzSimmons C, et al: Clinical characteristics and genotype analysis of patients with cystic fibrosis and nasal polyposis requiring surgery. *Arch Otolaryngol Head Neck Surg* 122:1209-1213, 1996.
17. Jorissen MB, DeBoeck K, Cuppens H: Genotype-phenotype correlations for the paranasal sinuses in cystic fibrosis. *Am J Respir Crit Care Med* 159:1312-1416, 1999.
18. Chmiel JF, Drumm ML, Konstan MW, et al: Pitfall in the use of genotype analysis as the sole diagnostic criterion for cystic fibrosis. *Pediatrics* 103:823-826, 1999.
19. Brihaye P, Clement PAR, Dab I, et al: Pathological changes of the lateral nasal wall in patients with cystic fibrosis (mucoviscidosis). *Int J Pediatr Otorhinolaryngol* 28:141-147, 1994.
20. Nishioka GJ, Barbero G, Konig P, et al: Symptom outcome following functional endoscopic sinus surgery in patients with cystic fibrosis: A prospective study. *Otolaryngol Head Neck Surg* 113:440-445, 1995.

21. Ravilly S, Robinson W, Suresh S, et al: Chronic pain in cystic fibrosis. *Pediatrics* 98:741-747, 1996.
22. Gentile VG, Isaacson G: Patterns of sinusitis in cystic fibrosis. *Laryngoscope* 106:1005-1009, 1996.
23. Coste A, Gilain L, Roger G, et al: Endoscopic and CT-scan evaluation of rhinosinusitis in cystic fibrosis. *Rhinology* 33:152-156, 1995.
24. Cuyler JP, Monaghan AJ: Cystic fibrosis and sinusitis. *J Otolaryngol* 18:173-175, 1989.
25. Ramsey B, Richardson MA: Impact of sinusitis in cystic fibrosis. *J Allergy Clin Immunol* 90:547-552, 1992.
26. Cuyler JP: Follow-up endoscopic sinus surgery on children with cystic fibrosis. *Arch Otolaryngol Head Neck Surg* 118:505-506, 1992.
27. Marks SC: Endoscopic sinus surgery in patients with cystic fibrosis. *Otolaryngol Head Neck Surg* 114:840, 1996.
28. Nishioka GJ, Parsons DS, Cook PR, et al: Endoscopic sinus surgery in patients with cystic fibrosis. *Otolaryngol Head Neck Surg* 114:840-841, 1996.
29. Marks SC, Kissner DG: Management of sinusitis in adult cystic fibrosis. *Am J Rhinol* 11:11-14, 1997.
30. Adinoff AD, Cummings NP: Sinusitis and its relationship to asthma. *Pediatr Ann* 18:785-790, 1989.
31. Umetsu DT, Moss RB, King VV, et al: Sinus disease in patients with severe cystic fibrosis: Relation to pulmonary exacerbation. *Lancet* 335:1077-1078, 1990.
32. Halvorson DJ, Dupree JR, Porubsky ES: Management of chronic sinusitis in the adult cystic fibrosis patient. *Ann Otol Rhinol Laryngol* 107:946-952, 1998.
33. Madonna D, Isaacson G, Rosenfeld RM, et al: Effect of sinus surgery on pulmonary function in patients with cystic fibrosis. *Laryngoscope* 107:328-331, 1997.
34. Jaffe BF, Strome M, Khaw KT, et al: Nasal polypectomy and sinus surgery for cystic fibrosis: A 10-year review. *Otolaryngol Clin North Am* 10:81-90, 1977.
35. Drake-Lee AB, Morgan DW: Nasal polyps and sinusitis in children with cystic fibrosis. *J Laryngol Otol* 103:753-755, 1989.
36. Crockett DM, McGill TJ, Healy GB, et al: Nasal and paranasal sinus surgery in children with cystic fibrosis. *Ann Otol Rhinol Laryngol* 96:367-372, 1987.
37. Schulte DL, Kasperbauer JL. Safety of paranasal sinus surgery in patients with cystic fibrosis. *Laryngoscope* 108:1813-1815, 1998.
38. Jones JW, Parsons DS, Cuyler JP: The results of functional endoscopic sinus (FES) surgery on the symptoms of patients with cystic fibrosis. *Int J Pediatr Otorhinolaryngol* 28:25-32, 1993.
39. Nishioka GJ, Barbero GJ, König P, et al: Symptom outcome after functional endoscopic sinus surgery in patients with cystic fibrosis: A prospective study. *Otolaryngol Head Neck Surg* 113:440-445, 1995.

40. Rowe-Jones JM, Mackay IS: Endoscopic sinus surgery in the treatment of cystic fibrosis with nasal polyposis. *Laryngoscope* 106:1540-1544, 1996.

41. Kosko JR, Hall BE, Tunkel DE: Acquired maxillary sinus hypoplasia: A consequence of endoscopic sinus surgery? *Laryngoscope* 106:1210-1213, 1996.

42. Moss RB, King VV: Management of sinusitis in cystic fibrosis by endoscopic surgery and serial antimicrobial lavage. *Arch Otolaryngol Head Neck Surg* 121:566-572, 1995.

43. Davidson TM, Morphy C, Mitchell M, et al: Management of chronic sinusitis in cystic fibrosis. *Laryngoscope* 105:354-358, 1995.

44. Ramsey BW, Pepe MS, Quan JM, et al: Intermittent administration of inhaled tobramycin in patients with cystic fibrosis. *N Engl J Med* 340:23-30, 1999.

45. Messner AH, Moran ML, Nepomuceno IB, Wagner JA: Tobramycin resistance: Patterns in cystic fibrosis patients with chronic sinusitis undergoing serial antimicrobial lavage. Unpublished data.

46. Yankaskas JR, Mallory GB, Consensus Committee: Lung transplantation in cystic fibrosis. *Chest* 113:217-226, 1998.

47. Nunley DR, Grgurich W, Iacono AT, et al: Allograft colonization and infections with *Pseudomonas* in cystic fibrosis lung transplant recipients. *Chest* 113:1235-1243, 1998.

48. Walter S, Gudowius P, Bosshammer J, et al: Epidemiology of chronic *Pseudomonas aeruginosa* infections in the airways of lung transplant recipients with cystic fibrosis. *Thorax* 51:318-321, 1997.

49. Lewiston N, King V, Umetsu D, et al: Cystic fibrosis patients who have undergone heart-lung transplantation benefit from maxillary sinus antrostomy and repeated sinus lavage. *Transplant Proc* 23:1207-1208, 1991.

50. Mendeloff EN, Huddleston CB, Mallory GB: Pediatric and adult lung transplantation for cystic fibrosis. *J Thorac Cardiovasc Surg* 115:404-414, 1998.

51. Konstan MW, Byard PH, Hoppel CL, et al: Effect of high-dose ibuprofen in patients with cystic fibrosis. *N Engl J Med* 332:848-854, 1995.

52. Eigen H, Rosenstein BJ, FitzSimmons S, et al: A multicenter study of alternate-day prednisone therapy in patients with cystic fibrosis. *J Pediatr* 126:515-523, 1995.

53. Oermann CM, Sockrider MM, Konstan MW: The use of anti-inflammatory medications in cystic fibrosis. *Chest* 115:1053-1058, 1999.

54. Balfour-Lynn IM, Klein NJ, Dinwiddie R: Randomised controlled trial of inhaled corticosteroids (fluticasone propionate) in cystic fibrosis. *Arch Dis Child* 77:124-30, 1997.

55. Van Haren EH, Lammers JW, Festen J, et al: The effects of the inhaled corticosteroid budesonide on lung function and bronchial hyperresponsiveness in adult patients with cystic fibrosis. *Respir Med* 89:209-214, 1995.

56. Nikolaizik WH, Schoni MH: Pilot study to assess the effect of inhaled corticosteroids on lung function in patients with cystic fibrosis. *J Pediatr* 128:271-274, 1996.

57. Fuchs HJ, Borowitz DS, Christiansen DH, et al: Effect of aerosolized recombinant human Dnase on exacerbations of respiratory symptoms and on pulmonary function in patients with cystic fibrosis. *N Engl J Med* 331:637-642, 1994.

58. Johnson LG, Olsen JC, Sarkadi B, et al: Efficiency of gene transfer for restoration of normal airway epithelial function in cystic fibrosis. *Nat Genet* 2:21-25, 1992.

59. Knowles MR, Hohneker KW, Zhou Z, et al: A controlled study of adenoviral-vector-mediated gene transfer in the nasal epithelium of patients with cystic fibrosis. *N Engl J Med* 333:823-831, 1995.

60. Rosenstein BJ, Zeitlin PL: Cystic fibrosis. *Lancet* 351:277-282, 1998.

61. Wagner JA, Moran ML, Messner AH, et al: Efficient and persistent gene transfer of AAV-CFTR in the CF maxillary sinus. *Laryngoscope* 109:266-274, 1999.

62. Wagner JA, Gardner P: Towards cystic fibrosis gene therapy. *Annu Rev Med* 48:203-216, 1997.

63. Boucher RC, Knowles MR: Gene therapy for cystic fibrosis using E1-deleted adenovirus: A phase I trial in the nasal cavity. *Hum Gene Ther* 5:615-639, 1994.

64. Wagner JA, Nepomuceno IB, Shah N, et al: Maxillary sinusitis as a surrogate model for CF gene therapy clinical trials. *J Gene Med* 1:13-21, 1999.

CHAPTER 4

Update on the Effects of Gastroesophageal Reflux Disease on Otolaryngologic Disorders in Infants and Children

Robert F. Yellon, MD
Assistant Professor of Otolaryngology, University of Pittsburgh School of Medicine; Co-director, Department of Pediatric Otolaryngology; Director of Clinical Services, Children's Hospital of Pittsburgh, Pa

Gastroesophageal reflux disease (GERD) contributes to many types of otolaryngologic conditions in infants and children. The problems may be intermittent and unresponsive to usual therapies such as antimicrobial treatments. A high level of suspicion for GERD and for the concept of "silent" GERD (GERD without overt symptoms) is necessary for accurate diagnosis and treatment of otolaryngologic manifestations of GERD for these patients. In this chapter, the literature on the effects of GERD on otolaryngologic disorders of infants and children is reviewed. In addition, results are discussed from a review of the records of 101 children who underwent esophagoscopy and biopsy as a diagnostic test for GERD at the time of other otolaryngologic procedures.

DIAGNOSIS

Although a child's symptoms may include rhinopharyngitis, sinusitis, cough, laryngitis, globus pharyngeus, oropharyngeal dysphagia, vocal cord granuloma, airway obstruction, apnea, asthma, recurrent croup, laryngomalacia, stridor, or subglottic stenosis, GERD may be an underlying etiologic factor. The diagnosis of GERD is straightforward in a child with otolaryngologic symptomatology that clearly coincides with episodes of spitting up and irritability, or in an older child with heartburn. In many cases, the diagnosis is less clear and additional diagnostic studies are required. A number of diagnostic studies are available and the following discussion may help to guide selection of the most appropriate test.

The 24-hour pH probe is considered the gold standard for the diagnosis of GERD.[1] The double-electrode pH probe with distal esophageal and pharyngeal or proximal esophageal electrodes is the gold standard for diagnosis of otolaryngologic manifestations of gastropharyngoesophageal reflux.[2]

Esophageal biopsy is another useful diagnostic test for GERD. Esophageal biopsy may be done during rigid or flexible esophagoscopy or by suction biopsy without esophagoscopy.[3,4] A positive esophageal biopsy with histologic evidence of esophagitis precludes the need for more costly and time-consuming pH probes or gastric scintiscans. This is a rapid way to make a diagnosis, especially if esophagoscopy is performed at the time of direct laryngoscopy, rigid bronchoscopy, or procedures such as adeno-tonsillectomy or tympanostomy tube placement. Bronchoalveolar lavage with measurement of lipid-laden macrophages may be performed at the time of bronchoscopy to document aspiration that may either be an independent event or related to GERD.[5] If the esophageal biopsy findings are negative and clinical suspicion of GERD is high, then pH probe or scintiscan may be required.

Scintiscans also have the advantage in the detection of aspiration, delayed gastric emptying, and nonacid reflux.[6] Modified barium swallows may show GERD, but a barium swallow with negative results does not preclude GERD because the swallow only helps detect the occurrence of GERD during a small window of time. The modified barium swallow can be used to provide information about the functional aspects of swallowing and the presence of strictures, webs, achalasia, other structural problems, and aspiration. Manometric studies may be required to characterize motility disorders or chronic low tone of the lower esophageal sphincter.

CHILDREN'S HOSPITAL OF PITTSBURGH STUDY

The Children's Hospital of Pittsburgh study was a review of the records of 101 infants and children undergoing rigid esophagoscopy with biopsies or suction biopsy[4] during otolaryngologic procedures. These procedures were performed by the Department of Pediatric Otolaryngology at the Children's Hospital of Pittsburgh between

January 1995 and June 1997.[7] The mean age of the participants was 1.8 years, with a range from 10 days to 17 years. There were 70 males and 31 females.

Esophageal biopsy specimens were taken from the distal one third of the esophagus with the use of up-biting cup forceps during rigid esophagoscopy. Suction biopsies[4] were performed by the pediatric gastroenterology service when it was judged that the airway was too tenuous for a rigid esophagoscopy, which might cause airway edema and further airway compromise. The suction esophageal biopsy catheter is small and causes less airway edema than the larger rigid esophagoscope.

All specimens were interpreted by board-certified pathologists on staff in the Department of Pathology of the Children's Hospital of Pittsburgh based on well-accepted published criteria.[8] Statistical analyses were performed by use of the paired *t* test.

The otolaryngologic procedures shown in Table 1 were performed along with the esophageal biopsies.

Table 2 shows the number of patients with selected pediatric problems and the number of esophageal biopsies that had positive or negative findings for esophagitis in children with each type of problem. Associations were found between the presence of histologic esophagitis and the child's history of asthma, recurrent croup, cough, apnea, sinusitis, and stridor. Associations also were found between the presence of histologic esophagitis and the endoscopic findings of laryngomalacia, subglottic stenosis, posterior glottic erythema, and posterior glottic edema. It must be noted that each association was evaluated statistically as an individual association.

TABLE 1.

Otolaryngologic Procedures Performed With Esophageal Biopsies in 101 Children at the Children's Hospital of Pittsburgh, January 1995 to June 1997

Procedure	Number
Direct laryngoscopy	92
Rigid bronchoscopy	87
Tympanostomy tubes	27
Adenotonsillectomy	19
Tracheotomy	12
Adenoidectomy	9
Maxillary sinus aspiration and irrigation	4
Other procedures	6

TABLE 2.
Number of Biopsies Positive or Negative for Histologic Esophagitis in 101
Children With Selected Problems and Endoscopic Findings Seen at the
Children's Hospital of Pittsburgh Between January 1995 and June 1997

Problem	Pos.	(%)	Neg.	(%)	Total	P value
Asthma	21	(75)	7	(25)	28	.006
Recurrent croup	12	(75)	4	(25)	16	.04
Cough	30	(81)	7	(19)	37	<.001
Apnea	33	(75)	11	(25)	44	<.001
Sinusitis	10	(100)	0	(0)	10	<.001
Stridor	42	(63)	25	(27)	67	.04
Laryngomalacia	21	(75)	7	(25)	28	.006
Subglottic stenosis	23	(68)	11	(32)	34	.02
Posterior glottic						
Erythema	20	(83)	4	(17)	24	<.001
Edema	17	(81)	4	(19)	21	.002

However, the data are confounded by individual patients who may
have had more than one of the signs or endoscopic findings. No
complications were associated with esophageal biopsy.

DISCUSSION AND REVIEW OF THE LITERATURE

The following literature review includes selected GERD-associated
problems in the pediatric population. It compares the incidence of
GERD in children with selected problems who were observed in
the Children's Hospital of Pittsburgh study with other studies in
the literature.

SANDIFER'S SYNDROME

Sandifer's syndrome occurs in children with GERD. Although it is
not a true otolaryngologic problem, it is included in this review
because awareness of it may aid in the diagnosis of GERD in
patients who have associated otolaryngologic problems. Children
with Sandifer's syndrome are irritable, have frequent regurgitation
after feeding, and often have episodes of arching, crying, and torti-
collis. It is believed to be related to esophageal discomfort induced
by GERD; the posturing may help to clear esophageal acid.[9]

REFLUX RHINOPHARYNGITIS AND CHRONIC SINUSITIS

Contencin and Narcy[2] performed nasopharyngeal pH monitoring
on 14 children with chronic rhinopharyngitis and GERD and 18

control subjects without rhinopharyngitis. The incidence of nasopharyngeal pH below 6 was significantly higher in the rhinopharyngitis group. It is provocative that all 10 patients with sinusitis in our study[7] had positive esophageal biopsies. Reflux of gastric contents into the nasal cavity is believed to cause chronic inflammation. Other mechanisms used to explain an association between GERD and sinusitis include GERD-induced alterations in mucosal bacterial adherence or lymphatic drainage. Children with chronic sinusitis have multiple etiologies for their disease, and GERD may be a component. However, viral upper respiratory infections, adenoid hypertrophy, allergic rhinitis, anatomical factors, and immunodeficiency also contribute to this complex problem. These other factors also must be addressed.

CHRONIC COUGH

Holinger and Sanders[10] studied 72 infants and children who had cough of at least 1 month's duration and normal chest radiographic findings. Diagnostic testing included complete blood count with differential, cytology of nasal and bronchial washings, upper gastrointestinal studies (barium esophagram, reflux scan, pH probe, or esophagoscopy), sinus and soft tissue upper airway radiography, pulmonary function testing, direct laryngoscopy, and bronchoscopy. For the overall group, cough variant asthma (32%) was the most common cause of chronic cough, followed by sinusitis (23%), GERD (15%), aberrant innominate artery with tracheal compression (12%), and psychogenic cough (10%). Among children younger than age 18 months, aberrant innominate artery was the most common cause of disease.

In our series,[7] the incidence of positive esophageal biopsy was 81% in 37 children with chronic cough. In the study by Holinger and Sanders, the 4 tests for GERD (barium esophagram, reflux scan, pH probe, and esophagoscopy) were used selectively and not uniformly. This may be the explanation for the low incidence of GERD among children with chronic cough in their study compared with ours. Uniform use of esophageal biopsy may have a higher sensitivity than the studies by Holinger and Sanders[10] in the detection of GERD.

REFLUX LARYNGITIS, HOARSENESS, VOCAL CORD NODULES, AND THROAT CLEARING

Reflux of gastric contents up to the glottis can lead to inflammation that may result in hoarseness or throat clearing. Putnam and Orenstein[11] reported a case of a child with hoarseness and GERD documented by esophagoscopy, esophageal biopsy, and pH probe. The child's hoarseness resolved with GERD pharmacotherapy. Hanson et al[12] reported a series of 182 adults with endoscopically documented chronic laryngitis; 96% responded to antireflux precautions, famotidine, or omeprazole. Endoscopically, a red and possibly edematous posterior glottis is noted. There may be vocal cord edema. With long-term throat clearing, hoarseness, and vocal abuse, vocal cord nodules may develop. Kuhn et al[13] reported an association between vocal cord nodules and GERD documented by pH probe, with a higher incidence of GERD in the vocal cord nodule group compared with control subjects. In our study, if an erythematous or edematous posterior glottis was noted, the esophageal biopsy was positive 83% and 81% of the time, respectively. Allergic rhinitis or sinusitis with postnasal drip, which also may contribute to these laryngeal problems, must be considered in the differential diagnosis.

GLOBUS PHARYNGEUS

Globus pharyngeus—the sensation of having a lump in the throat—may be caused by reflux pharyngitis in some patients. Curran et al[14] used 24-hour pH monitoring to document GERD in 8 of 21 adult patients with globus pharyngeus. The differential diagnosis includes osteophytes of the spine, foreign body, cricopharyngeal hyperactivity, large tonsils, goiter, postcricoid web, cervical lymph nodes, or mass in the pharynx or esophagus. Physical examination, anteroposterior and lateral films of the neck, barium swallow, and endoscopy may be helpful in making the diagnosis.

OROPHARYNGEAL DYSPHAGIA

Oropharyngeal dysphagia is a difficulty of passage of solids or liquids from the mouth to the upper esophagus. The etiologies include central neurologic problems, peripheral neurologic causes, primary muscular problems, cricopharyngeal dysfunction, and local factors. Local factors include those listed for globus pharyngeus. Donner[15] found that certain adults have an acid-sensitive esophagus in which acid barium promotes a motility disturbance with spastic contractions or an abnormally propagated peristaltic wave. Antacid was found to relax the esophagus.

CHRONIC SORE THROAT

Reflux of gastric contents into the pharynx with mucosal inflammation can be a cause of chronic sore throat in children. It usually is worse in the morning because the reflux occurs in the supine position during sleep. Erythema of the pharynx, tonsils, uvula, and larynx may be observed. The sore throat is unresponsive to antimicrobial therapy and throat culture findings are negative. Flexible laryngoscopy may reveal erythema and edema of the posterior glottis.

OTALGIA AND OTITIS
Referred otalgia may occur as a result of pharyngitis from reflux.[16] The differential diagnosis of chronic otalgia also includes otitis media and temporomandibular joint problems. Although there are anecdotal reports of otitis resulting from gastropharyngeal reflux with eustachian tube inflammation as the etiology, there is no conclusive evidence that reflux causes otitis.

VOCAL CORD GRANULOMAS AND ULCERS
Cherry and Margulies[17] reported 3 cases of refractory contact ulcer of the larynx that resolved only after treatment of GERD. In 1968, Delahunty and Cherry[18] reported a canine model in which they repeatedly painted the posterior glottis with gastric juice, resulting in posterior glottic ulcers and granulation tissue. Airway mucosal trauma, vocal abuse, and infection also are possible etiologies for vocal cord granulomas and ulcers. Surgical removal of vocal cord granulomas may be followed by recurrence if the associated GERD is not treated.

AIRWAY OBSTRUCTION AND GERD
There appears to be an association between airway obstruction and GERD. A study in rats showed that partial upper airway obstruction resulted in a powerful thoracoabdominal end-expiratory pressure gradient that may contribute to GERD by overcoming the antireflux barrier mechanism.[19] Thus, children with partial airway obstruction may progress to more severe airway obstruction if exposure of airway mucosa to gastric contents contributes to mucosal thickening. Also, coughing associated with aspiration that frequently occurs during airway obstruction increases intra-abdominal pressure, which further promotes GERD.

APNEA
GERD-induced apnea episodes may be life threatening. Herbst et al[20] and Gorrotxategi et al[21] used pH probes to document apnea associated with GERD in infants. There are two possible mechanisms of GERD-induced apnea. The first is related to GERD, followed by aspiration of stomach contents into the glottis, subglottis, or tracheo-

bronchial tree. This event will usually be followed by an episode of laryngospasm of varying duration. The second mechanism is reflex related. Herbst et al[20] have described the use of esophageal pH monitoring to document reflex apnea induced by acid reflux in the distal esophagus. In a recent abstract, Ing et al[22] reported a significant association between GERD and obstructive sleep apnea in adults. When the GERD was treated with medication, the apnea index decreased significantly. Additionally, when patients were treated with continuous positive airway pressure, both GERD and the apnea index significantly decreased. In our study, 33 of 44 (75%) children with apnea had esophageal biopsies with positive results, which suggested a strong association between apnea and GERD. Apneic episodes may respond to medical therapy, but severe, refractory, life-threatening episodes require fundoplication.

ASTHMA

Although asthma is not a true otolaryngologic problem, it is not uncommon in an otolaryngology practice to see patients with asthma that is possibly related to GERD. For example, it is not unusual to see a child with airway obstruction from adenoid hypertrophy who also has asthma and GERD. These children often improve after adenoidectomy with relief of airway obstruction and treatment of GERD. GERD is diagnosed with the use of esophagoscopy and esophageal biopsy showing histologic esophagitis. Several studies have documented an association between asthma and GERD. Instillation of acid into the esophagus was shown to induce bronchospasm and to decrease peak expiratory flow rates significantly in adults with and without both asthma and GERD.[23] Twenty-four hour pH probes were used to document GERD in 12 infants with persistent wheezing who improved significantly after medical or surgical treatment.[24] GERD was found with the use of pH probes in 27 of 36 (75%) asthmatic children who had no overt GERD symptomatology.[25] These results are in strong agreement with ours, in that 21 of 28 (75%) children with a history of asthma had positive esophageal biopsies. In a study of 186 adults with asthma, endoscopy and esophageal biopsy were used to document GERD in 39% of these patients; 58% were found to have hiatal hernia.[26]

RECURRENT CROUP/SPASMODIC CROUP

Spasmodic croup is supposedly caused by allergy and psychological causes; however, the etiology often is not clear in these difficult cases. It is likely that at least some cases of spasmodic croup are caused by recurrent bouts of reflux-induced stridor.

Waki et al[27] used scintiscan, pH probe, esophagoscopy, and barium swallow studies to document GERD in 15 of 32 children (47%) with recurrent coup. Contencin and Narcy[28] found pharyngeal and esophageal reflux with a double pH probe in 8 of 8 children with recurrent croup. In another series of 15 children with recurrent croup, GERD was documented through the use of a pH probe in 7.[29] In our study,[7] 12 of 16 children (75%) with a history of recurrent croup had a positive esophageal biopsy. The explanation for these observations may be that children with GERD and baseline airway inflammation, when challenged with a viral upper respiratory infection, have additional edema that causes significant obstruction. Endoscopy that is used to rule out associated anatomical airway anomalies is important in selected cases of recurrent croup. Waki et al[27] found that 8 of 32 patients (25%) had anatomical airway anomalies, including laryngomalacia and subglottic stenosis.

LARYNGOMALACIA

Laryngomalacia, which is caused by prolapse of floppy supraglottic tissues into the glottic airway during inspiration, is considered the most common cause of stridor in infants. The usual initial symptoms include inspiratory stridor that is worse while the infant is crying and in the supine position. It is usually improved by placing the child in the prone position.

Belmont and Grundfast[30] have reported that 16 of 20 children (80%) with laryngomalacia had GERD documented through the use of a barium esophagram. Polonovski et al[31] used a barium swallow and esophagoscopy to document a 50% incidence of GERD in 39 children with severe laryngomalacia requiring surgical intervention. We observed[7] that 21 of 28 children (75%) with endoscopically proven laryngomalacia had positive esophageal biopsies. If the duration and severity of the stridor have been impressive enough to warrant endoscopy, a complete airway evaluation in the operating room is indicated. Flexible nasopharyngolaryngoscopy with topical intranasal anesthesia is performed with the child awake or minimally sedated to evaluate for laryngomalacia and vocal cord mobility. Many of these children have erythematous and edematous supraglottic tissue.

Rigid bronchoscopy also is performed to assess the subglottis and tracheobronchial tree. The incidence of finding a second airway lesion that is synchronous with laryngomalacia is 17%,[32] and thus we prefer to perform rigid bronchoscopy for these patients to avoid missing a possible second, life-threatening airway lesion.

During bronchoscopy, bronchoalveolar lavage also is performed to look for increased lipid-laden macrophages that may indicate aspiration related to GERD.[5]

At the time of endoscopy, if the airway is normal in appearance, then rigid esophagoscopy and esophageal biopsy are performed to determine if there is gross or histologic esophagitis. If the airway is tenuous, then rigid esophagoscopy is deferred and the gastroenterology service is consulted for esophageal suction biopsy or pH probe, both of which are less traumatic. Arytenoid edema may result from rigid esophagoscopy, which should be avoided with a tenuous airway. Many of these children improve significantly as airway mucosal thickening resolves with pharmacotherapy for GERD. If the children have continued life-threatening airway obstruction or cannot gain weight, then laser supraglottoplasty or tracheotomy are performed.

REFLUX-INDUCED STRIDOR AND "PSEUDOLARYNGOMALACIA"

Several reports have documented that GERD can induce stridor. With laryngomalacia, the stridor tends to be consistent when the child is crying or lying supine, and it improves with prone positioning and cessation of crying. In contrast, with reflux-induced stridor or "pseudolaryngomalacia," the stridor may be intermittent; it has a variable temporal pattern and is not significantly affected by changes in position. This clinical picture, along with frequent spitting up and, possibly, irritability, is consistent with reflux-induced stridor.

Orenstein et al[33] and Nielson et al[34] have reported cases of infants who had intermittent stridor only during episodes of GERD. The reflux was documented through the use of an esophageal pH probe, and stridor resolved with pharmacotherapy. Henry and Mellis[35] reported on two children whose stridor resolved completely after Nissen fundoplication. Orenstein et al[36] also documented, with the modified Bernstein test, that esophageal instillation of acid could cause stridor in some children. Direct exposure of the glottis to gastric contents may result in laryngospasm; however, instillation of acid into the esophagus also has been reported to result in laryngospasm by reflex pathways.[20,37] Another mechanism of stridor may be related to agitation and more-rapid or forceful breathing associated with esophageal pain during GERD, leading to a "relative airway narrowing."[36] In our series, when children with a complaint of stridor, regardless of etiology, were combined, we observed that 42 of 67 (63%) had a positive esophageal biopsy.

If the history and physical findings are clear-cut and mild, empiric pharmacotherapy for GERD may be tried. For more severe airway obstruction, the workup would proceed as described under the section for laryngomalacia, above. The typical laryngoscopic findings with pseudolaryngomalacia are edema and erythema of the arytenoids and posterior commissure. Many of these children respond to dietary changes or pharmacotherapy, but fundoplication may be required.

SUBGLOTTIC STENOSIS

The etiology of subglottic stenosis in animal models has included trauma, infection,[38-40] and GERD.[41-44] In canine studies, trauma to the subglottic perichondrium resulted in subglottic stenosis[40] that was more severe when gastric juice was applied.[41] Wynne et al[42] developed a murine model in which animals that aspirated gastric juice had desquamation of the superficial tracheal cell layer and delayed regeneration, compared with control animals that aspirated saline and acid (pH = 1.5) without gastric juice. Gaynor[43] irrigated the rabbit trachea with synthetic gastric juice (pH = 4 or 1.4) for periods of 1 to 4 hours and observed ulceration and necrosis. Koufman[44] reported in a canine model that healing of subglottic mucosal injuries was delayed by repeated painting of the injury with an acid plus pepsin solution, compared with control animals receiving a saline and acid solution without pepsin.

We developed a porcine model in our laboratory to study the effects of brief gastric juice exposure on intact subglottic mucosa. Reverse transcriptase polymerase chain reaction was used to measure epidermal growth factor receptor messenger RNA.[45] In the gastric group, basal cell hyperplasia (80%), squamous metaplasia (80%), and moderate submucosal edema were seen, and two animals (40%) had ulceration of the mucosa. The saline control group did show squamous metaplasia (80%) and mild edema, but no basilar hyperplasia or ulceration was found. Messenger RNA measurement showed that application of gastric juice to the intact subglottis resulted in significantly lower expression of message for epidermal growth factor receptor compared with control animals. Thus, direct adverse effects of exposure of the intact subglottis to gastric juice were observed with changes including mucosal ulceration, epithelial basal hyperplasia, and down-regulation of epidermal growth factor receptor messenger RNA production.

Koufman[44] also demonstrated, with 24-hour esophageal pH monitoring, a 78% incidence of GERD in 32 adult patients with laryngeal and tracheal stenosis. Jindal et al[46] reported that 7 of 7 adult women with idiopathic subglottic stenosis required treatment of their GERD for resolution. In our series of 36 children with subglottic stenosis who underwent laryngotracheal reconstruction at the Children's Hospital of Pittsburgh, 21 of 26 tested (80%) had at least one positive test for GERD.[47] A diagnosis of GERD was made after a positive finding on at least one of the following: barium swallow, 24-hour pH probe, esophageal biopsy, or a radionuclide gastric emptying scan. The estimated incidence of pathologic infantile GERD is only 20%.[48] The fourfold increased incidence of GERD in patients with subglottic stenosis suggests that GERD plays a role in the etiology of subglottic stenosis. In our series,[7] we found that 23 of 34 (68%) children with subglottic stenosis had positive esophageal biopsies, suggesting a possible association between GERD and subglottic stenosis.

In a recent report concerning laryngotracheal reconstruction for subglottic stenosis by Zalzal et al,[49] the authors concluded that there was no benefit from GERD testing or treatment. That study was flawed because there were only 7 patients in the group with documented GERD who were not treated with anti-GERD medication. Thus, the absence of statistical significance may simply be a result of inadequate sample size. Other statistical analyses also were flawed in that groups of patients with and without positive tests for GERD, and with and without GERD treatment, were included in the same group for statistical purposes.

TREATMENT OF GERD

Conservative therapy for GERD in children includes elevation of the head of the bed or prone positioning, thickening of feeds, avoiding large meals (especially at bedtime), specific food avoidance (fatty foods, chocolate, peppermint, coffee), weight loss for obese children, and antacids as needed for symptomatic reflux.[1,50,51] Pharmacotherapy includes H_2 blockers such as ranitidine[52] or cimetidine.[53] Prokinetic agents include cisapride,[25,51,54] metoclopramide, and bethanechol.[1] Cisapride is considered the best prokinetic agent. It is less likely than bethanechol to worsen bronchospasm or than metoclopramide to cause extrapyramidal side effects.[50] Cases of prolonged Q-T interval and fatal arrhythmias have been associated with cisapride used along with certain other drugs. Administration of cisapride with macrolide antimicrobials or imidazole antifungal agents must be avoided to prevent these arrhythmias.[55-60] Parents should be given written notification to avoid potential adverse drug interactions. Electrocardiograms should be considered for patients receiving cisapride.

More refractory cases may require omeprazole, a proton-pump inhibitor.[50] A case of hyponatremia and hypokalemia associated with omeprazole use in a child has been reported.[61] Although omeprazole appears to be safe for short-term use, its long-term effects are not well known.[51,62,63] There is some concern regarding the safety of prolonged omeprazole use and resultant hypergastrinemia. These concerns are related to reports of development of gastric polyps, expansion of the parietal cell zone, dilatation of gland lumina, and lingular pseudohypertrophy of individual parietal cells in adults and children.[64-69] Cases still refractory to medical therapy will require surgical fundoplication.[70,71]

CONCLUSION

Associations between GERD and several other important pediatric problems are suggested by review of the literature, data concerning children with subglottic stenosis, data concerning esophageal biopsies performed together with other otolaryngologic procedures, and our porcine model results. Although GERD has not been shown definitively to cause all of these problems, the associations we have documented suggest that testing for GERD should be considered in selected children who have diagnoses of and endoscopic findings for asthma, recurrent croup, cough, apnea, sinusitis, stridor, laryngomalacia, subglottic stenosis, posterior glottic erythema, and posterior glottic edema. Further prospective clinical and basic studies are needed to demonstrate conclusively a cause and effect between GERD and these problems and to determine whether treatment improves the outcomes for these patients.

REFERENCES

1. Andze GO, Brandt ML, St Vil D, et al: Diagnosis and treatment of gastroesophageal reflux in 500 children with respiratory symptoms: The value of pH monitoring. *J Pediatr Surg* 26:295-300, 1991.
2. Contencin P, Narcy P: Nasopharyngeal pH monitoring in infants and children with chronic rhinopharyngitis. *Int J Pediatr Otorhinolaryngol* 22:249-256, 1991.
3. Black DD, Haggitt RC, Orenstein SR, et al: Esophagitis in infants: Morphometric histological diagnosis and correlation with measures of gastroesophageal reflux. *Gastroenterology* 98:1408-1414, 1990.
4. Putnam P, Orenstein S: Blind esophageal suction biopsy in children less than 2 years of age. II. *Gastroenterology* 102:A149, 1992.
5. Nussbaum E, Maggi JC, Mathis R, et al: Association of lipid-laden alveolar macrophages and gastroesophageal reflux in children. *J Pediatr* 110:190-194, 1987.

6. Ruth M, Carlsson S, Mansson I, et al: Scintigraphic detection of gastro-pulmonary aspiration in patients with respiratory disorders. *Clin Physiol* 13:19-33, 1993.

7. Yellon R, Coticchia J, Dixit S, et al: Esophageal biopsy for the diagnosis of gastroesophageal reflux-associated otolaryngologic problems in children. *Am J Med* 108 (Suppl 4a): 131S-138S, 2000.

8. Dahms BB: Reflux esophagitis and sequelae in infants and children, in Dahms BB, Qualman SJ (eds): *Gastrointestinal Diseases,* in: *Perspect Pediatr Pathol,* vol 20. Basel, Karger, 1997, pp 14-34.

9. Puntis JW, Smith HL, Buick RG, et al: Effect of dystonic movements on oesophageal peristalsis in Sandifer's syndrome. *Arch Dis Child* 64:1311-1313, 1989.

10. Holinger LD, Sanders AD: Chronic cough in infants and children: An update. *Laryngoscope* 101:596-605, 1991.

11. Putnam PE, Orenstein SR: Hoarseness in a child with gastroesophageal reflux. *Acta Paediatr* 81:635-636, 1992.

12. Hanson DG, Kamel PL, Kahrilas PJ: Outcomes of antireflux therapy for the treatment of chronic laryngitis. *Ann Otol Rhinol Laryngol* 104:550-555, 1995.

13. Kuhn J, Toohill R, Ulualp S, et al: Pharyngeal acid reflux events in patients with vocal cord nodules. *Laryngoscope* 108:1146-1149, 1998.

14. Curran AJ, Barry MK, Callanan V, et al: A prospective study of acid reflux and globus pharyngeus using a modified symptom index. *Clin Otolaryngol* 20:552-554, 1995.

15. Donner MW, Silbiger ML, Hookman P, et al: Acid barium swallows in the radiographic evaluation of clinical esophagitis. *J Laryngol Otol* 87:220-225, 1966.

16. Malherbe WD: Otalgia with esophageal hiatus hernia. *Lancet* 1:1368-1369, 1958.

17. Cherry J, Margulies SI: Contact ulcer of the larynx. *Laryngoscope* 1937-1940, 1967.

18. Delahunty JE, Cherry J: Experimentally produced vocal cord granulomas. *Laryngoscope* 78:1941-1947, 1968.

19. Wang W, Tovar J, Eizaguirre I, et al: Airway obstruction and gastroesophageal reflux: An experimental study on the pathogenesis of this association. *J Pediatr Surg* 28:995-998, 1993.

20. Herbst JJ, Minton SD, Book LS: Gastroesophageal reflux causing respiratory distress and apnea in newborn infants. *J Pediatr* 95:763-768, 1979.

21. Gorrotxategi P, Eizaguirre I, Saenz de Ugarte A, et al: Characteristics of continuous esophageal pH metering in infants with gastroesophageal reflux and apparent life-threatening events. *Eur J Pediatr Surg* 5:136-138, 1995.

22. Ing A: Obstructive sleep apnea and gastroesophageal reflux. Proceedings of the Second Multidisciplinary International Symposium on Supraesophageal Complications of Gastroesophageal Reflux Disease. Seattle, WA, August 6-8, 1998. *Am J Med,* 1999, in press.

23. Schan CA, Harding SM, Haile JM, et al: Gastroesophageal reflux-induced bronchoconstriction. *Chest* 106:731-737, 1994.
24. Eid NS, Shepherd RW, Thomson MA: Persistent wheezing and gastroesophageal reflux in infants. *Pediatr Pulmonol* 18:39-44, 1994.
25. Tucci F, Resti M, Fontana R, et al: Gastroesophageal reflux and bronchial asthma: Prevalence and effect of cisapride therapy. *J Pediatr Gastroenterol Nutr* 17:265-270, 1993.
26. Sontag SJ, Schnell TG, Miller TQ, et al: Prevalence of oesophagitis in asthmatics. *Gut* 33:872-876, 1992.
27. Waki EY, Madgy DN, Belenky WM, et al: The incidence of gastroesophageal reflux in recurrent croup. *Int J Pediatr Otorhinolaryngol* 32:223-232, 1995.
28. Contencin P, Narcy P: Gastropharyngeal reflux in infants and children. *Arch Otolaryngol Head Neck Surg* 118:1028-1030, 1992.
29. Andrieu-Guitrancourt J, Dehesdin D, Luyer BL, et al: Role due reflux gastro-esophagien au cours des dyspnees laryngees aigues recidivantes de l'enfant. *Ann Otolaryngol Chir Cervicofac* 101:141-149, 1984.
30. Belmont JR, Grundfast K: Congenital laryngeal stridor (laryngomalacia): Etiologic factors and associated disorders. *Ann Otol Rhinol Laryngol* 93:430-437, 1984.
31. Polonovski JM, Contencin P, Viala P, et al: Aryepiglottic fold excision for the treatment of severe laryngomalacia. *Ann Otol Rhinol Laryngol* 99:625-627, 1990.
32. Gonzales C, Reilly JS, Bluestone CD: Synchronous airway lesions in infancy. *Ann Otol Rhinol Laryngol* 96:77-80, 1987.
33. Orenstein SR, Orenstein DM, Whitington P: Gastroesophageal reflux causing stridor. *Chest* 84:301-302, 1983.
34. Nielson DW, Heldt GP, Tooley WH: Stridor and gastroesophageal reflux in infants. *Pediatrics* 85:1034-1039, 1990.
35. Henry RL, Mellis CM: Resolution of inspiratory stridor after fundoplication: Case report. *Aust Paediatr J* 18:126-127, 1982.
36. Orenstein SR, Kocoshis SA, Orenstein DM, et al: Stridor and gastroesophageal reflux: Diagnostic use of intraluminal esophageal acid perfusion (Bernstein Test). *Pediatr Pulmonology* 3:420-424, 1987.
37. Orenstein SR, Orenstein DM: Gastroesophageal reflux and respiratory disease in children. *J Pediatr* 112:847-858, 1988.
38. Sasaki CT, Horiuchi M, Koss N: Tracheostomy-related subglottic stenosis: Bacteriologic pathogenesis. *Laryngoscope* 89:857-865, 1979.
39. Squire R, Brodsky L, Rossman J: The Role of infection in the pathogenesis of acquired tracheal stenosis. *Laryngoscope* 100:765, 1979.
40. Borowiecki B, Croft CB: Experimental animal model of subglottic stenosis. *Ann Otol Rhinol Laryngol* 86:835-840, 1977.
41. Little FB, Koufman JA, Kohut RI, et al: Effect of gastric acid on the pathogenesis of subglottic stenosis. *Ann Otol Rhinol Laryngol* 94:516-519, 1985.

42. Wynne JW, Ramphal R, Hood CI: Tracheal mucosal damage after aspiration: A scanning electron Microscope study. *Am Rev Respir Dis* 124:728-732, 1981.

43. Gaynor EB: Gastroesophageal reflux as an etiologic factor in laryngeal complications of intubation. *Laryngoscope* 98:972-979, 1988.

44. Koufman JA: The otolaryngologic manifestations of gastroesophageal reflux disease (GERD): A clinical investigation of 225 patients using ambulatory 24-hour pH monitoring and an experimental investigation of the role of acid and pepsin in the development of laryngeal injury. *Laryngoscope* 101:1-78, 1991.

45. Yellon R, Szeremeta W, Grandis J, et al: Subglottic injury, gastric juice, corticosteroids, and peptide growth factors in a porcine model. *Laryngoscope* 108:854-862, 1998.

46. Jindal JR, Milbrath MM, Hogan WJ, et al: Gastroesophageal reflux disease as a likely cause of "idiopathic" subglottic stenosis. *Ann Otol Rhinol Laryngol* 103:186-191, 1994.

47. Yellon R, Parameswaran M, Brandom B: Decreasing morbidity following laryngotracheal reconstruction in children. *Int J Ped Otorhinolaryngol* 41:145-154, 1997.

48. Aronow E, Silverberg M: Normal and abnormal GI motility, in Silverberg M (ed): *Pediatric Gastroenterology.* New York, Medical Examination, 1983, p 214.

49. Zalzal GH, Choi SS, Patel KM: The effect of gastroesophageal reflux on laryngotracheal reconstruction. *Arch Otolaryngol Head Neck Surg* 122:297-300, 1996.

50. Orenstein SO: Management of GERD in childhood asthma. *Pediatr Pulmonol Suppl* 11:57-58, 1995.

51. Olafsdottir E: Gastro-oesophageal reflux and chronic respiratory disease in infants and children: Treatment with cisapride. *Scand J Gastroenterol* 30(Suppl 211): 32-34, 1995.

52. Cucchiara S, Minella R, Iervolino C, et al: Omeprazole and high dose ranitidine in the treatment of refractory reflux oesophagitis. *Arch Dis Child* 69:655-659, 1993.

53. Lambert J, Mobassaleh M, Grand RJ: Efficacy of cimetidine for gastric acid suppression in pediatric patients. *J Pediatr* 120:474-478, 1992.

54. Kamel PL, Hanson D, Kahrilas PJ: Omeprazole for the treatment of posterior laryngitis. *Am J Med* 96:321-326, 1994.

55. Klausner MA, Janssen Pharmaceutria Research Foundation. Dear Doctor letters. Feb 3, 1995, Oct 14, 1995.

56. Lewin MB, Bryant RM, Fenrich AL, et al: Cisapride-induced long QT interval. *J Pediatr* 128:279-281, 1996.

57. Bran S, Murray WA, Hirsch IB, et al: Long QT syndrome during high-dose cisapride. *Arch Intern Med* 155:765-768, 1995.

58. Ahmad SR, Wolfe SM: Cisapride and torsades de pointes. *Lancet* 345:508, 1995.

59. Olsson S, Edwards IR: Tachycardia during cisapride treatment. *BMJ* 305:748-749, 1992.

60. Wysowski DK, Bacsanyi J: Cisapride and fatal arrhythmia (letter). *N Engl J Med* 335:290-291, 1996.
61. Melville C, Shah A, Matthew D, et al: Electrolyte disturbance with omeprazole therapy. *Eur J Pediatr* 153:49-51, 1994.
62. Gunasekaran TS, Hassail EG: Efficacy and safety of omeprazole for severe gastroesophageal reflux in children. *J Pediatr* 123:148-154, 1993.
63. Karjoo M, Kane R: Omeprazole treatment of children with peptic esophagitis refractory to ranitidine therapy. *Arch Pediatr Adolesc Med* 149:267-271, 1995.
64. Hassall E: Wrap session: Is the Nissen slipping? Can medical treatment replace surgery for severe gastroesophageal reflux disease in children? *Am J Gastroenterol* 90:1212-1220, 1995.
65. Dent J, Yeomans ND, Mackinnon M, et al: Omeprazole v ranitidine for prevention of relapse in reflux oesophagitis: A controlled double blind trial of their efficacy and safety. *Gut* 35:590-598,1994.
66. Berlin RG: Omeprazole: Gastrin and gastric endocrine cell data from clinical studies. *Dig Dis Sci* 36:129-136, 1991.
67. Sachs G: The safety of omeprazole: True or false? *Gastroenterology* 106:1400-1140, 1994.
68. Graham JR: Gastric polyposis: Onset during long-term therapy with omeprazole. *Med J Aust* 157:287-288, 1992.
69. Stolte M, Bethke B, Ruhl G, et al: Omeprazole-induced pseudohypertrophy of gastric parietal cells. *Z Gastroenterol* 30:134-138,1992.
70. Fonkalsrud EW, Ellis DG, Shaw A, et al: A combined hospital experience with fundoplication and gastric emptying procedure for gastroesophageal reflux in children. *J Am Coll Surg* 180:449-455, 1995.
71. Leape LL, Ramenofsky ML: Surgical treatment of gastroesophageal reflux in children. *Am J Dis Child* 134:935-938, 1980.

CHAPTER 5

Advances in the Management of Cancer of the Thyroid Gland

Steven I. Sherman, MD
Associate Professor of Medicine and Associate Internist, University of Texas M. D. Anderson Cancer Center, Houston

Ann M. Gillenwater, MD
Assistant Professor of Medicine, University of Texas M. D. Anderson Cancer Center, Houston

Helmuth Goepfert, MD
Professor of Surgery and Chairman, Department of Head and Neck Surgery, University of Texas M. D. Anderson Cancer Center, Houston

In 1999, about 17,000 patients were diagnosed with carcinoma of the thyroid gland. Of these, 80% and 14%, respectively, have papillary or follicular carcinomas (differentiated carcinomas), 4% medullary carcinoma, and 2% anaplastic carcinoma. About 1200 persons will die of complications of these diseases or their treatments.[1,2] In this chapter, we review recent advances in the approaches to the diagnosis, staging, and treatment of differentiated and medullary carcinomas.

DIAGNOSTIC EVALUATION OF THE SOLITARY THYROID NODULE

The most common clinical presentation of a patient with thyroid carcinoma is with a solitary thyroid nodule.[3] In the setting of an unsuppressed serum thyroid-stimulating hormone (TSH) concentration, cytologic examination after a fine-needle aspiration (FNA) of the nodule is the most appropriate diagnostic procedure.[4] To minimize false-negative results from inadequate specimens, we recommend on-site cytologic review for adequacy of diagnostic material. Yet 15% of aspirations are inadequate or nondiagnostic, largely because of aspiration of cystic, hemorrhagic, or hypocellular colloid nodules. Subsequent reaspiration may reduce this frequency in half. For patients with repeated nondiagnostic aspirates, 5% of women and 30% of men may prove to have malignant nodules.[5] For nonpalpable lesions and those that have yielded inadequate material on previous attempts, ultrasound (US)-guided aspiration may improve the efficacy of the diagnosis.[6]

When surgical findings have been subsequently available, the likelihood of malignancy (or the false-negative rate) after a benign cytologic finding has been less than 5%.[7] Diagnoses of malignancy—particularly papillary, medullary, and anaplastic carcinomas, as well as lymphoma—can be made in about 5% of nodules. The false-positive rate is also less than 5%. If medullary thyroid carcinoma is suspected, a serum calcitonin determination is appropriate.[8]

Follicular tumors usually yield abnormal follicular epithelium of varying degrees of atypia and potential for malignancy.[4] Most cytopathologists agree that follicular adenomas and carcinomas cannot be adequately separated without a histologic demonstration of invasiveness. A similar diagnostic difficulty exists for oxyphilic or Hürthle cell neoplasms. For cytopathologically diagnosed follicular and oxyphilic neoplasms, the overall rate of carcinoma is about 20%. Among potential clinical and radiologic factors that might identify nodules at greater risk for malignancy, larger nodule size, older age, and male gender are significant predictors of carcinoma among follicular neoplasms, increasing the risk to as high as 80%.[9-11] An improved diagnosis may be expected as the molecular abnormalities associated with thyroid carcinomas are determined and this knowledge is incorporated into clinical practice (eg, galectin-3, telomerase, GLUT1, and the RET.[12-15]

By radionuclide scanning, malignant thyroid lesions are usually hypofunctioning, or "cold," but this finding is both nonspecific and nondiagnostic. On the other hand, a "hot" nodule—a hyperfunctioning lesion with suppression of uptake in surrounding normal thyroid tissue—is rarely associated with malignancy. The limiting of scanning to cytologically diagnosed follicular neoplasms yields hot nodules in up to 30% of patients.[7] When a nonoxyphilic follicular neoplasm is found, a radionuclide scan should be obtained to rule out a hyperfunctioning nodule. If the follicular lesion is hypofunctioning or oxyphilic, then a decision must be made on whether to operate.[11,16,17] Given the higher risk of malignancy among patients who are older than 50 years, who have larger nodules, or who are male, surgery should be performed for this subgroup. A similar recommendation for surgery may hold for men who have undergone multiple aspirations for whom the cumulative yield of specimens remains nondiagnostic.[5] Instead of immediately undergoing surgery, younger patients with smaller nodules, or those in whom a hyperplastic nodule cannot be distinguished from a follicular neoplasm, may be treated with levothyroxine to suppress serum TSH levels to less than 0.1 mU/L for 6 to 12 months. A nodule that does not completely resolve in this interval should then be excised. Patients should be advised of the relative risks and benefits of suppression therapy and surgery so that they may participate in this therapeutic decision.

US can be used to find solitary nodules in about 25% to 50% of asymptomatic persons, particularly lesions of less than 1 cm.[18,19] However, the significance of most of these nodules remains unclear, and most patients with asymptomatic nodules detected by means of US that are less than 1 cm can be followed up with serial palpation only.[19] The capability of US to aid in the accurate measurement of nodule dimensions does make it an appropriate test for longitudinal follow-up of small nodules. Other imaging procedures, such as computed tomography and magnetic resonance, have no role in the routine evaluation of thyroid nodules.

THYROID CANCER STAGING

Several classification and staging schemes have been introduced for thyroid carcinoma.[20] Each is characterized by assignment of patient stage on the basis of clinicopathologic parameters such as patient age, tumor size, tumor grade or differentiation, presence of local invasion, and regional or distant metastases.[21-27] The most commonly used classifications include AMES (*a*ge of patient, presence of distant *m*etastases, *e*xtent, and *s*ize of tumor—a binary classification that divides patients into low- and high-risk groups)[23]; TNM (the American Joint Commission on Cancer *t*umor-*n*ode-*m*etastasis classification system)[21,28]; AGES (*a*ge, *g*rade, *e*xtent, and *s*ize) and MACIS (*m*etastasis, *a*ge, *c*ompleteness of resection, *i*nvasion, and *s*ize), both devised at the Mayo Clinic[25,29-31]; Clinical Class (developed at The University of Chicago)[24]; and the Ohio State classification.[26] In 1986, a prospective multicenter thyroid cancer registry was created, in part to establish a broadly applicable staging classification for predicting the outcome of patients with thyroid carcinoma.[27] Parameters that were selected as key components for staging of papillary and follicular (including oxyphilic) carcinomas included patient age at diagnosis, tumor type, tumor size, presence of gross extraglandular invasion, and presence of regional or distant metastases. With a median follow-up of 40 months for about 1400 patients, this four-stage classification could stratify risk for survival and disease-free survival for both histologic subtypes.[27] Several factors predominated in the assignment of disease stage for each histologic subtype. In addition to age at diagnosis, the features that most commonly determined staging for a patient with papillary carcinoma were tumor size, gross extraglandular invasion, and metastases. For follicular carcinomas, age at diagnosis, tumor size, extracervical metastases, and poor differentiation were the most important staging factors.

How to select among these approaches to thyroid cancer risk stratification remains a significant challenge for the clinician. When used for the retrospectively identified cohort of patients with papillary carcinoma seen at the Princess Margaret Hospital, the TNM approach was demonstrated to have superior predictive value when compared with the University of Chicago, Ohio State, MACIS, and AMES strategies[32]—supporting findings reported by the Chicago group itself.[33] Based on the prospectively gathered multicenter data of the National Thyroid Cancer Treatment Cooperative Study (NTCTCS) Registry, short-term survival for patients with either papillary or follicular carcinomas was best predicted by either the NTCTCS or the TNM approaches, compared with the Chicago, Ohio State, MACIS, and AMES classifications.[27] The importance of histologic features, such as extrathyroidal invasion, underscores the need for pathologists to determine and report these data on each thyroidectomy specimen examined for differentiated thyroid carcinoma.

SURGICAL MANAGEMENT

The surgical management of well-differentiated thyroid carcinoma has not changed markedly in decades, yet some aspects remain controversial: the extent of initial thyroidectomy; the indications for, and type of, neck dissections; and the appropriate procedure for tumors invading the recurrent laryngeal nerve or aerodigestive tract. In addition, recent reports evaluated the surgical management issues of groups that require special considerations, such as children, adolescents, and pregnant women.

Most thyroid surgeons now agree that total (or near-total) thyroidectomy is the preferred initial surgical procedure for patients with high-risk differentiated thyroid carcinoma, although what constitutes a "high-risk" patient varies. An analysis of 700 patients treated between 1970 and 1995 found that for all patients with a tumor larger than 1 cm, cancer recurrence and mortality after unilateral lobectomy or subtotal thyroidectomy were significantly higher compared with what occurred after total or near-total thyroidectomy.[34] To address the question of surgical extent in AMES low-risk patients, researchers evaluated 1685 patients with papillary carcinoma for recurrence and cause-specific mortality.[35] These patients, selected from 1913 patients undergoing definitive primary surgical therapy at the Mayo Clinic from 1940 through 1991, had 20-, 30-, and 40-year cause-specific mortality rates of 0.9%, 2.2%, and 2.5%, respectively; recurrence rates (any site) were 10.0%, 11.5%, and 12.6%. There was no difference in the cause-specific mortality or distant metastasis rate between the patients who had undergone unilateral lobectomy and those receiving a bilateral procedure. However, the 20-year recurrence rate after a unilateral procedure was 22.2% compared with 8.3% ($P < .001$) for patients treated with a bilateral procedure. Given the high rate of radioiodine unresponsiveness and subsequent mortality among patients with recurrence, these findings strongly support the use of total or near-total thyroidectomy, even in AMES low-risk patients.[36]

The Mayo data contrast with a report from Memorial Sloan-Kettering that analyzed a series of 465 patients with differentiated carcinoma who were judged to be low-risk according to the following criteria: age less than 45 years, tumor smaller than 4 cm, low-grade histologic finding, absence of distant metastasis, and absence of extrathyroidal extension.[37] Four hundred three patients (87%) had papillary carcinoma, and 62 (13%) had follicular carcinoma. With a median follow-up of 20 years, the overall local, regional, and distant recurrence rates were 5%, 9%, and 2%, respectively. Not surprisingly, the investigators found a statistically significant increase in the local recurrence rate for patients treated with less than a unilateral lobectomy compared with patients who underwent at least a lobectomy. However, there was no significant difference in the local recurrence rates (4% vs 1%) or overall failure rates (13% vs 8%) for the 276 patients treated with unilateral lobectomy compared with the 90 treated with total thyroidectomy. The differences noted between the results of this series and the Mayo Clinic series may be related to differences in the criteria for inclusion as low-risk, the inclusion of follicular carcinoma patients, and a shorter follow-up period.

A resolution of the controversy concerning the extent of thyroidectomy might be achieved through a randomized trial comparing total thyroidectomy with ipsilateral lobectomy and isthmusectomy. However, with the use of data from published series, it has been estimated that a sample size of 3100 patients and at least 6 years of follow-up would be necessary to detect an improvement in cause-specific survival from 1.5% to 0.39%[38]; four times as many patients would be required for a comparison of complications. Clearly, given the relative rarity of the disease, it is highly unlikely that such a study would be completed.

In the absence of definitive prospective trial data, we favor total thyroidectomy for most patients with differentiated thyroid carcinoma. For patients with T1 N0 M0 disease, generally detected incidentally, unilateral lobectomy and isthmusectomy may be sufficient.

MANAGEMENT OF CERVICAL LYMPH NODES

The treatment of the regional lymphatics for patients with differentiated thyroid carcinoma is determined by the histologic diagnosis, extent of nodal involvement, and other clinical factors. Nodal metastases are common with papillary carcinoma but rare in follicular carcinoma; in papillary carcinoma, young patients are much more likely to be seen with nodal involvement than are older patients. Unlike most other malignancies, the presence of lymph node metastasis among patients with papillary carcinoma appears to be only a minor prognostic factor. In a matched-pair analysis of 100 patients, there was no survival difference between the node-positive and node-negative groups, although there was a slightly higher frequency of recurrence among node-positive patients older than 45 years.[39] A meta-analysis of 9 studies that specifically evaluated papillary carcinoma demonstrated no relationship between the lymph node status at presentation and survival; however, several of the studies did show an increased risk of tumor recurrence among patients with nodal metastases. In contrast, 2 of the 5 studies that looked at follicular carcinoma demonstrated decreased survival rates for patients with nodal disease at presentation.[40]

Given the evidence that regional nodal metastasis influences the risk of recurrence, a retrospective analysis was done to determine whether performing a neck dissection at the time of thyroidectomy affects recurrence rates.[41] In addition to total thyroidectomy with central nodal compartment dissection and adjuvant radioiodine, lateral neck dissection was performed when involvement of these nodal groups was suspected. Of the papillary carcinoma patients, 30 of 59 (51%) who were treated with total thyroidectomy alone had regional recurrence develop, compared with 15 of 82 (18%) who also had lateral neck dissection. This significant relationship existed for each group of patients when stratified by T stage. Although it is difficult to determine the effectiveness of the preoperative determination of nodal status for these patients, the results of this study suggest that performing lateral neck dissections at the time of initial thyroidectomy may decrease the incidence of regional recurrence. These results also support our practice of routinely using US preoperatively to evaluate regional lymphatics.

MANAGEMENT OF THE RECURRENT LARYNGEAL NERVE

A significant cause of morbidity, recurrent laryngeal nerve invasion (47%) was second in frequency only to muscle invasion (53%) for a series of patients with locally invasive papillary carcinoma.[42] However, for a series of 262 patients with invasive thyroid carcinoma, complete resection of the involved recurrent laryngeal nerve did not lead to improved survival over that seen among patients who underwent incomplete excision.[43] Our current practice is to preserve a functioning recurrent laryngeal nerve whenever it is technically feasible to dissect this structure out from the surrounding tumor. A functioning nerve should not be resected only to remove microscopic disease. If vocal cord paralysis is present preoperatively, however, no attempt should be made to preserve the nonfunctioning recurrent laryngeal nerve.

MANAGEMENT OF AERODIGESTIVE TRACT INVOLVEMENT

Thyroid carcinoma rarely invades the larynx, trachea, or esophagus—a situation that produces particular management difficulties and controversies. In situations with limited involvement of the larynx or trachea, there is controversy over whether a "shave excision," which may leave microscopic disease at the site, or a complete resection, which includes removal of a portion of these structures, is the better approach. In the case of more extensive involvement of upper aerodigestive tract structures by thyroid carcinoma, the most appropriate method of resection and reconstruction is also at issue. Most studies support the use of a conservative procedure that involves the removal of all gross tumor. Usually, a curative resection can be accomplished in patients with limited involvement of the larynx or trachea by shaving the tumor off the cartilage without resecting these structures. Radioactive iodine therapy and thyroid hormone suppression are administered postoperatively, and external beam radiotherapy also should be considered.[44]

A recent study examined 262 patients treated at the Mayo Clinic between 1940 and 1990 with invasive papillary carcinoma (including invasion of the muscle, laryngeal nerve, trachea, esophagus, larynx, and other sites).[42] Patients were divided into 3 groups according to the extent of the surgical resection: group I patients had complete surgical excision; group II patients underwent a shave excision that conserved upper aerodigestive structures, although microscopic residual disease was identified or suspected; and group III patients had an incomplete excision, with gross tumor left behind. The overall 5- and 15-year survival rates were 79% and 54%, respectively. There was no significant difference in the survival rate between group I and group II patients, but the survival rate was lower for group III patients. Multivariate analysis showed that invasion of the trachea or esophagus, but not of the larynx, was significantly associated with a decrease in survival. Based on these results, the authors recommended that aerodigestive tract structures be sacrificed only if it is necessary to eradicate all gross tumor. Similar findings were reported in a smaller cohort of patients.[45]

When thyroid carcinoma produces frank cartilage destruction or intraluminal involvement of the upper aerodigestive tract structures, a shave excision cannot be performed without leaving gross tumor behind. Of 16 patients whose tracheal cartilage invasions were managed with a cartilage-shaving procedure and either radioiodine or external radiation, only 4 were clinically free of disease at 49 to 112 months (mean, 71 months).[46] The remaining 12 patients had tumor relapse in the central compartment of the neck, with 7 eventually dying of their disease after a mean of 43 months. The most common cause of death was airway obstruction produced by local disease.

Failure to remove all gross disease from the central neck compartment leads to a significant decrease in tumor control and a decline in survival rates. The goal of surgery for patients with extensively invasive thyroid carcinoma should therefore be to remove all the tumor, but to retain as much airway, vocal, and digestive function as possible. However, given the variability in the presentation of each patient's tumor (including whether metastatic disease is present), the variability in the expertise of and the resources available to physicians, and the preferences of the patient, the most appropriate procedure must be determined on an individual basis. This notwithstanding, long-term disease-free survival can be achieved by patients who have extensive invasion of aerodigestive tract structures by differentiated thyroid carcinomas and who undergo an aggressive resection.[47-49] Only if the tumor is unresectable or the patient does not agree to a radical resection should gross tumor be left behind in the neck.

OUTPATIENT THYROIDECTOMY

Because of market pressure and other factors, hospital stays for a variety of illnesses and surgical procedures have progressively decreased. Historically, patients undergoing thyroidectomy remained hospitalized to detect the potentially life-threatening complications of bleeding/hematoma and hypocalcemia. Several recent studies have reported the feasibility of outpatient thyroid surgery, with acceptable short-term results.[50-53] It has been recommended that surgeons provide extensive preoperative counseling, carefully adhere to technical details to minimize the risk of bleeding (eg, avoiding tight closure of the strap muscles to allow the blood to decompress into the subcutaneous space), observe patients for 6 hours postoperatively, and advise patients to self-medicate with calcium tablets for symptoms of mild hypocalcemia.[54] Others argue that the real economic savings are small and that they are not worth the increased risk of inadequately treated life-threatening complications.

MANAGEMENT OF DIFFERENTIATED THYROID CARCINOMA IN CHILDREN AND ADOLESCENTS

Thyroid carcinoma in children and adolescents is uncommon; therefore, there have been few large series evaluating the long-term prognosis and appropriate therapy for young patients who have this malignancy develop. Despite a generally good short-term prognosis and survival, young patients can suffer from significant morbidity due to frequent local and regional disease recurrence, especially if inadequately treated initially.

A recent series described the extended follow-up of 112 young patients with differentiated thyroid carcinoma treated at the M.D. Anderson Cancer Center between 1944 and 1986.[55] One fourth of the 99 living patients had recurrent disease develop at some point. Six patients died of thyroid cancer, at a mean of 26 years after initial diagnosis. One, who had lung metastases at the time of diagnosis, died of progressive pulmonary disease after 36 years. The other 5 patients had lung and bone metastases develop and died after a 2- to 20-year disease-free interval. Three additional patients died of complications of radiation therapy, 1 with tracheal necrosis 26 years after diagnosis and 2 with cervical sarcomas more than 20 years after diagnosis. An additional 2 died of subsequent breast cancer, although it remains unclear if this was a complication of thyroid cancer therapy.[56] In another series of 61 young patients treated for thyroid cancer at one institution from 1952 to 1995, the 20-year survival rate was 97%.[57] Two patients died of progressive metastatic thyroid cancer within 10 years of the initial operations. Three of the 10 patients who had lobectomy or subtotal thyroidectomy had local recurrence develop in the residual thyroid gland, whereas none of the 51 patients who had total or near-total thyroidectomy had a local recurrence.

Given the high frequency of multifocal intrathyroidal disease and locoregional metastases, we advocate aggressive surgical management of the primary tumor and cervical lymphatics with adjuvant radiation iodine therapy for young patients with differentiated thyroid carcinoma. Lifelong close follow-up surveillance is warranted because of the risk of late recurrences and disease progression.

THYROID CARCINOMA IN PREGNANT WOMEN

Differentiated thyroid carcinoma has been estimated to develop in 1 in 1000 women who are pregnant.[58,59] There has been some concern that the hormonal factors associated with pregnancy might accelerate the progression of disease and necessitate a more aggressive management strategy.[60] However, a recent report that evaluated the outcomes of 61 pregnant women and 528 age-matched nonpregnant women with differentiated thyroid carcinoma disputed this concern.[61] Most (77%) of the pregnant women underwent thyroidectomy after delivery; 20% had the procedure performed during the second trimester. There was no significant difference in outcome between the 2 groups, despite a longer delay in treatment of the pregnant women, suggesting that the prognosis for pregnant women with differentiated thyroid carcinoma is similar to that of nonpregnant women. These findings support the results of an earlier, smaller study.[62] Therefore, in most cases, the treatment of thyroid cancer can be safely delayed until after delivery.

ADJUVANT TREATMENT

Once a patient with differentiated thyroid carcinoma has undergone surgical therapy, several possible adjuvant modalities can be considered, depending on the patient's extent of disease. Similarly, the published standard guidelines for long-term follow-up of these patients leave considerable room for variation in frequency and selection of monitoring procedures.[63,64]

RADIOIODINE

Adjuvant ablation of residual thyroid tissue after primary surgery has three rationales: (1) to destroy any residual microscopic foci of disease, (2) to increase the sensitivity of ^{131}I scanning for detection of recurrent or metastatic disease due to the elimination of uptake by residual normal tissue, and (3) to improve the value of measurements of serum thyroglobulin as a tumor marker. Combining retrospective data from multiple studies, radioiodine ablation may be associated with as much as a 50% reduction in locoregional relapse, and long-term disease-specific mortality is probably reduced for patients with primary tumors that are at least 1 to 1.5 cm in diameter, are multicentric, or have soft-tissue invasion at presentation.[24,26,65,66] Despite the common perception that adjuvant radioiodine is uniformly administered,[67] treatment is given to only one third of patients with differentiated carcinoma.[1] Nonetheless, adjuvant radioiodine should probably be administered to all patients with differentiated thyroid carcinoma who are at least age 45 at diagnosis, whose primary tumor is at least 1 cm in diameter, or who have evidence of extrathyroidal disease, either by direct invasion outside the gland or locoregional metastases. For patients with residual disease after primary surgery, particularly those with extracervical metastases, radioiodine therapy is commonly recommended.

The efficacy of radioiodine in both adjuvant and therapeutic settings depends on patient preparation, tumor-specific characteristics, sites of disease, and administered radioiodide activity. Iodide uptake by thyroid tissue is stimulated by TSH and is suppressed by increased endogenous iodide stores. After thyroidectomy, the patient's thyroid hormone levels must decline sufficiently to allow the TSH concentration to rise to more than 25 to 30 mU/L.[68] This period of hormone withdrawal should last for at least 4 to 5 weeks. To minimize the resulting symptoms of hypothyroidism, the shorter-acting hormone liothyronine (T3) is often administered at doses of 25 μg two times per day.[69] Lower doses are administered to elderly patients and those with ischemic heart disease. Therapy with liothyronine is then stopped at least 2 weeks before dosing for a radioiodine scan. Patients are also advised to avoid foods with high iodine content for at least 2 weeks before the scan.[70]

Other strategies can increase the efficiency of radioiodide uptake by the lesions. Lithium prolongs ^{131}I retention by thyroid cells, and the administration of lithium before ^{131}I administration can augment the radiation dose delivered to thyroid tissue, particularly in cells that are poor concentrators of radioiodine.[71] Reports have shown 13-*cis* retinoic acid to reverse the loss of radioiodine concentrating ability associated with tumor dedifferentiation.[72,73] However, a distinct tumor response from such retinoid therapy is less clear. Laxatives that do not contain iodine are routinely recommended to prevent hypothyroidism-induced constipation and prolonged nontherapeutic retention of ^{131}I in the gut.

Radioiodine scans for localization of uptake before ablation or therapy are usually performed with a diagnostic activity of 2 to 5 mCi of [131]I. Between 24 and 96 hours after oral administration of the diagnostic dose, whole-body scans and spot images of the neck and other areas of uptake are performed with a large-field-of-view gamma-scintillation camera. In some institutions, quantitative dosimetry is performed to determine lesion uptake and to predict effective tumor radiation dose; however, this requires specialized equipment and software.[74] Greater sensitivity for the detection of residual or metastatic tumor can be attained with the use of higher amounts of [131]I. There is, however, some risk involved with performing diagnostic scans, particularly with larger radioisotope activities. The scans can lead to "stunning," whereby uptake of the subsequent ablative or therapeutic dose is reduced as a result of sublethal radiation delivered by the diagnostic dose.[75,76] Use of ^{123}I, with a shorter physical half-life and lower radiation dose to thyroid tissue, may prevent stunning of therapeutic uptake after a diagnostic, preablation scan.[77]

Between 75% and 100% of residual differentiated thyroid carcinomas will demonstrate significant uptake of radioiodide within the thyroid bed after thyroidectomy. In contrast, only about 50% of metastatic lesions in the lungs or bones will concentrate [131]I.[68] Certain histologic subtypes, such as the oxyphilic variant (Hürthle cell carcinoma), tall cell variant of papillary carcinoma, and poorly differentiated lesions, concentrate radioiodide less frequently, especially in extracervical metastases. Older patients and women may also be less likely to have adequate uptake in metastases.

In the presence of postoperative radioiodine uptake in the thyroid bed, an empirically selected activity of ^{131}I is administered for adjuvant ablation, typically 100 mCi. A lower activity of radioiodine, 29 mCi, has also been used for adjuvant ablation, permitting treatment that does not require hospitalization for radiation safety precautions. Assuming that the 24-hour radioiodine uptake is less than 5%, this lower activity appears to have a reasonable efficacy of successful ablation.[78,79] However, there is scant evidence of long-term outcomes comparable to that seen with higher-activity therapy, and considerably more study is required.[26] Alternatively, quantitative dosimetry can be applied to estimate the radioiodine activity necessary to deliver an effective radiation dose to the tissue of at least 30,000 cGy.[80]

A posttreatment scan is routinely performed several days after administration of the radioiodine dose, although the diagnostic use of such scans immediately after ablative treatments is maximal for patients whose thyroid bed activity was previously ablated.[76,81]

THYROID HORMONE SUPPRESSION

After initial therapy with surgery, with or without radioiodine, patients require lifelong thyroid hormone treatment to prevent hypothyroidism and to minimize TSH stimulation to tumor growth. With TSH suppressive thyroid hormone therapy, disease-free survival may be improved 2-fold to 3-fold, particularly for "high-risk" patients.[82,83] However, potential morbidity from overly aggressive thyroid hormone suppression therapy may include acceleration of osteopenia[84,85] and provocation of cardiac tachyarrhythmias such as atrial fibrillation.[86] Although some studies have also suggested that TSH-suppressive therapy leads to induction of cardiac hypertrophy and dysfunction,[87-89] these findings have recently been disputed.[90,91]

It seems reasonable, therefore, to treat patients after initial therapy with suppressive doses of L-thyroxine, the degree of TSH suppression dependent on the patient's initial clinicopathologic features and disease status during follow-up[82]:

- T1 N0 M0 disease—the TSH can be maintained within the lower half of the normal range
- T2-T3 N0 M0 disease—the TSH can be maintained between 0.1 and 0.5 mU/L
- T2-T3 N1 M0 disease—the TSH can be maintained between 0.05 and 0.1 mU/L
- T4 or M1 disease—the TSH can be maintained below 0.05 mU/L

Patients who remain disease-free for 5 to 10 years may have their degree of TSH suppression reduced by lowering their doses of thyroid hormone. Other mitigating factors, such as concurrent cardiac disease, may also dictate a need for reduced hormone dosing.

EXTERNAL BEAM RADIATION THERAPY

The exact role of external beam radiotherapy in the treatment of differentiated carcinoma remains undetermined. The effectiveness of adjuvant external beam radiation therapy was questioned in earlier reports, but more recently its benefit in maintaining locoregional control has been supported for older patients with locally invasive papillary carcinoma.[92,93] A review of 282 patients with differentiated thyroid carcinoma treated at the Princess Margaret Hospital found that the administration of postoperative radiation therapy did not significantly affect the local regional control or disease-specific survival rates. However, in the subgroup of 155 patients with papillary histology and microscopic residual disease (evidence of disease at or within 2 mm of the resection margin or tumor that was shaved off adjacent structures in the neck), the use of external radiation therapy produced a significant improvement in 10-year local regional control (93% vs 78%) and in disease specific survival rates (100% vs 95%).[93] Another recent study reported an increased freedom from locoregional and distant failure for patients over the age of 40 with extrathyroidal extension and lymph node involvement from papillary carcinoma when treated with adjuvant external beam therapy in addition to total thyroidectomy, two courses of ^{131}I, and TSH suppression.[92] In neither study was a benefit of adjuvant radiotherapy demonstrated for patients with follicular carcinoma. Efforts to initiate a definitive randomized study to determine the effectiveness of adjuvant external radiation are under way, although such a study will require a large number of patients and prolonged follow-up.

Patients with gross residual disease or inoperable tumors may also benefit from the addition of external beam radiation therapy. In one series involving 33 patients with gross residual disease who received postoperative external radiation therapy, the 5-year local control and disease-specific survival rates were about 65%.[93]

Although there is variation among treatment centers, the dosages for adjuvant external radiation therapy for differentiated thyroid cancer are in the range of 40 to 50 Gy.[94] Adjuvant radiotherapy should be considered for older patients with locally invasive papillary cancer with questionable margins or residual microscopic disease after surgical excision and radioiodine, and for patients with multiply recurrent disease after surgical resection and radioiodine. Similarly, palliative radiation should be offered to patients with significant residual disease or inoperable tumors, and to those with bony metastases either causing pain or risking pathologic fracture.

LONG-TERM FOLLOW-UP

Recurrence of differentiated thyroid carcinoma can occur decades after initial therapy, mandating the need for careful monitoring to detect and treat recurrence to reduce morbidity and mortality. No single diagnostic tool will detect all recurrences or evidence of disease, and therefore combinations of modalities must be used. In addition to radioiodide scans, routine monitoring can include measurement of serum thyroglobulin (Tg), chest radiographs, and neck US.

RADIOIODINE SCANNING

After initial ablation, we perform radioiodine scanning annually until at least two negative whole-body scans are obtained. In a recent study, the predictive value for 10-year relapse-free survival of one negative radioiodide scan was about 90%, whereas two consecutive negative scans had a predictive value greater than 95%.[95]

Traditionally, these scans are performed after thyroid hormone withdrawal, permitting endogenous elevation of serum TSH levels. However, the recent introduction of thyrotropin alfa (recombinant human TSH) permits radioiodine scanning without induction of hypothyroidism.[96] Whole-body radioiodine scans performed after two injections of thyrotropin alfa are somewhat less sensitive than those obtained after thyroid hormone withdrawal but are associated with significantly fewer symptoms of hypothyroidism.[97,98] If a patient is identified as requiring radioiodine therapy, thyroid hormone withdrawal can then be initiated after the scan is completed.

SERUM THYROGLOBULIN

The synthesis and secretion of Tg is a differentiated characteristic of thyroid follicular cells. In the long-term follow-up of patients, measurement of the serum concentration of Tg aids the detection of residual, recurrent, or metastatic disease, particularly given the rough correlation between tumor size and Tg level. Once the thyroid gland has been resected and completely ablated with radioiodine, serum Tg concentrations should approach the limits of assay detectability.[99] The Tg level may take 1 or more years to decline to an undetectable nadir after primary therapy.[100] One important factor in the interpretation of Tg concentrations is the concurrent level of TSH, given the dependence on TSH for Tg production. Thus, like radioiodine scanning, the sensitivity for detection of residual cancer is enhanced by elevation of the serum TSH during thyroid hormone withdrawal.[100,101] The sensitivity of detecting disease by measurement of Tg during thyroid hormone withdrawal is 85% to 95%, but it may be as low as 50% during TSH suppression.[102] False-negative results can occur, however, particularly for patients with small nodal metastases of papillary carcinoma, or in the setting of tumor dedifferentiation. A detectable Tg level even during TSH-suppressive thyroid hormone therapy likely signifies disease, but the absence of detectable Tg during TSH stimulation suggests the absence of disease. Thyroid hormone withdrawal to obtain TSH stimulation of Tg levels may be avoided by the use of thyrotropin alfa.[103] The maximum sensitivity for detecting residual thyroid tissue or disease after thyrotropin alfa stimulation depends on simultaneous measurement of the serum Tg and performance of a whole-body radioiodine scan, with a diagnostic accuracy approaching that of diagnostic studies done after thyroid hormone withdrawal.[97,104] However, the utility of stimulated Tg measurements in the absence of scanning remains to be determined.

Despite the enhanced sensitivity of currently available Tg immunoassays, problems remain in their clinical application. In immunometric assays, reported Tg concentrations can be falsely lowered by autoantibodies that bind Tg and prevent antigen interaction with the assay's antibodies.[105] For the 25% of the differentiated thyroid cancer population with anti-Tg autoantibodies, serum Tg levels must be interpreted with caution or not used at all in patient management. Notably, the persistence of anti-Tg autoantibodies in a differentiated thyroid cancer patient after thyroidectomy and radioiodine ablation likely indicates the presence of residual thyroid tissue and may predict an increased risk for recurrence.[106] Use of sensitive polymerase chain reaction methods allows the detection of messenger RNA circulating in the peripheral blood of patients with thyroid cancer, presumably contained within circulating tumor cells.[107] Besides permitting assessment of disease status in the presence of antithyroglobulin antibodies, such assays may also be more sensitive, particularly for patients whose TSH levels are suppressed due to thyroid hormone therapy.[107]

OTHER DIAGNOSTIC MODALITIES

US of the thyroid bed and cervical node compartments can be used to accurately identify locoregional metastases and disease recurrence measuring several millimeters in diameter.[108] Additionally, identification of suspicious lesions can be followed by US-guided FNA. In one study, 50% of patients with locoregional disease diagnosed through the use of high-resolution US had undetectable Tg levels, and 80% had negative radioiodine scans.[109] Computed tomography is probably not as sensitive for detecting such small lesions, but the technique is more readily standardized and less operator-dependent. Routine chest radiographs are of limited sensitivity, particularly in the setting of micronodular metastases, but they may be used to identify macronodular metastases that do not concentrate radioiodine. Other imaging modalities may be beneficial in evaluating patients with elevated or rising Tg levels and negative radioiodine scans, such as scintigraphy with indium In 111 DTPA-Phe-octreotide,[110] technetium Tc 99m tetrofosmin,[111] or thallium-201,[112] positron emission tomography,[113] computed tomography, or magnetic resonance imaging. Given the propensity of follicular thyroid carcinoma to metastasize to bones, skeletal imaging with technetium Tc 99m pyrophosphate may also be of value.

In summary, individual clinicopathologic features may allow development of a routine follow-up strategy as follows:

- Years 1-3: clinical examination and serum-free T4 estimate, TSH, and thyroglobulin every 6 months; chest radiograph annually; neck US annually (if N1 or T4 disease at presentation); radioiodine scans (possibly with thyrotropin alfa stimulation) and potential therapy annually until two successive negative scans (every 6 months for M1 disease)
- Years 4-10: clinical examination, serum-free T4 estimate, TSH, thyroglobulin, and chest radiograph annually; neck US every 2 years (if N1 or T4 disease at presentation); radioiodine scan if thyroglobulin rising or recurrence suspected
- Years 11-20: clinical examination, serum-free T4 estimate, TSH, and thyroglobulin annually; chest radiograph every 3 years; neck US every 3 years (if N1 or T4 disease at presentation); radioiodine scan if thyroglobulin rising or recurrence suspected
- Years 21+: clinical examination, serum-free T4 estimate, TSH, and thyroglobulin annually; chest radiograph every 3 to 5 years; neck US every 3 to 5 years (if N1 or T4 disease at presentation); radioiodine scan if thyroglobulin rising or recurrence suspected

MEDULLARY THYROID CANCER

Medullary thyroid carcinoma (MTC) is a neuroendocrine malignancy that is derived from the parafollicular or C cells of the thyroid. Sporadic MTC accounts for 80% of all cases of the disease, with the remainder of patients having inherited tumor syndromes such as multiple endocrine neoplasia (MEN) type 2A, MEN 2B, or familial medullary carcinoma (FMTC). The most common presentation of sporadic MTC is that of a palpable thyroid nodule, occurring in about 75% to 95% of patients.[114] Because the C cells are predominantly located in the upper portion of each thyroid lobe, patients with sporadic disesae typically have upper pole nodules.

Metastatic cervical adenopathy is noted in about 50% of patients at initial presentation, and symptoms of upper aerodigestive tract compression or invasion such as dysphagia or hoarseness are reported by up to 15% of patients with sporadic disease.[115] Symptoms from distant metastases in lungs or bones may be elicited from 5% to 10% of patients at presentation. The ability of the tumor to oversecrete measurable quantities of calcitonin, occasionally accompanied by hormonally active peptides such as adrenocorticotrophic hormone or calcitonin-gene related peptide, leads to unexplained diarrhea, symptoms of Cushing syndrome, or facial flushing for many patients with advanced disease. MTC is rarely suggested by the presence of dense calcifications seen on radiologic imaging of the anterior neck or sites of metastatic disease. The typical age of a sporadic presentation is in the fifth or sixth decade, and there may be a slight female preponderance.

The diagnosis of sporadic MTC is usually suspected after a FNA of a solitary nodule (or a dominant nodule within a multinodular goiter). Routine measurement of the serum calcitonin concentration is not recommended as a screen for MTC for a patient with a solitary nodule. However, recent reports suggest that as many as 3% of patients with nodular thyroid disease will have an elevated serum calcitonin level when measured in a sensitive immunometric assay; of those, 40% will prove to have MTC at thyroidectomy.[8,116,117] At an estimated cost of $12,500 per diagnosed case that would not otherwise be identified by FNA, and because of the lack of widespread availability of such a sensitive immunoassay, routine measurement of serum calcitonin levels for all patients with nodular thyroid disease cannot be recommended.[64,118]

For patients in known kindreds with inherited MTC, prospective family screening increasingly identifies disease carriers long before clinical symptoms or signs are noted. Using the traditional approach of stimulated secretion of calcitonin by either pentagastrin or calcium infusion, 65% of MEN 2A gene carriers will have abnormal calcitonin levels by age 20 years, and 95% by age 35.[119] Compared with sporadic disease, the typical age of presentation for familial disease is the third decade, without gender preference. In MEN 2A, it is uncommon for the signs or symptoms of hyperparathyroidism or pheochromocytoma to present before those of MTC, even in the absence of prospective screening.[120] All familial forms of MTC and MEN 2 are inherited in an autosomal dominant fashion. In at least 95% of known kindreds, the disease is associated with (and likely caused by) a germline mutation in the *ret* proto-oncogene, a 21 exon gene located near the centromere on chromosome 10. *Ret* codes for a cell membrane–associated tyrosine kinase receptor for glial cell line–derived neurotrophic factor, a circulating ligand that promotes development of various central and peripheral nervous system neurons.[121,122] Mutations associated with MEN 2A and FMTC have been primarily identified in several codons of the cysteine-rich extracellular domains of exons 10, 11, and 13, whereas MEN 2B and some FMTC mutations are found within the intracellular exons 15 and 16 (Table 1).[123] Somatic mutations in exons 11, 13, and 16 have also been found in at least 25% of sporadic MTC tumors, particularly the codon 918 mutation that activates the tyrosine kinase function of the receptor and is associated with poorer patient prognosis.[124,125] Further, about 6% of patients with clinically sporadic MTC carry a germline mutation

TABLE 1.

ret Proto-oncogene Mutations in Hereditary Medullary Thyroid Carcinoma[123]

Mutated Codon/Exon	Clinical Syndrome
609/10	FMTC; MEN 2A with or without Hirschsprung disease
611/10	FMTC; MEN 2A
618/10	FMTC; MEN2A with or without Hirschsprung disease
620/10	FMTC; MEN 2A with or without Hirschsprung disease
630/11	FMTC; MEN 2A
634/11	FMTC; MEN 2A; MEN 2A with cutaneous lichen amyloidosis
635/11	MEN 2A
637/11	MEN 2A
768/13	FMTC
790/13	FMTC; MEN 2A
791/13	FMTC
804/13	FMTC; MEN 2A
883/15	MEN 2B
891/15	FMTC
918/16	MEN 2B
922/16	MEN 2B

in *ret*, leading to identification of new kindreds with multiple previously undiagnosed affected individuals.[124,126] Genetic testing for *ret* proto-oncogene mutations should be offered to all patients newly diagnosed with clinically apparent sporadic MTC; it should also be used to screen children and adults in known kindreds with inherited forms of MTC. Given the frequency of mutations in certain exons, a sensible strategy for mutational analysis would start with examination of exon 11, followed sequentially by exons 10, 16, 13, 14, and 15.[123] Although common mutations can be identified by broadly available commercial testing sources, only a limited number of sites perform the more thorough analyses that are required to identify the less common mutations. Presently, a 5% error rate is generally reported, underscoring the importance of repeat testing of at least two independently obtained blood samples in more than one laboratory to minimize the likelihood of both false-positive and false-negative results.[127]

Three approaches to staging of medullary carcinoma are in common use: TNM,[128,129] Clinical Class,[115,130] and the NTCTCS Registry.[27] Important prognostic factors are lacking from these staging classifications. Notably absent is consideration of age at diagnosis. Patients less than 40 years of age at diagnosis have 5- and 10-year disease-specific survival of about 95% and 75%, respectively, compared with 65% and 50% for those older than 40 years.[115] Controlling for this effect of age at diagnosis, the prognosis of patients with inherited disease, who typically are diagnosed at an earlier age, is probably similar to that of patients with sporadic disease.[120,131] Yet, despite an even younger typical age at diagnosis, patients with MTC in MEN 2B are more likely than those with either MEN 2A or FMTC to have locally aggressive disease.[120] Other factors that may be important for predicting a worse prognosis include the heterogeneity and paucity of calcitonin immunostaining of the tumor,[132] rapidly rising serum carcinoembryonic antigen (particularly in the setting of a stable calcitonin level),[133] and postoperative residual hypercalcitoninemia.[129] With more study, specific germline or somatic mutations in *ret* may also be useful predictors of disease outcome; certainly, presence of an exon 16 mutation either within a sporadic tumor or associated with MEN 2B is associated with more aggressive disease.[126]

Even among patients with apparently sporadic disease, the possibility of MEN 2 should be considered, and serum calcium and 24-hour urinary excretion of metanephrines and catecholamines should be measured.

INITIAL SURGICAL MANAGEMENT

Total thyroidectomy is indicated for all patients with MTC, especially given the high frequency of bilateral disease in both sporadic and familial disease.[115] Once an MTC tumor is large enough to be palpated, there is a high frequency of metastasis to adjacent nodal tissue. Therefore, even in the absence of clinically detectable nodal metastases, central compartment dissection from the hyoid bone to the innominate veins and medial to the jugular veins should be performed for all patients, and ipsilateral lateral neck or mediastinal dissections should be strongly considered when the primary tumor is greater than 2 cm or central compartment disease is present.[134] Disfiguring radical node dissections do not improve prognosis and are not indicated. In the presence of grossly invasive disease, more extended procedures with resection of involved neck structures may be appropriate, but function-preserving approaches are preferred.

ADJUVANT RADIATION THERAPY

External beam radiation therapy should be considered for patients after maximal surgical therapy who are considered at high risk for locoregional recurrence. A recent study retrospectively reviewed the outcome of 40 MTC patients with microscopic residual disease, extraglandular invasion or lymph node metastases.[135] The locoregional relapse-free rate at 10 years was 86% for the 25 patients who received postoperative radiotherapy, compared with 52% for those patients who did not receive adjuvant therapy. We currently recommend radiotherapy to the neck and upper mediastinum after primary surgery for patients with extrathyroidal disease or extensive nodal metastases who do not undergo curative dissection. A typical treatment regimen would be 40 Gy administered in 20 fractions to the cervical, supraclavicular, and upper mediastinal lymph nodes over 4 weeks, with subsequent booster doses of 10 Gy in five fractions to the thyroid bed.[136] In addition, radiotherapy can be given to palliate painful bone metastases.

PERSISTENTLY ELEVATED CALCITONIN

Six months postoperatively, serum concentrations of calcitonin and carcinoembryonic antigen should be measured.[137] The patient whose calcitonin level is less than 10 pg/mL should undergo stimulation testing with either calcium or pentagastrin. About 80% of patients with palpable MTC and 50% of those with nonpalpable but macroscopic MTC who undergo supposedly curative resection have stimulated serum calcitonin values of at least 10 pg/mL, indicative of residual disease.[138,139] Those with near-normal values can be followed up, but those with values above 100 pg/mL should be evaluated for either residual resectable disease in the neck or the presence of distant metastases, including careful review of the initial operative report, physical examination, and high-resolution US of the neck. Patients with a basal serum calcitonin value of more than 1000 pg/mL and no obvious MTC in the neck and upper mediastinum probably have distant metastases, most likely in the liver. The prognosis for patients with such postoperative hypercalcitoninemia depends primarily on the extent of disease at the time of initial surgery. In a study of 31 patients (10 patients with apparently sporadic disease, 15 with MEN 2A, and 6 with MEN 2B), the 5- and 10-year survival rates were 90% and 86%, respectively.[140] Two recent studies have reported higher mortality rates for patients with high postoperative serum calcitonin values, with more than half of the patients having a recurrence during a mean follow-up of 10 years.[129,141]

Given the general failure of routine lymphadenectomy or excision of palpable tumors to normalize the serum calcitonin concentrations of such patients, attention has been directed toward detection and eradication of microscopic tumor deposits in an attempt to improve outcome. Microdissection techniques to remove all nodal and perinodal tissue from the neck and upper mediastinum were first reported to normalize the stimulated serum calcitonin levels in 4 of 11 patients at least 2 years postoperatively.[142] In subsequent larger studies, 20% to 40% of patients undergoing microdissection of the central and bilateral neck compartments were biochemically cured, with minimal perioperative morbidity.[143,144] Preoperative assessment should include US of the neck, computed tomography of the chest, magnetic resonance imaging of the abdomen, bone scintigraphic imaging, and localization of disease by catheterization of the hepatic veins, both internal jugular veins, and the innominate veins, with measurements of serum calcitonin before and after stimulation.[145] Laparoscopic assessment of the liver can be performed if distant metastases are not detected by this diagnostic approach.[144] However, in the absence of long-term outcomes, the application of this approach should probably be limited to those centers experienced in this procedure; only patients with overt disease in the neck and no distant metastases should undergo reoperative neck surgery.

PROPHYLACTIC SURGERY FOR GENE CARRIERS

Prophylactic thyroidectomy has been recommended for at-risk family members who are identified as carriers of a familial *ret* mutation.[146] Of 18 patients who underwent prophylactic thyroidectomy at a median age of 14 years, nearly 80% had a histologic diagnosis of MTC but none had evidence of nodal metastases. For the 13 patients evaluated 3 years after surgery, all stimulated plasma calcitonin levels were normal. Given identification of patients with malignant disease as early as age 6, most experts advocate prophylactic thyroidectomy before the age of 6 years in MEN 2A carriers.[134,143] Surveillance with stimulated calcitonin measurements rather than surgery is still suggested by some investigators for young gene carriers without evidence of MTC, although this approach should probably be avoided in children with the more virulent *ret* mutations in exons 10 and 11.[123]

REFERENCES

1. Hundahl SA, Fleming ID, Fremgen AM, et al: A National Cancer Data Base report on 53,856 cases of thyroid carcinoma treated in the U.S., 1985-1995. *Cancer* 83:2638-2648, 1998.
2. Landis SH, Murray T, Bolden S, et al: Cancer statistics, 1999. *CA Cancer J Clin* 49:8-31, 1999.
3. Mazzaferri EL: Management of a solitary thyroid nodule. *N Engl J Med* 328:553-559, 1993.
4. Hamburger JI: Diagnosis of thyroid nodules by fine needle biopsy: Use and abuse. *J Clin Endocrinol Metab* 79:335-339, 1994.
5. McHenry CR, Walfish PG, Rosen IB: Non-diagnostic fine needle aspiration biopsy: A dilemma in management of nodular thyroid disease. *Am Surg* 59:415-419, 1993.
6. Cochand-Priollet B, Guillausseau PJ, Chagnon S, et al: The diagnostic value of fine-needle aspiration biopsy under ultrasonography in nonfunctional thyroid nodules: A prospective study comparing cytologic and histologic findings. *Am J Med* 97:152-157, 1994.
7. Gharib H, Goellner JR: Fine-needle aspiration biopsy of the thyroid: An appraisal. *Ann Intern Med* 118:282-289, 1993.
8. Ozgen AG, Hamulu F, Bayraktar F, et al: Evaluation of routine basal serum calcitonin measurement for early diagnosis of medullary thyroid carcinoma in seven hundred seventy-three patients with nodular goiter. *Thyroid* 9:579-582, 1999.
9. Schlinkert RT, van Heerden JA, Goellner JR, et al: Factors that predict malignant thyroid lesions when fine-needle aspiration is "suspicious for follicular neoplasm." *Mayo Clin Proc* 72:913-916, 1997.
10. Tuttle RM, Lemar H, Burch HB: Clinical features associated with an increased risk of thyroid malignancy in patients with follicular neoplasia by fine-needle aspiration. *Thyroid* 8:377-383, 1998.
11. Tyler DS, Winchester DJ, Caraway NP, et al: Indeterminate fine-needle aspiration biopsy of the thyroid: Identification of subgroups at high risk for invasive carcinoma. *Surgery* 116:1054-1060, 1994.

12. Haber RS, Weiser KR, Pritsker A, et al: GLUT1 glucose transporter expression in benign and malignant thyroid nodules. *Thyroid* 7:363-367, 1997.

13. Haugen BR, Nawaz S, Markham N, et al: Telomerase activity in benign and malignant thyroid tumors. *Thyroid* 7:337-342, 1997.

14. Inohara H, Honjo Y, Yoshii T, et al: Expression of galectin-3 in fine-needle aspirates as a diagnostic marker differentiating benign from malignant thyroid neoplasms. *Cancer* 85:2475-2484, 1999.

15. Takano T, Miyauchi A, Matsuzuka F, et al: Preoperative diagnosis of medullary thyroid carcinoma by RT-PCR using RNA extracted from leftover cells within a needle used for fine needle aspiration biopsy. *J Clin Endocrinol Metab* 84:951-955, 1999.

16. Belfiore A, La Rosa GL, La Porta GA, et al: Cancer risk in patients with cold thyroid nodules: Relevance of iodine intake, sex, age, and multinodularity. *Am J Med* 93:363-369, 1992.

17. Gharib H: Fine-needle aspiration biopsy of thyroid nodules: Advantages, limitations, and effect. *Mayo Clin Proc* 69:44-49, 1994.

18. Ezzat S, Sarti DA, Cain DR, et al: Thyroid incidentalomas: Prevalence by palpation and ultrasonography. *Arch Intern Med* 154:1838-1840, 1994.

19. Tan GH, Gharib H: Thyroid incidentalomas: Management approaches to nonpalpable nodules discovered incidentally on thyroid imaging. *Ann Intern Med* 126:226-231, 1997.

20. Sherman SI: Toward a standard clinicopathologic staging approach for differentiated thyroid carcinoma. *Semin Surg Oncol* 16:12-15, 1999.

21. Beahrs OH, Henson DE, Hutter RVP: *Manual for Staging of Cancer, American Joint Commission on Cancer* (3rd ed). Philadelphia, JB Lippincott, 1988.

22. Byar DP, Green SB, Dor P, et al: A prognostic index for thyroid carcinoma: A study of the E.O.R.T.C. Thyroid Cancer Cooperative Group. *Eur J Cancer* 15:1033-1041, 1979.

23. Cady B, Rossi R: An expanded view of risk-group definition in differentiated thyroid carcinoma. *Surgery* 104:947-953, 1988.

24. DeGroot LJ, Kaplan EL, McCormick M, et al: Natural history, treatment, and course of papillary thyroid carcinoma. *J Clin Endocrinol Metab* 71:414-424, 1990.

25. Hay ID, Bergstralh EJ, Goellner J, et al: Predicting outcome in papillary carcinoma: Development of a reliable prognostic scoring system in a cohort of 1779 patients treated surgically at one institution during 1940 through 1989. *Surgery* 114:1050-1058, 1993.

26. Mazzaferri EL, Jhiang SM: Long-term impact of initial surgical and medical therapy on papillary and follicular thyroid cancer. *Am J Med* 97:418-428, 1994.

27. Sherman SI, Brierley JD, Sperling M, et al: Prospective multicenter study of treatment of thyroid carcinoma: Initial analysis of staging and outcome. *Cancer* 83:1012-1021, 1998.

28. Hermanek P, Sobin LH: *TNM Classification of Malignant Tumours* (4th ed, 2nd rev). Berlin, Springer-Verlag, 1992.
29. Davis NL, Bugis SP, McGregor GI, et al: An evaluation of prognostic scoring systems in patients with follicular thyroid cancer. *Am J Surg* 170:476-480, 1995.
30. Hay ID: Papillary thyroid carcinoma. *Endocrinol Metab Clin North Am* 19:545-576, 1990.
31. Hay ID, Grant CS, Taylor WF, et al: Ipsilateral lobectomy versus bilateral lobar resection in papillary thyroid carcinoma: A retrospective analysis of surgical outcome using a novel prognostic scoring system. *Surgery* 102:1088-1095, 1987.
32. Brierley JD, Panzarella T, Tsang RW, et al: A comparison of different staging systems predictability of patient outcome: Thyroid carcinoma as an example. *Cancer* 79:2414-2423, 1997.
33. DeGroot LJ, Kaplan EL, Straus FH: Does the method of management of papillary thyroid carcinoma make a difference in outcome? *World J Surg* 18:123-130, 1994.
34. Loh KC, Greenspan FS, Gee L, et al: Pathological tumor-node-metastasis (pTNM) staging for papillary and follicular thyroid carcinomas: A retrospective analysis of 700 patients. *J Clin Endocrinol Metab* 82:3553-3562, 1997.
35. Hay ID, Grant CS, Bergstralh EJ, et al: Unilateral total lobectomy: Is it sufficient surgical treatment for patients with AMES low-risk papillary thyroid carcinoma? *Surgery* 124:958-964; discussion 964-956, 1998.
36. Vassilopoulou-Sellin R, Schultz PN, Haynie TP: Clinical outcome of patients with papillary thyroid carcinoma who have recurrence after initial radioactive iodine therapy. *Cancer* 78:493-501, 1996.
37. Shaha AR, Shah JP, Loree TR: Low-risk differentiated thyroid cancer: The need for selective treatment. *Ann Surg Oncol* 4:328-333, 1997.
38. Udelsman R, Lakatos E, Ladenson P: Optimal surgery for papillary thyroid carcinoma. *World J Surg* 20:88-93, 1996.
39. Hughes CJ, Shaha AR, Shah JP, et al: Impact of lymph node metastasis in differentiated carcinoma of the thyroid: A matched-pair analysis. *Head Neck* 18:127-132, 1996.
40. Grebe SK, Hay ID: Thyroid cancer nodal metastases: Biologic significance and therapeutic considerations. *Surg Oncol Clin N Am* 5:43-63, 1996.
41. Simon D, Goretzki PE, Witte J, et al: Incidence of regional recurrence guiding radicality in differentiated thyroid carcinoma. *World J Surg* 20:860-866, 1996.
42. McCaffrey TV, Bergstralh EJ, Hay ID: Locally invasive papillary thyroid carcinoma: 1940-1990. *Head Neck* 16:165-172, 1994.
43. Falk SA, McCaffrey TV: Management of the recurrent laryngeal nerve in suspected and proven thyroid cancer. *Otolaryngol Head Neck Surg* 113:42-48, 1995.

44. Gillenwater AM, Goepfert H: Surgical management of laryngotracheal and esophageal involvement by locally advanced thyroid cancer. *Semin Surg Oncol* 16:19-29, 1999.
45. Melliere DJ, Ben Yahia NE, Becquemin JP, et al: Thyroid carcinoma with tracheal or esophageal involvement: Limited or maximal surgery? *Surgery* 113:166-172, 1993.
46. Park CS, Suh KW, Min JS: Cartilage-shaving procedure for the control of tracheal cartilage invasion by thyroid carcinoma. *Head Neck* 15:289-291, 1993.
47. Ballantyne AJ: Resections of the upper aerodigestive tract for locally invasive thyroid cancer. *Am J Surg* 168:636-639, 1994.
48. Grillo HC, Zannini P: Resectional management of airway invasion by thyroid carcinoma. *Ann Thorac Surg* 42:287-298, 1986.
49. Ishihara T, Kobayashi K, Kikuchi K, et al: Surgical treatment of advanced thyroid carcinoma invading the trachea. *J Thorac Cardiovasc Surg* 102:717-720, 1991.
50. Marohn MR, LaCivita KA: Evaluation of total/near-total thyroidectomy in a short-stay hospitalization: Safe and cost-effective. *Surgery* 118:943-947; discussion 947-948, 1995.
51. McHenry CR: "Same-day" thyroid surgery: An analysis of safety, cost savings, and outcome. *Am Surg* 63:586-589; discussion 589-590, 1997.
52. Mowschenson PM, Hodin RA: Outpatient thyroid and parathyroid surgery: A prospective study of feasibility, safety, and costs. *Surgery* 118:1051-1053, 1995.
53. Samson PS, Reyes FR, Saludares WN, et al: Outpatient thyroidectomy. *Am J Surg* 173:499-503, 1997.
54. Schwartz AE, Clark OH, Ituarte P, et al: Therapeutic controversy: Thyroid surgery—the choice. *J Clin Endocrinol Metab* 83:1097-1105, 1998.
55. Vassilopoulou-Sellin R, Goepfert H, Raney B, et al: Differentiated thyroid cancer in children and adolescents: Clinical outcome and mortality after long-term follow-up. *Head Neck* 20:549-555, 1998.
56. Vassilopoulou-Sellin R, Palmer L, Taylor S, et al: Incidence of breast carcinoma in women with thyroid carcinoma. *Cancer* 85:696-705, 1999.
57. Segal K, Shvero J, Stern Y, et al: Surgery of thyroid cancer in children and adolescents. *Head Neck* 20:293-297, 1998.
58. Akslen LA, Haldorsen T, Thoresen SO, et al: Incidence of thyroid cancer in Norway 1970-1985: Population review on time trend, sex, age, histological type and tumour stage in 2625 cases. *Apmis* 98:549-558, 1990.
59. Donegan WL: Cancer and pregnancy. *CA Cancer J Clin* 33:194-214, 1983.
60. Hod M, Sharony R, Friedman S, et al: Pregnancy and thyroid carcinoma: A review of incidence, course, and prognosis. *Obstet Gynecol Surv* 44:774-779, 1989.

61. Moosa M, Mazzaferri EL: Outcome of differentiated thyroid cancer diagnosed in pregnant women. *J Clin Endocrinol Metab* 82:2862-2866, 1997.
62. Herzon FS, Morris DM, Segal MN, et al: Coexistent thyroid cancer and pregnancy. *Arch Otolaryngol Head Neck Surg* 120:1191-1193, 1994.
63. Schlumberger MJ: Papillary and follicular thyroid carcinoma. *N Engl J Med* 338:297-306, 1998.
64. Singer PA, Cooper DS, Daniels GH, et al: Treatment guidelines for patients with thyroid nodules and well-differentiated thyroid cancer. *Arch Intern Med* 156:2165-2172, 1996.
65. Taylor T, Specker B, Robbins J, et al: Outcome after treatment of high-risk papillary and non-Hürthle-cell follicular thyroid carcinoma. *Ann Intern Med* 129:622-627, 1998.
66. Wong JB, Kaplan MM, Meyer KB, et al: Ablative radioactive iodine therapy for apparently localized thyroid carcinoma: A decision analytic perspective. *Endocrinol Metab Clin North Am* 19:741-760, 1990.
67. Cady B: Staging in thyroid cancer (editorial). *Cancer* 83:844-847, 1998.
68. Schlumberger M, Tubiana M, De Vathaire F, et al: Longterm results of treatment of 283 patients with lung and bone metastases from differentiated thyroid carcinoma. *J Clin Endocrinol Metab* 63:960-967, 1986.
69. Goldman JM, Line BR, Aamodt RL, et al: Influence of triiodothyronine withdrawal time on ^{131}I uptake postthyroidectomy for thyroid cancer. *J Clin Endocrinol Metab* 50:734-739, 1980.
70. Lakshmanan M, Schaffer A, Robbins J, et al: A simplified low iodine diet in I-131 scanning and therapy of thyroid cancer. *Clin Nucl Med* 13:866-868, 1988.
71. Koong SS, Reynolds JC, Movius EG, et al: Lithium as a potential adjuvant to ^{131}I therapy of metastatic, well differentiated thyroid carcinoma. *J Clin Endocrinol Metab* 84:912-916, 1999.
72. Grünwald F, Pakos E, Bender H, et al: Redifferentiation therapy with retinoic acid in follicular thyroid cancer. *J Nucl Med* 39:1555-1558, 1998.
73. Simon D, Koehrle J, Reiners C, et al: Redifferentiation therapy with retinoids: Therapeutic option for advanced follicular and papillary thyroid carcinoma. *World J Surg* 22:569-574, 1998.
74. Maxon HR, Thomas SR, Samaratunga RC: Dosimetric considerations in the radioiodine treatment of macrometastases and micrometastases from differentiated thyroid cancer. *Thyroid* 7:183-188, 1997.
75. Muratet JP, Daver A, Minier JF, et al: Influence of scanning doses of iodine-131 on subsequent first ablative treatment outcome in patients operated on for differentiated thyroid carcinoma. *J Nucl Med* 39:1546-1550, 1998.
76. Sherman SI, Tielens ET, Sostre S, et al: Clinical utility of posttreatment radioiodine scans in the management of patients with thyroid carcinoma. *J Clin Endocrinol Metab* 78:629-634, 1994.

77. Park HM, Park YH, Zhou XH: Detection of thyroid remnant/metastasis without stunning: an ongoing dilemma. *Thyroid* 7:277-280, 1997.

78. Bal C, Padhy AK, Jana S, et al: Prospective randomized clinical trial to evaluate the optimal dose of 131 I for remnant ablation in patients with differentiated thyroid carcinoma. *Cancer* 77:2574-2580, 1996.

79. Logue JP, Tsang RW, Brierley JD, et al: Radioiodine ablation of residual tissue in thyroid cancer: Relationship between administered activity, neck uptake and outcome. *Br J Radiol* 67:1127-1131, 1994.

80. Maxon HR, Englaro EE, Thomas SR, et al: Radioiodine-131 therapy for well-differentiated thyroid cancer—A quantitative radiation dosimetric approach: Outcome and validation in 85 patients. *J Nucl Med* 33:1132-1136, 1992.

81. Reynolds JC: Percent ^{131}I uptake and post-therapy ^{131}I scans: Their role in the management of thyroid cancer. *Thyroid* 7:281-284, 1997.

82. Cooper DS, Specker B, Ho M, et al: Thyrotropin suppression and disease progression in patients with differentiated thyroid cancer: Results from the National Thyroid Cancer Treatment Cooperative Registry. *Thyroid* 8:737-744, 1998.

83. Pujol P, Daures J-P, Nsakala N, et al: Degree of thyrotropin suppression as a prognostic determinant in differentiated thyroid cancer. *J Clin Endocrinol Metab* 81:4318-4323, 1996.

84. Diamond T, Nery L, Hales I: A therapeutic dilemma: Suppressive doses of thyroxine significantly reduce bone mineral measurements in both premenopausal and postmenopausal women with thyroid carcinoma. *J Clin Endocrinol Metab* 72:1184-1188, 1990.

85. Stall GM, Harris S, Sokoll LJ, et al: Accelerated bone loss in hypothyroid patients overtreated with L-thyroxine. *Ann Intern Med* 113:265-269, 1990.

86. Sawin CT, Geller A, Wolf PA, et al: Low serum thyrotropin concentrations as a risk factor for atrial fibrillation in older persons. *N Engl J Med* 331:1249-1252, 1994.

87. Biondi B, Fazio S, Carella C, et al: Cardiac effects of long term thyrotropin-suppressive therapy with levothyroxine. *J Clin Endocrinol Metab* 77:334-338, 1993.

88. Biondi B, Fazio S, Cuocolo A, et al: Impaired cardiac reserve and exercise capacity in patients receiving long-term thyrotropin suppressive therapy with levothyroxine. *J Clin Endocrinol Metab* 81:4224-4228, 1996.

89. Fazio S, Biondi B, Carella C, et al: Diastolic dysfunction in patients on thyroid-stimulating hormone suppressive therapy with levothyroxine: Beneficial effect of β-blockade. *J Clin Endocrinol Metab* 80:2222-2226, 1995.

90. Shapiro LE, Sievert R, Ong L, et al: Minimal cardiac effects in asymptomatic athreotic patients chronically treated with thyrotropin-suppressive doses of L-thyroxine. *J Clin Endocrinol Metab* 82:2592-2595, 1997.

91. Sherman SI, Chiu AC, Kopelen H, et al: Minimal resting cardiac effects of TSH-suppressive doses of L-thyroxine. *Thyroid* 7:S58, 1997.

92. Farahati J, Reiners C, Stuschke M, et al: Differentiated thyroid cancer: Impact of adjuvant external radiotherapy in patients with perithyroidal tumor infiltration (stage pT4). *Cancer* 77:172-180, 1996.
93. Tsang RW, Brierley JD, Simpson WJ, et al: The effects of surgery, radioiodine, and external radiation therapy on the clinical outcome of patients with differentiated thyroid carcinoma. *Cancer* 82:375-388, 1998.
94. Brierley JD, Tsang RW: External radiation therapy in the treatment of thyroid malignancy. *Endocrinol Metab Clin N Amer* 25:141-157, 1996.
95. Grigsby PW, Baglan K, Siegel BA: Surveillance of patients to detect recurrent thyroid carcinoma. *Cancer* 85:945-951, 1999.
96. Meier CA, Braverman LE, Ebner SA, et al: Diagnostic use of recombinant human thyrotropin in patients with thyroid carcinoma (phase I/II study). *J Clin Endocrinol Metab* 78:188-196, 1994.
97. Haugen BR, Pacini F, Reiners C, et al: A comparison of recombinant human thyrotropin and thyroid hormone withdrawal for the detection of thyroid remnant or cancer. *J Clin Endocrinol Metab* 84:3877-3885, 1999.
98. Ladenson PW, Braverman LE, Mazzaferri EL, et al: Comparison of administration of recombinant human thyrotropin with withdrawal of thyroid hormone for radioactive iodine scanning in patients with thyroid carcinoma. *N Engl J Med* 337:888-896, 1997.
99. Spencer CA, Wang C-C: Thyroglobulin measurement: Techniques, clinical benefits, and pitfalls. *Endocrinol Metab Clin N Amer* 24:841-863, 1995.
100. Ozata M, Suzuki S, Miyamoto T, et al: Serum thyroglobulin in the follow-up of patients treated with differentiated thyroid cancer. *J Clin Endocrinol Metab* 79:98-105, 1994.
101. Pacini F, Lari R, Mazzeo S, et al: Diagnostic value of a single serum thyroglobulin determination on and off thyroid suppressive therapy in the follow-up of patients with differentiated thyroid cancer. *Clin Endocrinol* 23:405-411, 1985.
102. Mueller-Gaertner HW, Schneider C: Clinical evaluation of tumor characteristics predisposing serum thyroglobulin to be undetectable in patients with differentiated thyroid cancer. *Cancer* 61:976-981, 1988.
103. Ladenson PW: Strategies for thyrotropin use to monitor patients with treated thyroid carcinoma. *Thyroid* 9:429-433, 1999.
104. Spencer CA, LoPresti JS, Fatemi S, et al: Detection of residual and recurrent differentiated thyroid carcinoma by serum thyroglobulin measurement. *Thyroid* 9:435-441, 1999.
105. Mariotti S, Barbesino G, Caturegli P, et al: Assay of thyroglobulin in serum with thyroglobulin autoantibodies: An unobtainable goal? *J Clin Endocrinol Metab* 80:468-472, 1995.
106. Spencer CA, Takeuchi M, Kazarosyan M, et al: Serum thyroglobulin autoantibodies: Prevalence, influence on serum thyroglobulin measurement, and prognostic significance in patients with differentiated thyroid carcinoma. *J Clin Endocrinol Metab* 83:1121-1127, 1998.

107. Ringel MD, Ladenson PW, Levine MA: Molecular diagnosis of residual and recurrent thyroid cancer by amplification of thyroglobulin messenger ribonucleic acid in peripheral blood. *J Clin Endocrinol Metab* 83:4435-4442, 1998.

108. Antonelli A, Miccoli P, Fedeghini M, et al: Role of neck ultrasound in the follow-up of patients operated on for thyroid cancer. *Thyroid* 5:25-28, 1995.

109. Franceschi M, Kusic Z, Franceschi D, et al: Thyroglobulin determination, neck ultrasonography and iodine-131 whole-body scintigraphy in differentiated thyroid carcinoma. *J Nucl Med* 37:446-451, 1996.

110. Baudin E, Schlumberger M, Lumbroso J, et al: Octreotide scintigraphy in patients with differentiated thyroid carcinoma: Contribution for patients with negative radioiodine scan. *J Clin Endocrinol Metab* 81:2541-2544, 1996.

111. Lind P, Gallowitsch HJ, Langsteger W, et al: Technetium-99m-tetrofosmin whole body scintigraphy in the follow-up of differentiated thyroid carcinoma. *J Nucl Med* 38:348-352, 1997.

112. Burman K, Anderson J, Wartofsky L, et al: Management of patients with thyroid carcinoma: Application of thallium-201 scintigraphy and magnetic resonance imaging. *J Nucl Med* 31:1958-1964, 1990.

113. Wang W, Macapinlac H, Larson SM, et al: [18F]-2-fluoro-2-deoxy-D-glucose positron emission tomography localizes residual thyroid cancer in patients with negative diagnostic (131)I whole body scans and elevated serum thyroglobulin levels. *J Clin Endocrinol Metab* 84:2291-2302, 1999.

114. Ball DW, Baylin SB, de Bustros AC: Medullary thyroid carcinoma, in Braverman LE, Utiger RD (eds): *Werner and Ingbar's The Thyroid* (ed 7th). Philadelphia, Lippincott-Raven, 1996, pp 946-960.

115. Saad MF, Ordonez NG, Rashid RK, et al: Medullary carcinoma of the thyroid. *Medicine* 63:319-342, 1984.

116. Niccoli P, Wion-Barbot N, Caron P, et al: Interest of routine measurement of serum calcitonin: Study in a large series of thyroidectomized patients. *J Clin Endocrinol Metab* 82:338-341, 1997.

117. Pacini F, Fontanelli M, Fugazzola L, et al: Routine measurement of serum calcitonin in nodular thyroid diseases allows the preoperative diagnosis of unsuspected sporadic medullary thyroid carcinoma. *J Clin Endocrinol Metab* 78:826-829, 1994.

118. Horvit PK, Gagel RF: Editorial: The goitrous patient with an elevated serum calcitonin: What to do? *J Clin Endocrinol Metab* 82:335-337, 1997.

119. Ponder BA, Ponder MA, Coffey R, et al: Risk estimation and screening in families of patients with medullary thyroid carcinoma. *Lancet* 1:397-401, 1988.

120. O'Riordain DS, O'Brien T, Weaver AL, et al: Medullary thyroid carcinoma in multiple endocrine neoplasia types 2A and 2B. *Surgery* 116:1017-1023, 1994.

121. Durbec P, Marcos-Gutierrez CV, Kilkenny C, et al: GDNF signalling through the Ret receptor tyrosine kinase. *Nature* 381:789-791, 1996.
122. Trupp M, Arenas E, Fainzilber M, et al: Functional receptor for GDNF encoded by the c-ret proto-oncogene. *Nature* 381:785-789, 1996.
123. Gagel RF, Cote GJ: Pathogenesis of medullary thyroid carcinoma, in Fagin JA (ed): *Thyroid Cancer.* Endocrine Updates. Boston, Kluwer Academic Publishers, 1998, pp 85-103.
124. Wohllk N, Cote GJ, Bugalho MMJ, et al: Relevence of RET proto-oncogene mutations in sporadic medullary thyroid carcinoma. *J Clin Endocrinol Metab* 81:3740-3745, 1996.
125. Zedenius J, Larsson C, Bergholm U, et al: Mutations of codon 918 in the RET proto-oncogene correlate to poor prognosis in sporadic medullary thyroid carcinomas. *J Clin Endocrinol Metab* 80:3088-3090, 1995.
126. Romei C, Elisei R, Pinchera A, et al: Somatic mutations of the ret protooncogene in sporadic medullary thyroid carcinoma are not restricted to exon 16 and are associated with tumor recurrence. *J Clin Endocrinol Metab* 81:1619-1622, 1996.
127. Gagel RF, Cote GJ, Martins Bugalho MJ, et al: Clinical use of molecular information in the management of multiple endocrine neoplasia type 2A. *J Intern Med* 238:333-341, 1995.
128. Head and Neck Tumors: Thyroid, in Beahrs OH, Henson DE, Hutter RVP, et al (eds): *Manual for Staging of Cancer* (ed 4th). Philadelphia, J.B. Lippincott, 1992, pp 53-54.
129. Dottorini ME, Assi A, Sironi M, et al: Multivariate analysis of patients with medullary thyroid carcinoma: Prognostic significance and impact on treatment of clinical and pathologic variables. *Cancer* 77:1556-1565, 1996.
130. DeGroot LJ: Thyroid carcinoma. *Med Clin North Am* 59:1233-1246, 1975.
131. Samaan NA, Schultz PN, Hickey RC: Medullary thyroid carcinoma: Prognosis of familial versus sporadic disease and the role of radiotherapy. *J Clin Endocrinol Metab* 67:801-805, 1988.
132. Lippman SM, Mendelsohn G, Trump DL, et al: The prognostic and biological significance of cellular heterogeneity in medullary thyroid carcinoma: A study of calcitonin, L-dopa decarboxylase, and histaminase. *J Clin Endocrinol Metab* 54:233-240, 1982.
133. Mendelsohn G, Wells SA, Baylin SB: Relationship of tissue carcinoembryonic antigen and calcitonin to tumor virulence in medullary thyroid carcinoma. *Cancer* 54:657-662, 1984.
134. Chi DD, Moley JF: Medullary thyroid carcinoma: genetic advances, treatment recommendations, and the approach to the patient with persistent hypercalcitoninemia. *Surg Oncol Clin N Am* 7:681-706, 1998.
135. Brierley J, Tsang R, Simpson WJ, et al: Medullary thyroid cancer: Analyses of survival and prognostic factors and the role of radiation therapy in local control. *Thyroid* 6:305-310, 1996.

136. Brierley J, Maxon HR: Radioiodine and external radiation therapy in the treatment of thyroid cancer, in Fagin JA (ed): *Thyroid Cancer. Endocrine Updates.* Boston, Kluwer Academic Publishers, 1998, pp 285-317.

137. Stepanas AV, Samaan NA, Hill CSJ, et al: Medullary thyroid carcinoma: Importance of serial serum calcitonin measurements. *Cancer* 43:825-837, 1979.

138. Jackson CE, Talpos GB, Kambouris A, et al: The clinical course after definitive operation for medullary thyroid carcinoma. *Surgery* 94:995-1001, 1983.

139. Wells SA Jr., Dilley WG, Farndon JA, et al: Early diagnosis and treatment of medullary thyroid carcinoma. *Arch Intern Med* 145:1248-1252, 1985.

140. van Heerden JA, Grant CS, Gharib H, et al: Long-term course of patients with persistent hypercalcitoninemia after apparent curative primary surgery for medullary thyroid carcinoma. *Ann Surg* 212:395-401, 1990.

141. Scopsi L, Sampietro G, Boracchi P, et al: Multivariate analysis of prognostic factors in sporadic medullary carcinoma of the thyroid. *Cancer* 78:2173-21883, 1996.

142. Tisell LE, Hansson G, Jansson S, et al: Reoperation in the treatment of asymptomatic metastasizing medullary thyroid carcinoma. *Surgery* 99:60-66, 1986.

143. Evans DB, Fleming JB, Lee JE, et al: The surgical treatment of medullary thyroid carcinoma. *Semin Surg Oncol* 16:50-63, 1999.

144. Moley JF, Debenedetti MK, Dilley WG, et al: Surgical management of patients with persistent or recurrent medullary thyroid cancer. *J Intern Med* 243:521-526, 1998.

145. Abdelmoumene N, Schlumberger M, Gardet P, et al: Selective venous sampling catheterisation for localisation of persisting medullary thyroid carcinoma. *Br J Cancer* 69:1141-1144, 1994.

146. Wells SA, Jr., Skinner MA: Prophylactic thyroidectomy, based on direct genetic testing, in patients at risk for the multiple endocrine neoplasia type 2 syndromes. *Exp Clin Endocrinol Diabetes* 106:29-34, 1998.

CHAPTER 6

Diagnosis and Management of Temporomandibular Joint Syndrome

Jonathan J. Park, DMD, MD
Chief Resident, Department of Oral and Maxillofacial Surgery,
University of Pittsburgh Medical Center, Pittsburgh, Pa

Thomas W. Braun, DMD, PhD
Interim Dean, School of Dental Medicine, University of Pittsburgh;
Professor and Chairman, Department of Oral and Maxillofacial Surgery,
University of Pittsburgh Medical Center, Pittsburgh, Pa

The correct approach to diagnosing and managing disorders of the temporomandibular joint (TMJ) remains controversial for health care professionals in medicine, public health, clinical dentistry, behavioral science, physical therapy, bioengineering, and the insurance industry. The etiologies and pathogenesis of temporomandibular joint disorders (TMD) are still poorly understood, and there is a lack of consistent data to illustrate the roles of dental occlusion, psychosocial stress, and parafunctional habits in the development of TMD. The result is a variety of confusing terminologies and diagnostic and treatment approaches. No well-defined consensus has emerged on which TMDs should be treated and when and how they should be treated.[1] This is further complicated by the diagnostic dilemma of separating disorders of the joint from headaches, disorders of the muscle, and craniofacial pain disorders. The historical failure of various treatments using TMJ alloplastic implants and artificial total joint replacements have further added to this confusion. This chapter presents a brief overview of the issues involved in the diagnosis and management of TMD.

In the past, it was common to refer to any (if not all) of the clinical complaints, signs, and symptoms caused by the dysfunction of the temporomandibular joint and associated dental relations (such as malocclusions and parafunctional habits) as, simply, temporomandibular joint syndrome. In addition, because the symptoms involving pain of the facial region often seemed to involve the adjacent anatomical structures of the TMJ (muscles, fascia), but seemed not to be directly caused by the joint itself, "myofascial pain dysfunction syndrome" and "myofascial pain syndrome" were used to describe this facial pain. During the 1950s, TMJ syndrome was often characterized as a single entity reflecting a subset of facial pain resulting from parafunctional habits such as clenching, grinding, or bruxism. During the 1960s and 1970s, emotional stress, in addition to malocclusion, was considered a major etiologic factor in TMJ syndrome. During the 1980s, the term *craniomandibular disorder* came into use, and it is still used by some clinicians. Some studies indicated that different etiologies, often in combination, can produce similar clinical complaints, signs, and symptoms related to TMJ problems.[2-12] To better reflect the wide range of etiologies based on scientific understanding of pathophysiology and anatomical abnormalities, the term temporomandibular joint disorder was adopted and is now used. TMD is a collective term that includes a variety of intracapsular and extracapsular disorders affecting structures intrinsic to the TMJ such as the disk and capsular joint spaces, and the musculoskeletal anatomical structures extrinsic and adjacent to the joint. "Internal derangement" is used to define the mechanical instability or interference with normal, smooth articulation of the disk between the mandibular condyle and glenoid fossa.[13] Internal derangements frequently involve disk displacement with or without degeneration of the disk. *Myofascial pain and dysfunction (MPD)* is also a term used to describe the multifactorial extracapsular TMJ disorders causing myogenic pain, tenderness, and subsequent mandibular dysfunction, which are often caused by abnormal masticatory muscle function or hyperactivity.

EMBRYOLOGY AND ANATOMY

The TMJ shares a common embryologic derivation with the mandible and the middle ear structures (incus and malleus) from the first branchial arch (also called the mandibular arch). The TMJ is a diarthroidal synovial joint found between the mandibular condyle and the glenoid fossa of the temporal bone, with its articular surfaces covered by avascular fibrocartilage. It is bisected by a biconcave densely fibrous disk (meniscus) consisting of an anterior band, a central or intermediate zone, and the posterior band, which lies at the 11- to 12-o'clock position to the mandibular condyle. The disk is attached posteriorly to the condyle and fossa by a densely neurovascular tissue with layers of collagen and elastin. This disk divides the joint space into separate inferior and superior joint compartments that allow rotation (hinging movement), translation (gliding and protrusive movement), and lateral excursions of mandibular condyles in relation to the glenoid fossa and articular eminence. In an average fully dentate adult, approximately 20 to 30 mm of maximal incisor opening is achieved by rotation, and approximately 15 to 25 mm of additional mandibular opening is achieved by translation. At physiologic rest, there is a 1.3- to 3.0-mm "freeway space" between the maxillary and mandibular anterior dentition.[14] The collateral ligaments attach the disk at the medial and lateral poles of the condyle. The TMJ derives its vascular supply from the superficial temporal and maxillary arteries posteriorly, and the masseteric artery anteriorly. Innervation by the mandibular branches of the trigeminal nerve consists of (1) auriculotemporal nerves (TMJ, retrodiskal tissue, posterior band, lateral ligament) and (2) masseteric and posterior deep temporal nerves (anterior band). The temporomandibular ligament attaches to the TMJ laterally. The mandibular range of motion is derived from a total of 12 muscles, including the supramandibular (muscles of mastication), inframandibular and infrahyoid muscle groups, all present bilaterally.[15]

SYMPTOMS, SIGNS, AND PATHOGENESIS OF TMD

The most common clinical symptoms in patients with TMD are pain and tenderness in the region of the TMJ. Intracapsular TMJ pain is reported to be associated with the presence of (1) inflammatory mediator substances such as interleukin-1β, interleukin-6, and tumor necrosis factor α, and (2) matrix metalloproteinases that can cause local joint degeneration.[16-18] Other common clinical symptoms are pain and tenderness in the preauricular, temporal, or frontal regions of the head. In addition to joint pain, various TMJ sounds during mandibular movement, earache, headache, neck pain, shoulder pain, and subsequent discomfort, even during speaking, can be present. Referred TMJ pain presenting as complaints of otalgia or other otologic symptoms such as tinnitus, sensation of "stuffiness" or "water in the ear," and vertigo are not uncommon.

The onset of TMD pain may be acute or chronic and can occur during mandibular function or at rest. Dental malocclusion may be observed in TMD patients. Acute TMJ pain is characterized by recent onset with limited duration; signs and symptoms lasting 3 or more months that are regular or frequent are considered chronic pain. TMD patients frequently report that the pain is associated with anxiety and depression.[19] A positive correlation between TMD complaints and habitual behavioral abnormalities or an inability to cope with environmental or social stress is thought to exist.

Common signs of TMD include limited jaw opening, asymmetric mandibular movement, and joint noises (including clicking, popping, and crepitus). These may or may not be associated with partial or complete locking of TMJ at open or closed positions. Other signs include myofascial pain or tenderness associated with trigger points. Dental occlusal trauma and wearing of dentition are often present, which may be interpreted by the TMD patients as toothache. Limited opening of the mouth can greatly affect the patient's daily activities such as mastication, nutrition, speech, and phonation.

Joint noise is not always pathologic. Many studies have found that sounds made by the joints, such as clicking, popping, and crepitus, occur in 5% to 65% of different study groups.[20] Clicking, popping, the sensation of catching or binding, and closed or open lock of the mandible—all can be results of internal derangement. On mandibular opening, the disk can be displaced anteriomedially or anteriorly off the condyle because of the stretched elastic fibers and the laxity of redundant retrodiskal tissue. Anteriomedial displacement of the disk is most common, and disk displacement without any significant clinical symptom can occur in up to 28% of the general population.[21] The anteriorly displaced disk may reduce itself to a proper position on condylar translation, resulting in clicking, popping, and sensation of TMJ catching. If the anteriorly displaced disk does not reduce, the disk may become deformed and further hinder translation of the condyle, resulting in closed lock. This is manifested by limitation of maximal opening to approximately 20 mm or less, corresponding with hinge motion only. On the other hand, an open lock occurs at the fully opened mandibular position when the condyle with or without the disk is locked anteriorly beyond the articular eminence. Crepitus is observed when the disk and retrodiskal tissue are perforated, which allows direct bone-to-bone contact between the condyle and articulating surface of the glenoid fossa during mandibular movement, or when severe degeneration (often with osteoid formation) occurs in the disk.

Symptoms and signs of TMD arise from heterogeneous local and systemic factors that can be broadly categorized as traumatic, muscular, inflammatory, infectious, congenital, and neoplastic (Box 1). However, it must be noted that such classifications of etiologies and pathogenesis are artificial, and no standard classification has been developed.

TMD symptoms and signs originating from intracapsular etiologies are often the result of direct TMJ trauma, which can be categorized as microtrauma or macrotrauma. Microtrauma involves persistent and repetitive functional stress to the joint that ultimately contributes to the TMJ degeneration. Causes of microtrauma include parafunctional habits (grinding, clenching, bruxism) that involve concomitant musculoskeletal straining and hyperactivity involving the muscles of mastication. Macrotrauma consists of high-impact, energy, and force directed to the TMJ such as occur in sports accidents, motor vehicle accidents, whiplash, mandibular overmanipulation during dental and anesthesia procedures, and hyperextension of the mandible. Both types of trauma can cause temporary or permanent damage to (1) the disk (disk degeneration and disk perforation), (2) the condyle (bony and cartilaginous erosion and bony sclerosis), (3) the joint space (capsular injury, joint effusion), or (4) the relationship between the disk, condyle, and fossa (TMJ dislocation, luxation, and subluxation).

Intracapsular TMJ trauma can lead to osteoarthritis, synovial adhesions, capsular fibrosis, and limited mandibular opening.

TMD symptoms and signs of extracapsular origin broadly include orofacial and cervical muscles. Pain in the temporal, preauricular, and masseteric regions may be the consequence of masticatory muscle spasm and trismus, myositis, and myofascial pain and dysfunction with trigger points (trapezius, sternocleidomastoid, and masticatory muscles).

Local and systemic inflammatory, rheumatologic, and autoimmune disorders may manifest as both intracapsular and extracapsular TMD. A notable iatrogenic inflammatory cause of TMD was caused by surgically placed alloplastic implants (Silastic and Proplast-Teflon disk replacements) that fragmented and induced a foreign body reaction and bony erosion. Inflammatory disorders involving primarily the soft tissues (collagen vascular diseases) cause diffuse regional pain with limitation of range of motion, swelling, erythema, and calor. Similar, but more localized, clinical findings can be observed in septic TMJ arthritis, which is uncommon in the United States.[22] Adult and juvenile forms of rheumatoid arthritis affect both soft and hard tissues, creating observable clinical and radiographic degenerative changes including synovitis, capsulitis, disk degeneration, crepitus, and condylar head

---

BOX 1.
Intracapsular and Extracapsular Etiologies of TMD

I. Intracapsular
  Articular disk
    Displacement/deformity
    Intrinsic degeneration
    Injury/contusion
    Perforation
    Anomalous development
  Disk attachment
    Inflammation (capsulitis)
    Injuries (crushing, avulsion, disruption, laceration, hematoma,
      contusion)
    Perforation
  Synovium
    Inflammation/effusion (synovitis)
    Synovial hypertrophy/hyperplasia
    Granulomatous inflammation
    Infection
    Synovial chondromatosis
    Neoplasia (pigmented villonodular synovitis, synovial sarcoma)
    Hemarthrosis
    Adhesion/scar formation
    Arthritides (rheumatoid, degenerative)
  Articular fibrocartilage
    Hypertrophy/hyperplasia
    Degeneration (chondromalacia): fissuring, fibrillation, blistering,
      erosion
  Mandibular condyle and glenoid fossa
    Fibrous and bony ankylosis
    Implant arthropathy (foreign body reactions, Silastic/Proplast-
      Teflon implants)
    Hypertrophy
    Fracture (intracapsular)
    Degenerative joint disease (osteoarthrosis)
    Avascular necrosis
II. Extracapsular
  Musculoskeletal
    Bony defects
    Anomalous bony development   *(continued)*

BOX 1. (continued)

    (hypoplasia, hyperplasia, malformation, condylar agenesis, hemifacial hypertrophy, bifid condyle, coronoid impingement, Pierre Robin and Treacher-Collins syndromes)
Fracture (condylar neck)
Osteoporosis
Metabolic disease
Systemic inflammatory disease (connective tissue/arthritides)
Dislocation/subluxation (traumatic, voluntary, transient)
Infection
Dysplasias
Neoplasia
    (osteoma, osteochondroma, chondroma, chondroblastoma, fibromyxoma, giant cell granuloma, chondrosarcoma, fibrosarcoma, osteosarcoma, and, rarely, metastatic lesions)
Masticatory muscles and tendons
Anomalous development
    (hypoplasia, hypertrophy)
Injury
    (avulsion, crushing, laceration, contusion, hematoma)
Inflammation
    (myositis, tendinitis, collagen vascular disease, spondyloarthropathies, myofascial pain disorders, masticatory muscle spasm)
Atrophy (denervation/disuse)
Fibrosis/contracture
Metabolic disease
Infection
Dysplasias
Neoplasia
Fibromyalgia

(Adopted and modified, with permission, from Meyers RA, Schellhas KP, Hall HD, et al: Guidelines for diagnosis and management of disorders involving the temporomandibular joint and related musculoskeletal structures. American Society of Temporomandibular Joint Surgeons. *Northwest Dent* 71:21-27, 1992. [Approved by the American Society of Temporomandibular Surgeons, February 1992].)

deformation (bony erosions, osteophyte formation, bony sclerosis, loss in vertical dimension). Myositis ossificans can cause diffuse regional pain, tenderness, muscular calcification, and secondary TMJ dysfunction. Spondyloarthropathy and lupus can present with TMD complaints.

Congenital and developmental abnormalities of the TMJ include condylar agenesis, condylar hypoplasia, condylar hypertrophy/hyperplasia, hemifacial hypertrophy, bifid condyle, coronoid impingement, Pierre Robin and Treacher Collins syndromes, benign hypermobile joint syndrome, and connective tissue disorders (Ehlers-Danlos syndrome). TMJ hypoplasia and hypertrophy are the most common developmental defects.[23-24] Condylar agenesis may be idiopathic or the result of radiation exposure during early condylar development. Condylar hyperplasia occurs in hyperpituitarism and in acromegaly. Both hypoplasia and hyperplasia of the condyles are characterized by an asymmetic dimensional defect. The unilateral developmental problem of condylar asymmetry is more common than bilateral abnormal growth. However, abnormal progressive mandibular asymmetry, malocclusion, and mandibular dysfunction characterize both unilateral and bilateral developmental TMJ defects. Benign hypermobile joint syndrome and connective tissue disorders (such as Ehlers-Danlos syndrome) involve laxity and hyperextension of the TMJ that predispose the patient to recurrent joint subluxation or dislocation.[25]

Primary neoplasms of the TMJ are rare, although osteochondroma, chondroma, chondroblastoma, fibromyxoma, and giant cell granuloma have been reported. Osteoma is the most common benign TMJ tumor.[26] The TMJ can be invaded by tumors from adjacent anatomical structures and metastatic neoplasms. In 1990, Bavits and Chewning[27] reported that many patients with neoplastic diseases have symptoms of TMD such as swelling, trismus, auditory changes, paresis or paresthesia, and dental occlusal changes. These diseases include schwannoma, multiple myeloma, fibrous histocytoma, squamous cell carcinoma, synovial cell sarcoma, adenocystic carcinoma, hypophyseal carcinoma, transitional cell carcinoma, synovial fibrosarcoma, metastatic breast and lung lesions, chondrosarcoma of TMJ, adenoid cystic carcinoma, prostatic adenocarcinoma, mucoepidermoid carcinoma, metastatic adenocarcinoma, undifferentiated carcinoma, intracranial metastatic melanoma, and nasopharyngeal and oropharyngeal carcinoma.

Psychosocial etiologies associated with physical symptoms and signs of TMD involve interactions between emotional stress, TMJ functional stress, and the subsequent TMJ/mandibular anatomical defects. Emotional stress is often associated with functional stress in the form of bruxism in many TMD patients. The average clenched jaw generates up to 280 psi of pressure, whereas a TMD patient with bruxism can generate up to 6 times the masticatory force of nonbruxers.[14] This force then contributes to accelerated deterioration of normal TMJ anatomy (eg, joint inflammation, disk perforation, condylar change during remodelling, and subsequent joint adhesion development).

Finally, it is important to note that there are many other conditions that may mimic clinical signs and symptoms of TMD. Laskin[28] reported that conditions such as dental pulpitis, pericoronitis, otitis media, parotitis, maxillary sinusitis, trigeminal neuralgia, atypical (vascular) neuralgia, temporal arteritis, Trotter's syndrome, and Eagle's syndrome, can mimic pain originating from TMJ or the muscles of mastication. Additional conditions—such as myositis, scleroderma, hysteria, myositis ossificans, chronic odontogenic and nonodontogenic infections, extrapyramidal reactions with use of medications such as phenothiazines, depressed zygomatic arch, fractures and hypertrophy of the coronoid process—may result in mandibular dysfunction.

EVALUATION AND DIFFERENTIAL DIAGNOSIS

Arriving at a correct differential diagnosis of TMD patients can be difficult because of the multifactorial nature of the etiologies. Successful treatment of TMD depends on the accurate evaluation of clinical presenting signs and symptoms and arrival at a correct diagnosis. The latter can be achieved by good history taking and physical examination, along with judicious use of laboratory and imaging studies.

HISTORY

A description of TMD pain based on its onset, location, quality, intensity, duration, referral pattern, exacerbating factors, accompanying symptoms and signs, and previous medical and surgical therapy are essential. Particular attention should be paid to general health, systemic diseases, neurologic/chronic pain disorders, psychosocial problems, traumatic injuries, and a history of benign or malignant neoplasm. The influence of TMD pain on quality of life and nutrition status is important. The patient interview and patient self-report using questionnaires and assessment instruments (visual analog scales, head and neck diagram marking) can be effectively used.

PHYSICAL EXAMINATION

The physical examination should include evaluation of the patient's general appearance, the TMJ, muscles of mastication and other muscles of the head and neck region, the dental occlusion, and a comprehensive head and neck examination. Careful observation of general appearance can indicate problems with mandibular posturing, head and neck posturing, parafunctional habits, facial symmetry, systemic conditions (eg, degenerative joint disease [DJD], collagen vascular diseases, and benign hypermobile joint syndrome), and the patient's level of distress. The TMJ examination begins with assessing the active and passive range of motion of the mandible, deviation of mandibular midline on function, and coexisting pain and joint noises. TMJ and external auditory meatus palpation for pain, tenderness, joint swelling, clicking, popping, and crepitus may reveal intracapsular joint problems. The muscles of mastication should be palpated for tenderness, spasm, trismus, and hypertrophy. Palpation of head and neck muscles may reveal trigger points for myofascial disorders. Dental examination may reveal malocclusion or edentulism, parafunctional habits (eg, wear facets), and sources of referred dental pain. Comprehensive head and neck examination including the sinuses, salivary glands, lymph nodes and cranial nerves is important.

LABORATORY STUDIES

No ideal scheme for ordering laboratory studies during diagnostic workup of TMD exists. Laboratory studies are indicated based on the patient's chief complaint, symptoms and signs, and the index of suspicion for a particular definitive diagnosis. For example, adjunctive laboratory studies may include complete blood cell count with differential, erythrocyte sedimentation rate, rheumatoid factors, various immune factors (eg, antinuclear antibody), C-reactive protein, uric acid, biopsies and electrophysiological studies. Laboratory studies can be helpful in differentiating disorders associated with TMD, such as gout, pseudogout, septic joint, Reiter's syndrome, scleroderma, psoriatic arthritis, osteoarthritis, sickle cell anemia, ankylosing spondylitis, neuromuscular disorders, polyarteritis nodosa, systemic lupus erythematosus, and adult and juvenile rheumatoid arthritis.

IMAGING STUDIES

Although the significance of imaging studies is often overlooked, diagnostic imaging can aid in accurate assessment of joint status, and is of high importance in differentiating various intracapsular and extracapsular TMDs. No study is ideal, and different modalities are indicated depending on clinical presentations. Each TMD may be associated with specific anatomical changes shown on baseline and follow-up imaging studies. Plain skull film series (posterior-anterior, lateral, Waters, open mouth Towne's views), panoramic views, arthrograms, CT scans, MRI, and nuclear bone scans may be beneficial. The studies most commonly used for diagnosis are panoramic views as screening studies, and MRI for further soft tissue resolution. Bone pathology involving significant condylar and temporal bone erosion, flattening of the condyle ("bird beak deformity"), overly steep articular eminence, condylar hyperplasia and hypoplasia, osteophyte formation, and narrowing of joint space is best detected in plain films and CT. Characteristic radiographic changes are associated with rheumatoid arthritis, osteoarthritis, acute and chronic traumatic injuries, congenital abnormalities, and neoplasms. Internal derangement such as disk perforation or anterior displacement can be demonstrated with arthrograms and MRI. However, because of the potential risks of infection, allergic reaction to contrast, pain of the procedure, and the superiority of MRI, arthrograms are rarely used today. MRI has progressively become more popular because of its superior soft tissue resolution (for disk thickness, position, pathology, perforation), absence of radiation exposure, and availability. Myofascial pain disorders limited to muscular dysfunction do not show typical radiographic characteristics. Occasionally bone scans may be indicated. Serial bone scans using technetium 99m–labeled diphosphonates can indicate when overly active osteoblastic activity at the condyle is "burned out," thus determining the optimum time for TMJ surgical intervention to correct condylar hyperplasia and asymmetry. Both developmental and neoplastic condylar hyperplasia cause facial asymmetry, but may be distinguished from each other by scintigraphy using gallium citrate.[29]

TREATMENT APPROACHES

The goals of TMD treatments are to reduce functional stress to TMJ and muscles, provide pain management, and optimize range of motion. It is extremely important that a definitive diagnosis be made since each etiology requires different treatment. Most important, not all TMD patients require treatment; and patient education and reassurance may be sufficient. Surgical disease necessitates surgical treatment; however, most patients with TMD require noninvasive reversible treatment.

MEDICAL AND NONSURGICAL TREATMENTS

The initial approach to the management of nonsurgical disorder should begin with medical treatment, consisting of patient education, mechanical soft diet, occlusal appliances (splint therapy), pharmacotherapy, physical therapy, and psychological and behavioral therapies. Two main treatments are used for myofascial pain dysfunction: mechanical soft diet and splint therapy. The mechanical soft diet regimen eliminates all foods with hard or fibrous consistency, and occasionally requires the use of liquid or pureed diet. Additional rest to the TMJ is achieved by minimizing talking and eliminating some everyday habits (eg, chewing gum). Occlusal splints of various designs are also commonly used to help patients guide their jaw posturing, become aware of parafunctional habits, and eliminate occlusal trauma. The use of soft diet and splint therapy are generally tried for a minimum duration of 2 weeks.

Pain management of TMD can generally be achieved by pharmacotherapy, which includes discrete use of four types of medications depending on the etiology: nonsteroidal anti-inflammatory drugs (NSAIDs), narcotics, muscle relaxants, and antidepressants. Acetaminophen and other miscellaneous medications may also be used occasionally. Different medications used for TMD pain management are listed in Box 2. Initial use of NSAIDs has the advantage of anti-inflammatory effects, satisfactory pain relief, and absence of potentially serious side effects. The disadvantages include potential gastrointestinal upset and antiplatelet properties. New pharmacologic agents (eg, celecoxib and rofecoxib) minimize such complications. The benefit of NSAIDs occurs with continuous dose regimen for approximately 2 weeks rather than on an as-needed schedule. Narcotic medications are indicated for TMD pain of high intensity and acute nature. Muscle relaxants are indicated for myogenic hyperactivity and spasms contributing to TMD symptoms. The side effects of respiratory depression, sedation, and addiction can arise; thus, the use of muscle relaxants should be limited to short-term treatment of myogenic symptoms. Low-dose antidepressants are often indicated for TMD patients with chronic neurogenic TMD pain and parafunctional habits (ie, nocturnal bruxism).

In TMD patients with limited jaw opening (TMJ and soft tissue fibrosis), or myogenic pain and tension, physical therapy may be helpful. Physical therapy includes jaw exercise by active and passive range of motion, the use of hot or cold compresses, and muscle relaxation by massage. Although the mechanism is not well understood, use of hot or cold compresses and massage often

---

BOX 2.
Example of Medications Available That May Be Helpful in Managing
TMD Pain

NSAIDs
  Aspirin, celecoxib, diclofenac, diflunisal, etodolac, flurbiprofen,
  ibuprofen, indomethacin, ketoprofen, ketorolac, nabumetone,
  naproxen, oxaprozin, piroxicam, rofecoxib, salsalate, trilisate, other
NSAID analgesic combination drugs
Acetaminophen and its combination drugs
Tramadol
Steroids
  Betamethasone, cortisone, dexamethasone, hydrocortisone, methyl
  prednisolone, prednisolone, prednisone, triamcinolone
Narcotics
  Codeine, hydromorphone, meperidine, morphine sulfate, oxy-
  codone, propoxyphene, other narcotic analgesic combination drugs
Muscle Relaxants
  Baclofen, carisoprodol, cyclobenzaprine, dantrolene, diazepam,
  metaxalone, methocarbamol, orphenadrine, tizanidine
Antidepressants
  Amitriptyline, desipramine, doxepin, imipramine, nortriptyline,
  fluoxetine

---

yields subjective symptomatic improvements. Use of finger pressures, jaw exercise devices (eg, Therabite [Therabite Corporation,
Newtown Square, Pa]), or stacking wooden tongue blades between
the maxillary and mandibular dentition can aid passive range of
motion jaw exercise.

The clinical benefits of psychological and behavioral therapies
are gained by teaching patients psychological stress reduction
techniques and behavioral modification.[30-32] Often biofeedback is
used to teach muscle relaxation techniques. Treatment of clinical
depression, anxiety disorders, and other psychiatric problems
(conversion disorders, hypochondriasis) may be appropriate.

SURGICAL TREATMENTS

Patients for whom medical treatments fail, in conjunction with
clearly diagnosed pathology and anatomical abnormalities, may
benefit from surgical intervention. Different surgical procedures

have specific indications, and each procedure has limitations. The majority of patients with temporal, parietal, and frontal headaches, as well as preauricular and masticatory muscle pain and tenderness, are not surgical candidates. No surgical intervention is indicated for myofascial pain involving spasm and inflammatory processes in cervical musclatures. Patients with neuralgia or other neurologic pain may benefit from specific surgical procedures such as rhizotomy, gamma knife procedures, retromastoid craniotomy and microvascular decompression. Specific intracapsular and extracapsular TMJ disorders may be treated with TMJ arthroscopy/arthrocentesis, disk repositioning surgery for internal derangement, or arthroplasty with or without joint reconstruction. TMJ reconstruction with autogenous grafts and total joint replacement with an artificial prosthesis are occasionally employed, especially for severe anatomical abnormalities and ankylosis. Although still performed, diskectomy without replacement of interpositional disk material[33] and condylotomy are becoming less favored by TMJ surgeons. Alloplastic disk replacement is no longer performed because of a lack of acceptable disk replacement material.[34] Detailed goals, indications, standard of care, outcome assessment, and factors affecting risk and complications for each of the intracapsular and extracapsular TMJ surgical procedures are defined in a book (currently under revision) by the American Association of Oral and Maxillofacial Surgeons.[35]

Arthroscopy with arthrocentesis for treating certain types of internal derangement, hypomobility, hypermobility, and DJD is the least invasive procedure available that is both diagnostic and therapeutic. Arthroscopy enables the operator to visually evaluate intracapsular TMJ pathologies such as disk adhesion, disk perforation, fibrillation, synovitis, condylar roofing, and increased vascularity. Adhesion lysis by arthroscopy and lavage of inflammatory substances during arthrocentesis can yield good results in patients with TMJ closed lock caused by severe adhesion, or mandibular dysfunction caused by chronic joint pain and inflammation.[36—39]

Disk repositioning surgery (for internal derangement) is performed with the goal of restoring the normal intracapsular anatomic relationship of the condyle, disk, and the fossa. It is quite successful in restoring a good functional disk-condyle relationship, but is not successful in restoring a "normal" position. Arthrotomy, repair of the damaged disk, removal of redundant retrodiskal tissue, and plication are readily accomplished. Anterior disk displacement with or without reduction, disk perforation, or disk adhesion is best corrected by this procedure.

Arthroplasty with temporalis myofascial reconstruction or dermal grafting is indicated for ankylosis in which the temporalis myofascial flap or dermal graft serve as interpositional material to replace the severely damaged disk and maintain vertical dimension of mandible. These procedures are performed to prevent recurrence of bony ankylosis between the mandible and temporal bone. Temporalis myofascial flap is the most favored interpositional autogenous graft disk replacement.[40,41] However, interpositional disk replacement with autogenous grafts such as dermal graft and auricular cartilage remain as options.[42,43]

In cases of TMJ pathologies with severe destruction of joint structures, autogenous TMJ reconstruction[44] or artificial total joint replacement can be performed. The main goal of these procedures is to replace the irreparably damaged anatomical structures, thus relieving TMD pain and restoring mandibular function. Autogenous TMJ reconstruction and artificial total joint replacement is reserved for treating the most severe cases of DJD, TMJ ankylosis, postresection of neoplasm, posttraumatic joint deformity, multiply treated and failed joint procedures, and congenital abnormalities. Autogenous TMJ reconstruction is most often performed using costochondral bone grafts where the severe joint destruction is limited to the condyle and disk portion excluding the fossa. Artificial total joint replacement involves replacement of condyle and fossa as a whole unit. It is reserved for treating failed autogenous TMJ reconstruction cases, and for the same indications applied for autogenous TMJ reconstruction. Standard stock artificial total joint replacement systems (Christensen system) were used prior to 1976. However, custom-fit artificial total joint replacement systems (Christensen/Garret system, TMJ Concepts System) using three-dimensional CT models are now used.[45]

CONCLUSION

Basic scientific and clinical understanding of diagnostic and treatment approaches of TMD are still evolving. There is a great need for better and more accurate use of terminology, characterization of different TMD subtypes, understanding of pathogenesis, and development and application of treatment approaches. Improved and safer artificial disk and joint replacement materials are desirable, but care must be taken to assure long-term, well-designed laboratory and clinical trials. Better education of TMD patients and better understanding by health care providers may prove to be the best and the most significant preventive and conservative treatment values.

REFERENCES

1. *Management of Temporomandibular Disorders. National Institutes of Health Technology Assessment Conference Statement*, Apr 29-May 1, 1996; pp 1-33.
2. Chase DC, McCoy JM: Histologic staging of internal derangement of the temporomandibular joint, in Merril RG (ed): *Oral and Maxillofacial Surgery Clinics of North America: Disorders of the TMJ II: Arthrotomy*, volume 1:2. Philadelphia, WB Saunders, 1989, pp 249-259.
3. Laskin DM: Etiology of the pain-dysfunction syndrome. *JADA* 79:147, 1968.
4. McNeil C, Mohl ND, Rugh JD, et al: Temporomandibular disorders: Diagnosis, management, education and research. *JADA* 120:253, 1990.
5. Merril RG, ed: *Oral and Maxillofacial Surgery Clinics of North America: Disorders of the TMJ I: Arthroscopy*, vol 1:1. Philadelphia, WB Saunders, 1989.
6. Moses JJ, Sartoris D, Glass R, et al: The effect of arthroscopic surgical lysis and lavage of the superior joint space on TMJ disc position and mobility. *J Oral Maxillofac Surg* 47:674, 1989.
7. Murakami K-I, Matsuki M, Iizuak T, et al: Diagnostic arthroscopy of the TMJ: Differential diagnosis in patients with limited jaw opening. *J Craniomand Pract* 4:117, 1986.
8. Quinn JH, Bazan NG: Identification of prostaglandins E2 and leukotriene B4 in the synovial fluid of painful, dysfunctional temporomandibular joints. *J Oral Maxillofac Surg* 48:1029, 1990.
9. Scapino RP: Histopathology associated with malpositions of the human temporomandibular joint disc. *Oral Surg Oral Med Oral Path* 55:382, 1983.
10. Scellhas KP: Internal derangement of the temporomandibular joint: Radiologic staging with clinical, surgical and pathologic correlation. *Magn Reson Imaging* 7(5):495, 1989.
11. Westesson PL, Rohlin M: Internal derangement related to osteoarthrosis in temporomandibular autopsy specimens. *Oral Surg Oral Med Oral Pathol* 57:17, 1984.
12. Wilkes CH: Internal derangements of the temporomandibular joint: pathologic variations. *Arch Otolaryngol Head Neck Surg* 115:469, 1989.
13. Dolwick MF: Diagnosis and etiology, in Helms CA, Katzberg RW, Dolwick MF (eds): *Internal Derangements of the Temporomandibular Joint*. San Francisco, University of California Press, 1983.
14. Bell WE: Normal craniomandibular function, in Bell WE (ed): *Temporomandibular Disorders: Classification, diagnosis and management*, 3rd ed. Chicago, Year Book Medical Publishers, 1990, pp 1-395.
15. DuBrul EL: *Sicher's Oral Anatomy*, ed 7. St. Louis, CV Mosby, 1980, pp 146-161; 174-209.
16. Kubota E, Imamura H, Kubota T, et al: Interleukin-1 beta and stromelysin (MMP3) activity of synovial fluid as possible markers of

osteoarthritis in the temporomandibular joint. *J Oral Maxillofac Surg* 55:20, 1997.

17. Fu K, Ma X, Zhang Z, et al: Interleukin-6 in synovial fluid and HLA-DR expression in synovium from patients with temporomandibular disorders. *J Orofacial Pain* 9:131-137, 1995.

18. Schafer DM, Assael L, White LB, et al: Tumor necrosis factor-alpha as a biochemical marker of pain and outcome in temporomandibular joints with internal derangements. *J Oral Maxillofac Surg* 52:786, 1994.

19. Kinney RK, Gatchel RJ, Ellis E, et al: Major psychologic disorders in TMD patients: Implications for successful management. *JADA* 123: 49-54, 1992.

20. Bush FM, Dolwick MF: Epidemiology, in Bush FM, Dolwick MF (eds): *The temporomandibular joint and related orofacial disorders.* Philadelphia, JB Lippincott, 1995, pp 131-222.

21. Helms CA, Katzberg R, Dolwick MF: *Internal Derangement of the Temporomandibular Joint.* San Francisco, Radiology Research and Education Foundation, 1983.

22. Leighty SM, Spach DH, Myall RW, et al: Septic arthritis of the temporomandibular joint: Review of literature and report of two cases in children. *Int J Oral Maxillofac Surg* 22:292, 1993.

23. Becker MH, Coccaro PJ, Converse JM: Antegonial notching of the mandible: An often overlooked mandibular deformity in congenital and acquired disorders. *Radiology* 121:149-151, 1976.

24. Blaschke DP: The temporomandibular joint, in Bergeron RT (ed): *Head and Neck Imaging Excluding the Brain.* St Louis, CV Mosby, 1984, p 251.

25. Ochs MW, Dolwick MF: Condylar injuries and their sequelae, in Zarb GA, et al (eds): *Temporomandibular Joint and Masticatory Muscle Disorders.* Copenhagen, Mosby, Munksgaard, 1994.

26. Keith D: *Surgery of the TMJ.* Boston, Blackwell Scientific, 1988, p 246.

27. Bavitz J, Chewning LC: Malignant disease as temporomandibular joint dysfunction: Review of the literature and report of case. *JADA* 1990:120:163.

28. Laskin DM: *Diagnosis and etiology of myofascial pain and dysfunction*, vol 7. Oral and Maxillofacial Surgery Clinics of North America, 1995, pp 3-78.

29. Benson BW, Otis LL: *Disorders of the Temporomandibular Joint. The Clinical Approach to Radiologic Diagnosis*, vol 38. Dental Clinics of North America, 1994, pp 167-185.

30. LeResche L, Massoth DL: Psychologic aspects of treating myofascial pain and dysfunction, in Laskin DM (ed): *Oral and Maxillofacial Surgery Clinics of North America: Medical Management of Temporomandibular Disorders*, vol 7. Philadelphia, WB Saunders, 1995, pp 113-127.

31. Gale EN: Biofeedback and relaxation therapy for the treatment of myofascial pain and dysfunction, in Laskin DM (ed): *Oral and Maxillofacial Surgery Clinics of North America: Medical Management of Temporomandibular Disorders*. Philadelphia, WB Saunders, 1995, pp 107-112.

32. Scott D, Gregg J: Myofascial pain of the temporomandibular joint: A review of the behavioral relaxation therapies. *Pain* 9:231, 1980.

33. Eriksson L, Westesson P: The need for disc replacement after discectomy, in Laskin DM (ed): *Oral and Maxillofacial Surgery Clinics of North America: Current Controversies in Surgery for Internal Derangement of the Temporomandibular Joint*, vol 6. Philadelphia, WB Saunders, 1994, pp 295-305.

34. Ryan DE: Alloplastic disc replacement, in Laskin DM (ed): *Oral and Maxillofacial Surgery Clinics of North America: Current Controversies in Surgery for Internal Derangements of the Temporomandibular Joint*, vol 6. Philadelphia, WB Saunders, 1994.

35. Helfrick JF, Kelly JF, Carberry A (eds): *Parameters of Care for Oral and Maxillofacial Surgery*. American Association of Oral and Maxillofacial Surgeons, 1995.

36. Murakami KI, Matsuki M, Iizuka T, et al: Recapturing the persistent anterior displaced disk by mandibular manipulation after pumping and hydraulic pressure to the upper joint cavity of the temporomandibular joint. *Journal of Craniomandibular Practice* 5:18, 1987.

37. Sanders B: Arthroscopic surgery of the temporomandibular joint: Treatment of internal derangement with persistent closed lock. *Oral Surg* 62:361, 1986.

38. Sanders B, Buoncristiani R: Diagnostic and surgical arthroscopy of the temporomandibular joint: Clinical experience with 137 procedures over a 2-year period. *J Craniomandib Disord* 1:202, 1987.

39. Nitzan DW, Dolwick MF, Martinez GA: Temporomandibular joint arthrocentesis: A simplified treatment for severe limited mouth opening. *J Oral Maxillofac Surg* 48:1163, 1991.

40. Albert TW, Merrill RG: Temporalis myofascial flap for reconstruction of the temporomandibular joint, in Merril G(ed): *Oral and Maxillofacial Surgery Clinics of North America: Disorders of TMJ II: Arthrotomy*, vol 1:2. Philadelphia, WB Saunders, 1989, 341-349.

41. Feinberg SE: Use of composite temporalis muscle flaps for disc replacement, in Laskin DM (ed): *Oral and Maxillofacial Surgery Clinics of North America: Current Controversies in Surgery for Internal Derangements of the Temporomandibular Joint*, vol 6:2. Philadelphia, WB Saunders, 1994.

42. Tucker MR: Use of autogenous dermal grafts in treating internal derangements of the temporomandibular joint, in Laskin DM (ed): *Oral and Maxillofacial Surgery Clinics of North America: Current Controversies in Surgery for Internal Derangements of the Temporomandibular Joint*, vol 6. Philadelphia, WB Saunders, 1994.

43. Waite PD, Matukas VJ: Use of auricular cartilage as a disc replacement, in Laskin DM (ed): *Oral and Maxillofacial Surgery Clinics of North America: Current Controversies in Surgery for Internal Derangements of the Temporomandibular Joint*, vol 6. Philadelphia, WB Saunders, 1994.

44. MacIntosh RB: Costochondral and dermal grafts in temporomandibular joint reconstruction, in Merril RG (ed): *Oral and Maxillofacial Clinics of North America: Disorders of the TMJ II: Arthrotomy*, vol 1:2. Philadelphia, WB Saunders, 1989.

45. Mercuri LG: Considering Total Temporomandibular Joint Replacement. *J Craniomandibular Practice* 17(1):44-48, Jan 1999.

46. Meyers RA, Schelhas KP, Hall HD, et al: Guidelines for diagnosis and management of disorders involving the temporomandibular joint and related musculoskeletal structures. *Northwest Dent* 71(5):24, 1992. (Approved by the American Society of Temporomandibular Joint Surgeons in February, 1992.)

CHAPTER 7

Stereotactic Advances in Otolaryngology–Head and Neck Surgery*

Michael J. O'Leary, MD
Clinical Assistant Professor, Uniformed Services University of the Health Sciences, and Chief of Neurotology/Skull Base Surgery, Naval Medical Center, San Diego, Calif

Perhaps the greatest influence for change over the last decade has been the application of computer technology to almost every area of human endeavor. In medicine, imaging advances with computerized tomography (CT), magnetic resonance imaging (MRI), and positron emission technology (PET) have markedly enhanced the accuracy of clinical diagnosis. The benefits of this technology have now extended to the operating room in the form of minimally invasive stereotactic surgery, which affords the surgeon precise anatomical image localization without the morbidities associated with broad, open exposures. Derived from the Greek *stereos,* which means "3-dimensional," and the Latin *tactic,* meaning "to touch," the term *stereotactic surgery* encompasses a wide variety of eponyms including image-guided surgery, neuronavigation, and computer-assisted surgery.

Although stereotactic devices have been around for more than a century, the recent coupling with computer technology has revolutionized the field, leading to a growing number of systems available for intraoperative guidance. This chapter examines the evolution of modern stereotaxis, followed by a review of the stereotactic principles integral to this new technology. We then divide the field in two, looking first at frame-based systems with a focus on stereotactic radiosurgery (SRS) and illustrated by case examples using the

---

*The views expressed in this chapter are those of the author and do not reflect the official policy or position of the Department of the Navy, Department of Defense, nor the US Government.

gamma knife. Newer, frameless stereotactic systems are then discussed, again with specific clinical illustrations. We conclude with a review of promising future developments likely to make stereotactic guidance a welcome addition to the surgical repertoire of every otolaryngologist and head and neck surgeon.

HISTORICAL DEVELOPMENTS

The earliest localization devices were developed, with the use of animals, more than a century ago to assist in neurophysiologic research. In 1873, Dittmar[1] introduced a mechanical device for instrument insertion in the rat medulla oblongata. The first human application was by the Russian surgeon D. N. Zernov[2] in 1889, using an arc-based "encephalometer" to drain a CNS abscess and localize a seizure focus.

In 1906, Sir Victor Horsley, a neurophysiologist and surgeon, joined Robert Henry Clarke, a mathematician, and applied a Cartesian coordinate system to their animal frame for the first, true "stereotactic" instrument.[3] Three perpendicular frame axes determined dimensions: the midsagittal plane, the axial plane through the orbital-meatus line, and the coronal plane through the external auditory meatus (Fig 1). Together, they also produced the first stereotactic atlas. Ironically, their partnership dissolved when Clarke pushed to extend the technique from monkeys to patients, and despite a subsequent patent for a human version of the device, their technique was never performed in humans. It was not until 30 years later that the accuracy improved enough to safely apply stereotactic techniques in human patients.

In 1936, Henry Wycis, a Temple University medical student, was prompted to pursue training in neurosurgery after working in the laboratory of neurologist Ernst Spiegel, a refugee from Nazi Germany. Wycis went on to join his mentor for a long and productive collaboration. Switching from external to intracranial landmarks, their technique incorporated x-ray image technology using pneumoencephalography, and later, iodine contrast ventriculograms matched to the first human stereotactic atlas, based on the cerebral ventricles.[4] Coupled with a greater understanding of the anatomy and neurophysiology produced by the interim stereotactic work in animals, their "stereoencephalotome" stimulated a myriad of interventions for movement disorders, epilepsy, intractable pain, and psychiatric diseases—a field now known as functional stereotactic surgery.[5-7]

Enthusiasm for these procedures waned with the introduction of successful medical therapies for Parkinson's disease in the

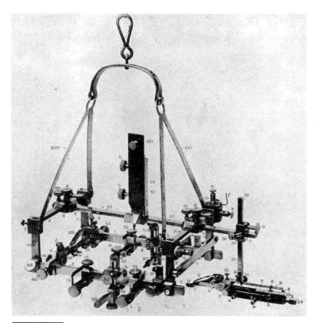

FIGURE 1.
Horsley and Clarke's stereotactic frame (1920).

1960s; however, the field was reinvigorated in the next decade by the application of CT to the guidance frames.[8] Computer workstations introduced the modern era by facilitating the move from frame-based to frameless stereotactic systems.

STEREOTACTIC PRINCIPLES

An understanding of fundamental stereotactic principles is useful before an evaluation of the features of any of the specific systems. The technological forces driving the rapid modern stereotactic advances are unprecedented. The mathematical concepts behind spatial Cartesian coordinates and the "registration" of two volumes to one another are inherent to all forms of stereotaxis.

TECHNOLOGY

In 1965, Gordon Moore, the cofounder of Intel Corporation, was preparing slides for a lecture when he noted that, up to that time, the number of transistors per microchip had doubled on a yearly basis since the invention of the integrated circuit years earlier. At this rate, he predicted computer power would increase exponentially over a brief time. Indeed, transistor density per chip has increased over the past quarter century more than 3200 times, from 2300 transistors on the 4004 chip to 7.5 million on the Pentium II processor (Fig 2). This observation, now known as Moore's Law, has held over the past 3 decades with predictions to continue through 2020. As a result, today's small stereotactic workstations can handle the complex equations required for real-time intraoperative localization, all with the power of yesterday's huge mainframe computers. Imaging systems have also improved rapidly, with the recent capability for "on-the-fly" instant conversion from CT to MRI images during surgery. Software innovations include the introduction of voice commands and the promise of surface recognition algorithms to make the process of "registering" image and anatomical space invisible to the surgeon. The exponential growth of the digital technology fueling these unique innovations is responsible for the rapid improvements that will likely make intraoperative stereotaxis commonplace in the near future.

CARTESIAN COORDINATES

Fundamental to all modern stereotactic systems is the ability to mathematically define a specific point in 3-dimensional (3-D)

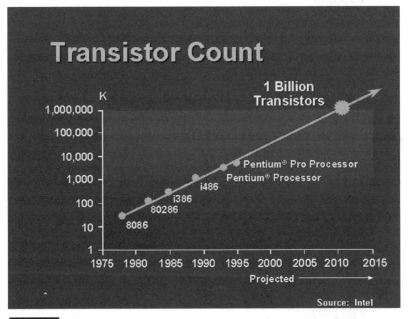

FIGURE 2.
Moore's Law graph depicting the exponential growth of computer power over the past 3 decades. (Reprinted by permission of Intel Corporation. Copyright Intel Corporation, 1996.)

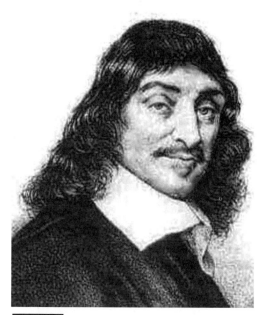

FIGURE 3.
Exploration of the mathematics of 3-D perception was by René Descartes.

space. The 17th century philosopher-scientist-mathematician René Descartes introduced the concept that two perpendicular lines can define any point in a plane (Fig 3). Similarly, coordinates on three perpendicular axes—conventionally labeled with "x," "y," and "z"—can uniquely identify points in a volume of 3-D space. From an anatomical and radiologic perspective, we are more familiar with these planes in terms of the vertical or axial view, anteroposterior (AP) or coronal view, and the lateral or sagittal plane.

As mentioned, linkage with CT images dramatically improved stereotactic precision. Early axial tomogram slices were 2-D planes composed of a collection of points, or *pixels,* which could be described by unique coordinates along the x- and y-axes (Fig 4). By using a geometric transformation, a series of individual slices were "stacked" to create a 3-D image volume in which each point, or *voxel,* is defined by three unique coordinates along the x-, y-, and z-axis. Specific volume targets and trajectories were calculated, and these formed the basis for most of the earlier, frame-based applications. Newer CT, MRI, and PET scanners obtain their images via volume acquisition, further reducing the time and error inherent in the "slice-stacking" transformation and opening the

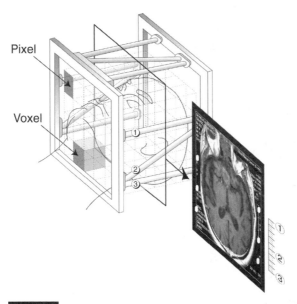

Pixel

Voxel

FIGURE 4.
Registration process: connecting image space with physical space.

possibilities for frameless stereotactic surgery. Portable workstations provide the intense processing power required by multiple
algebraic transformations, which allow rapid tracking of an array
of "anatomical localizers" within the entire volume.

Although the majority of stereotactic systems employ rectilin-
ear, Cartesian coordinates, there are other coordinate systems also
in use. Several popular frame-based systems employ an arc system, in which the target is always at the center of the arc and is
thus defined by a unique angle and distance. The Brown-Roberts-
Wells (BRW) and Leksell frames are examples of such arc-based, or
polar, coordinate systems. Regardless of the coordinates used, all
stereotactic systems require the accurate alignment of images and
anatomy through a process called registration.

REGISTRATION

In stereotactic surgery, the process of linking the volume of image
space to physical anatomical space is called registration. In framed
stereotactic systems, imaging is accomplished with a frame in place
to orient the slices in the volume. An "N-shaped" frame is commonly used, and the position of the diagonal rod is unique to each image
plane, indicating the correct slice depth in the image volume (Fig 4).

The frame is left in place or replaced exactly at the time of surgery for accurate registration—image volume linked to frame volume, frame to anatomy, thus image to anatomy. Although adequate for biopsy or radiosurgery, a head frame is clearly cumbersome for both the patient who must wear it and the surgeon who must operate around it. Frameless systems attempt to remove this impediment, while maintaining the precision characterized by frame-based systems.

Frameless stereotactic systems currently rely on three different methods for registration: external anatomical landmarks, prosthetic fiducials, and surface-mapping algorithms. External anatomical landmarks such as the nasion, the medial canthi, the external auditory canal, and specific interdental spaces have been used since the advent of stereotaxy, but these lead to inaccuracies outside the tolerances required by modern microsurgical procedures. The great leap in precision accompanying the introduction of Spiegel and Wycis's stereoencephalotome was founded on the switch from external to internal anatomical landmarks. Prosthetic external devices, known as *fiducials*, are visible by imaging techniques and offer a more discreet external point compared to the more diffuse anatomical landmarks. Radiopaque adhesive fiducials are noninvasive but can be accidentally moved during surgery or "drift" when left in place for hours or days between imaging and intervention. Implantable fiducials, such as titanium screws or markers, remain in place but require an invasive procedure and can also be inconvenient if considerable time transpires between the imaging and the intervention.

More recently, contour-matching software similar to that used in satellite mapping of the earth's surface has been adapted to mapping the facial skin contours unique to each individual. Sonic, magnetic, or video analysis of the physical surface is matched to computer analysis of the image surface.[9] Although the present accuracy of these systems is less than that of extrinsic fiducials, surface-mapping techniques hold the greatest potential for a rapid, noninvasive, and behind-the-scenes registration. Further developments in this area may expand the possibility of stereotaxis outside the confines of the head and neck with real-time continuous registration taking into account even the smallest intervening patient movements. Regardless of the method or the combination of methods used, once a number of unique points can be identified on both the image and the physical space, the remainder of the volumes can be precisely linked, or "registered." This process is central to all stereotactic systems, whether frame-based or frameless.

FRAME-BASED STEREOTACTIC SURGERY

Although the technology has advanced dramatically, Horsley and Clarke's basic concept of frame-based stereotaxis—external guidance to a specific intracranial target—has changed little. Current applications can be divided, according to pathology, into two main categories: treatment of functional neurologic disorders and the treatment of tumors. Following the introduction of powerful pharmaceutical agents such as L-dopa for Parkinson's disease in the 1960s, interest in functional stereotactic surgery waned. A recent resurgence has been based on several factors including:

- Improved understanding of the pathogenic mechanisms involved with various functional disorders
- Better "maps" of the neurophysiologic routes involved in various functional disorders, including advanced stereotactic atlases, data collected from intraoperative electrical stimulation, and newer physiologic targeting methods
- Increased precision in target localization as a result of improved scanning and stereotactic accuracy, combined with improved discrete lesioning modalities

The future impact of these improvements on chronic pain and movement disorders seen by otolaryngologists will be significant.

Although framed stereotactic biopsy of tumors and other intracranial lesions is common, the majority of the applications involve radiation therapy. In addition to traditional forms of external beam therapy, radiation therapy can be administered stereotactically in several ways. A variety of radionucleotides can be placed intracranially as interstitial implants similar to those used in the head and neck. Intracavitary injection using a stereotactic trajectory has also been performed. Stereotactic radiotherapy (SRT) is used to describe fractionated treatments to an intracranial target area under stereotactic guidance, usually performed over a series of days to weeks. This is in distinction to SRS, which is a single application of high-dosage radiation focused on a discreet target. The radiation sources used in SRS are commonly high-energy photons derived from either a linear accelerator (LINAC, Varian, Palo Alto, Calif) or from the cobalt 60 sources of a gamma knife unit. Less commonly, heavy charged particles created by a cyclotron can also be applied stereotactically (Table 1).

Linear accelerators are already in use at many hospitals where traditional radiation therapy is performed, and they can be adapted to framed stereotactic treatments. This economy of scale is unfortunately complicated by a lack of mechanical tolerances tight

TABLE 1.
Framed SRS Systems

System	Company	Technology	Software
LINAC	Varian, Palo Alto, Calif	Linear accelerator	X Knife
Gamma knife	Elekta, Atlanta, Ga	Cobalt 60	Gamma Plan
Charged particles	Varies by center	Cyclotron	Varies by center

enough to ensure the millimeter precision available in framed stereotactic systems. In addition, the cost and effort to recalibrate the LINAC unit each time it is adapted to framed stereotactic techniques is another major impediment to widespread adoption. Dedicated stereotactic LINAC systems have been developed to address these problems, but here the costs parallel those of a gamma knife center.

Cyclotron generators can produce "heavy" charged particles such as helium or hydrogen ions (protons)that can be also be delivered to a specific tumor target. These particles are characterized by maximal release of energy at the end of their beam in a phenomenon described as the Bragg Peak.[10] As a result, tissues along the beam path and beyond the release point have minimum radiation exposure. The great expense associated with the required cyclotron has restricted this technology to a limited number of research centers.

GAMMA KNIFE RADIOSURGERY

Lars Leksell was a Swedish pioneer in stereotactic surgery and is known as "the father of radiosurgery" for his development of the gamma knife in 1971. Previous attempts at mounting an orthovoltage collimator to his arc-based stereotactic frame were unsuccessful, as was a short collaboration with a radiation therapist using a cyclotron. His innovative concept of the gamma knife was to apply multiple cobalt 60 sources directed at a target at the center of the spherical frame through collimators that fixed the width of the beams. While concentrated at the target, the dosage decreases exponentially immediately outside the target area, sparing adjacent tissues. Intended by Leksell for use in functional stereotactic surgery, his first gamma knife case was actually treatment of a patient with a craniopharyngioma. Subsequently, the technique has been widely applied to benign tumors, including meningiomas, pituitary adenomas, and acoustic neuromas.

TECHNOLOGY AND RADIOBIOLOGY

A modern gamma knife unit (Elekta Instruments, Atlanta, Ga) has 201 cobalt 60 sources arranged in a large, shielded sphere. Sliding into the sphere is a precisely coupled external "helmet" with 201 matching collimators, 4, 8, 14, or 18 mm in size (Fig 5). The dose of radiation applied to the target reflects the size and number of open collimators, the age or decay of the cobalt sources, and the length of exposure time. Multiple "isocenters" (up to 28) can be applied to maximize the conformational fit for irregularly sized tumors such as some acoustic neuromas or skull base neoplasms. The Gamma Plan (Elekta Instruments) software and workstation perform the large number of calculations required to predict the isodose lines. These calculations become particularly intense when multiple shots are planned—combined with variable collimator sizes, age of the cobalt sources, etc.

The goal of radiosurgery is to apply a discrete, high dose of ionizing radiation to interfere with further tumor growth. Benign tumors do not share the radiosensitivity typical of rapidly growing malignancies, which have a therapeutic window optimized by traditional fractionated techniques. Instead, normal tissue sparing is accomplished through the exponential decrease in exposure out-

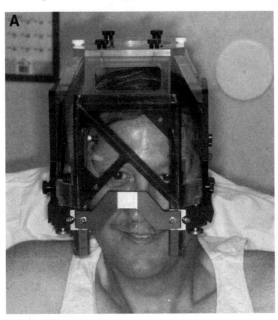

FIGURE 5.
Gamma knife radiosurgery. **A,** Head frame placed.

(continued)

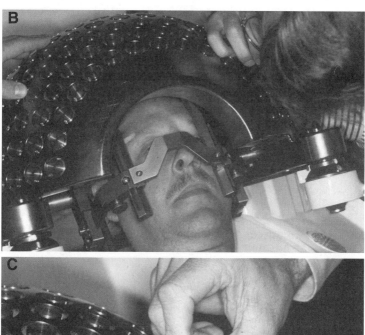

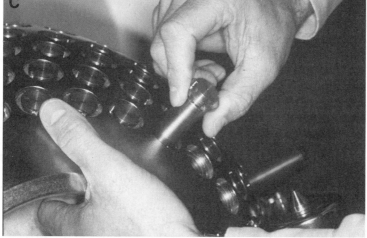

FIGURE 5. (continued)
B, Collimator helmet applied. **C,** Variable collimator port size.

(continued)

side the focal target. The dose is large enough within the target to interfere with the replication potential of cells that are not in the mitotic process at the time of exposure. Growth inhibition within the target, rather than cell death or necrosis, defines success.

TECHNIQUE
On the day of radiosurgery, a fiducial headframe is placed on the patient via pin fixation using local anesthesia, supplemented with

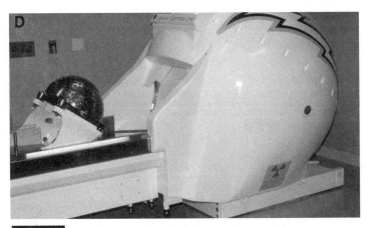

FIGURE 5. (continued)
D, Gamma knife unit.

an anticholinergic agent for vasovagal prophylaxis and intra-venous (IV) sedation. A high-resolution, volume acquisition MRI sequence with gadolinium is performed that provides 1-mm over-lapping slices. Physical verification of the fiducial distances con-firms the absence of significant magnetic field distortions, and the digital image is transferred over a rapid local area network to the gamma knife computer workstation.

The time for dose planning varies depending on the number of isocenters used to get the best conformation of the desired isodose line to the tumor margin. Because this correlates directly with the surrounding cranial nerve morbidity,[11] early tumor margin doses of 20 Gy have been reduced to the 14- to 16-Gy range and, in some small intracanalicular lesions and tumors larger than 2.5 cm, to 12 Gy. The surgeon "fits" the desired treatment level to the tumor margin on the computer workstation, the degree of conformity being very much dependent on the operator.

Before radiation is delivered, the measurements are double-checked by two physicians to reduce the potential for human error. The collimators for the first isocenter are placed, and beams that would travel through key structures, such as the optic nerve, are blocked. All personnel then leave the room and the patient is advanced into the unit with video and physiologic monitoring. Treatment time varies primarily by the age of the radiation sources but is usually on the order of 15 to 30 minutes. The patient is then removed from the unit and the process is repeated for each isocen-ter to be administered. On completion of the procedure, the head frame is removed and a dose of IV steroid is administered. The patient is observed for several hours but can usually be discharged the same day.

CASE REPORTS
Acoustic Neuroma

A 43-year-old man was referred with a 10-year history of right-sided hearing loss and intermittent tinnitus. There was a history of noise exposure (aircraft), but symptoms had progressed over the past year in a low-noise environment. The results of a physical examination were unremarkable, and an audiogram revealed uni-

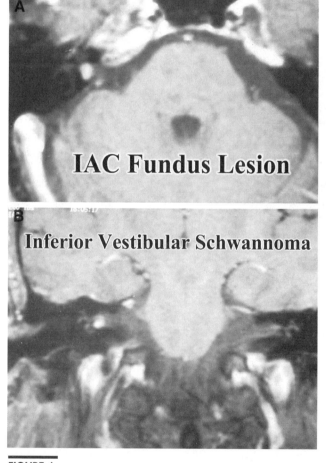

FIGURE 6.
Gamma knife case report 1: IAC acoustic neuroma. **A** and **B,** Lateral inferior IAC lesion.

(continued)

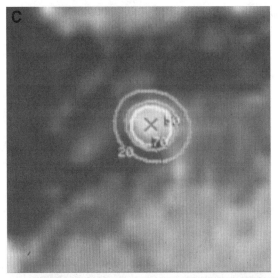

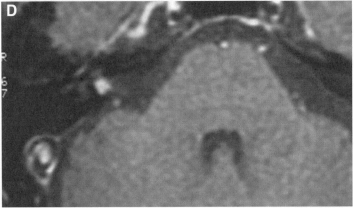

FIGURE 6. (continued)
C, Gamma plan with isodore lines. D, Lesion at 3.5 years after radio-surgery.

(continued)

lateral sensorineural hearing loss on the right side. Auditory brainstem responses were delayed on the right side, and MRI revealed a mass in the lateral inferior aspect of the right internal auditory canal (IAC) (Fig 6, A and B). Calorics were normal, supporting the likelihood of an inferior vestibular nerve schwannoma. After a thorough discussion of the available alternatives, including the various surgical approaches, observation, or radiosurgery, the patient opted for radiosurgery, despite counseling

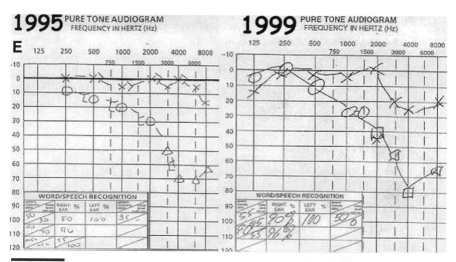

FIGURE 6. (continued)

E, Audiograms at presentation **(left)** and follow-up at 3.5 years **(right)**.

that surgical excision was the best selection in this healthy patient.

The patient underwent gamma knife radiosurgery treatment with one isocenter and 14 Gy to the tumor margin (Fig 6, C). He was released the same day. The patient tolerated the intervention without complications. Annual follow-up imaging at 3½ years reveals no tumor enlargement (Fig 6, D) and stable hearing (Fig 6, E).

Comments: Although this patient declined surgical excision, at present his results remain optimal. The lateral location at the fundus of the IAC makes surgical removal with hearing preservation by retrosigmoid approach more challenging, particularly if a direct view for complete tumor removal is desired. A "hearing preservation" middle cranial fossa approach, which was recommended, may have been theoretically more difficult due to the proximity of the inferior vestibular nerve tumor to the cochlear nerve and the need to repeatedly transit past the facial nerve while removing tumor. The question of tumor regression clearly cannot be answered, especially in light of the fact that a significant percentage of untreated small acoustic neuromas are observed to remain stable in size over time.[12] A critical feature of his ongoing management will be precise tumor size measurements[13] and further MRI scans to assess the intermediate and long-term results.

Recurrent Papillary Meningioma

A 24-year-old woman came in with a slowly enlarging right-side neck mass refractory to antimicrobial therapy for a presumed branchial cleft cyst. Fine-needle aspirate revealed "a low-grade carcinoma," and a CT scan demonstrated a jugular foramen mass extending into the neck. MRI confirmed the mass filling the right internal jugular vein from the thoracic inlet inferiorly (Fig 7, A) to the junction of the transverse and sigmoid sinuses superiorly (Fig 7, B). A CT-directed biopsy of the neck mass was used to diagnose

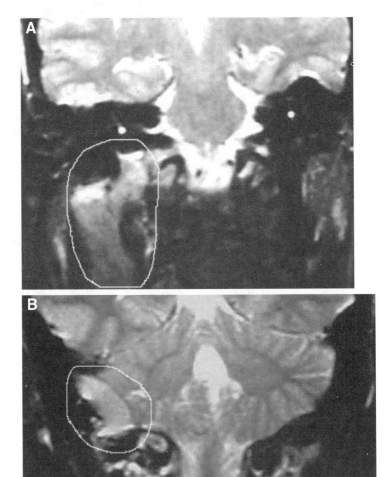

FIGURE 7.
Gamma knife case report 2: recurrent papillary meningioma. **A,** Preoperative MRI inferior extent. **B,** Preoperative MRI superior extent.

(continued)

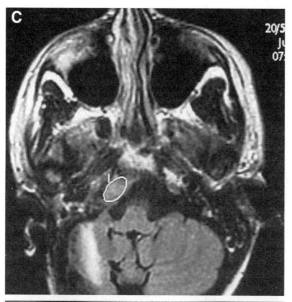

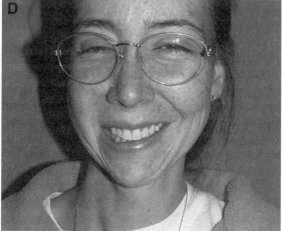

FIGURE 7. (continued)
C, Recurrent tumor. **D,** Patient 5 years postoperative, 1 year after gamma knife procedure.

papillary meningioma. The patient underwent excision of the mass by a far lateral transcondylar approach with modified radical neck dissection and postoperative external beam radiation therapy.

The patient recovered and exhibited no evidence of disease on annual imaging. After an episode of meningitis 3 years later, imaging revealed recurrence of the disease extending anteriorly in the region of the clivus (Fig 7, C). The volume of the lesion was calculated to be 3.82 mm^3. The patient opted for an attempt at tumor control with the gamma knife, chosen over surgical resection via a transcochlear approach. This was performed using a complex dose plan including 28 isocenters. The patient tolerated the extended treatment without complications. Five months after the gamma knife procedure, the patient developed trigeminal neuralgia, which responded to anti-inflammatory medications and resolved over a 3-week period. She has remained asymptomatic and is now 18 months out from her radiation (Fig 7, D).

Comments: This case illustrates the role radiosurgery plays as a potential adjunct in the treatment of skull base tumors. The prognosis remains grim based on the papillary variant classification of this meningioma, for which recurrence rates range as high as 80%.[14] Using multiple isocenters for treatment planning, the irregular contours of this skull base lesion were "fit" to the desired isodose lines. Previous fractionated radiotherapy required precise dose planning but did not preclude radiosurgery.

DISCUSSION

There are several problems that make the evaluation of gamma knife results rather complex in cases of benign tumors. Since the tumors persist, only long-term data can be used to determine the efficacy of treatment. On the other hand, the technology forces mentioned earlier have produced such rapid advances that the technique is often changed before it is possible to collect adequate long-term data. The transition from CT to MRI for dose planning, for example, had a dramatic impact on reduction of cranial nerve complications (including hearing loss). Extrapolating radiobiological research data suggesting that lower radiation levels may still cause tumor regression,[15] marginal doses have been reduced from 20 Gy to between 16 and 18 Gy, and now, even down to 12 Gy. Although this reduced marginal exposure has decreased the number of facial nerve morbidities, it does not insure maintenance of earlier, higher-dose tumor control rates. In many ways, we are trying to evaluate a moving target. A final critique is the paucity of controlled, long-term data, despite the growing number of institutions now providing SRS with gamma knife.

With the above caveats in mind, a group at the University of Pittsburgh recently published their results of 162 consecutive patients with acoustic neuroma, of which 149 had at least 5 years follow-up with imaging.[16] Tumor control was reported as 98%, with only four patients having increased growth requiring surgical salvage. Of interest, an additional five patients had growth demonstrated on imaging after 2 years, which then decreased in size during the subsequent years in a pattern consistent with postradiation edema versus bona fide tumor activity. Normal facial nerve function (House Brackmann Grade 1[17]) was preserved in 85% of patients who had normal function before receiving therapy. In the 20% of patients with serviceable hearing (Gardner Robertson Grade 1-2[18]), almost half retained grade 2 or better. These results compared well with most surgical series, particularly in the absence of any perioperative complications such as meningitis, wound infection, or cerebral spinal fluid leak.

The central issue for radiosurgery is whether early "control" of tumor growth will remain a long-term result. Despite the wording of the title ("Long-term outcomes...") in the recent Pittsburgh prospective series, the 5- to 10-year data of greatest interest is compromised by a lack of imaging in 52 of the 149 patients, half of which were lost to follow-up or refused imaging, and the other half of which simply weren't studied! In the 97 patients who were imaged more than 5 years after treatment, however, there were no cases of tumor enlargement. This is also consistent with the results reported by Noren et al,[19] which show an extremely low rate (estimated at 0.1%) of delayed tumor growth in patients who have been without growth over a 5-year period. Unfortunately, without greater efforts in the daunting task of true long-term follow-up in these patients, we may never adequately know the efficacy of the gamma knife in the treatment of acoustic neuroma.

It is critical to understand that radiosurgery cranial nerve morbidities are usually late, occurring 6 to 12 months after the intervention, and as such do not necessarily indicate disease progression. Similarly, half of the patients with measurable increases in tumor size at the 2-year follow-up imaging likely represent radiation side effects versus tumor growth. Controversy remains with regard to the difficulty of surgical salvage in these cases,[20] the theoretical risks of malignant transformation or secondary malignancies after radiation, and the vestibular consequences of persistent labyrinthine asymmetry.

Framed SRS is clearly a useful adjunct in the management of patients with benign intracranial tumors, particularly those who are at high rish for surgical complications. Others must consider weighing the perioperative microsurgery risks against tumor persistence and the need for repeated imaging when there is some uncertainty as to the long-term efficacy. As with the improved hearing preservation results noted on the switch from CT to MRI, further technological advances will only improve the contribution that framed SRS makes to the treatment of benign intracranial tumors.

FRAMELESS STEREOTACTIC SURGERY

A major paradigm shift occurred when advancing computer technology facilitated the intense calculations required to omit the stereotactic frame. Instead of focusing on a central target within a known volume, as occurs with the framed systems, the entire volume is the target in frameless stereotaxy. Instead of defining the physical location from image space, the surgical position is tracked in physical space and displayed in image space. Without frame restraints, the surgeon is free to navigate the anatomical region using real-time image feedback within tolerances under a few millimeters. The entire approach and peripheral anatomy are as available as the area of central pathology and, once the coordinates are registered, any number of instruments can be actively tracked. Although multiple systems abound, the type of 3-D localizing system can usually distinguish them from one another.

TECHNOLOGY

Localizing systems used in frameless stereotactic surgery are based on mechanical articulated arms or, more commonly, on a variety of wireless emitters (Table 2). Articulated arms are composed of multiple joints between linkages of known length. Mechanical potentiometers or optical encoders determine precise angles at each joint, which the computer uses to calculate the exact tip position. Much of this technology was extrapolated from the field of industrial robotics. Performance standards include *accuracy*—the measure of error in reaching any particular point—and *precision*—the repeatability of returning to a single point in the volume. The first commercially available device, the ISG Viewing Wand (ISG Tech, Mississauga, Ont), coupled an articulated arm device with CT or MRI images displayed in traditional axial, coronal, and sagittal views.[21,22] Mounted on the operating table, the mechanical arm consists of three joints, each with 2° of freedom. Joint angles created by placement of the arm tip in the operative field are sent to the computer workstation, which calculates the trigonometric transformation to produce the corresponding images. Being the first to market, the Wand has been applied to a large number of procedures with good results. Although it is definitely an ergonomic leap forward from the framed systems, the articulated arm has been largely eclipsed by a variety of frameless systems featuring freehand triangulating emitters.

TABLE 2.
Frameless Stereotactic Systems

Product	Company	Technology
InstaTrak	VTI, Cambridge, Mass	Electromagnetic
Magellan	Biosense, Israel	Electromagnetic
Regulus Navigator	Compass, Rochester, Minn	Electromagnetic
Easy Guide	Philips, Shelton, Conn	Optical
Optical Tracking System	Radionics, Burlington, Mass	Optical
PinPoint	Picker, Cleveland, Ohio	Optical
SMN	Carl Zeiss, Thornwood, NY	Optical
Stealth Station	Sofamor Danek, Memphis, Tenn	Optical
Vector Vision	BrainLAB, Heimstetten, Germany	Optical
Viewing Wand	ISG Tech, Mississauga, Ont	Optical

Triangulation involves at least three detectors in a rigid array forming the base of a pyramid, the tip of which is an emitter attached to the localizing device or instrument. Some detectors are unidirectional, requiring clear "line-of-sight" to the emitter, such as optical light emitting diodes, often in the infrared spectrum.[23] Since the instrument tips are blocked when inside the patient, a minimum of three infrared spectrums must be placed along the handle to allow triangulated calculation of the instrument's direction. Multidirectional localizers require fewer emitters, and include spark gap ultrasonic and electromagnetic systems.[24]

Electromagnetic systems use a transmitter to create three magnetic fields oriented in the x-, y-, and z-planes. The localizer instrument acts as an antenna whose position can be tracked in all three planes since field strength is inversely proportional to the cube of the radius distance between the transmitter and receiver. The accuracy and precision of the magnetic field system are in the 1- to 2-mm range which, combined with facility of use, make it an attractive adjunct to functional endoscopic sinus surgery and certain skull base procedures.

TECHNIQUE

The InstaTrak system (Visualization Technology Inc, Cambridge, Mass) can register images using external fiducials or a flexible headset fitted to the medial orbital rims and the external auditory canals for "autoregistration" (Fig 8). The device is worn during preoperative scanning and is then replaced after anesthesia induction in cases involving the sinuses. Embedded in the plastic headset are six magnetic fiducials; at surgery, calibration takes less than a minute. The films are fed to the computer workstation. In the operating room, sensors in the suction device and headset feed tracking information to the workstation. Images appear in the three primary planes, and a quarter of the screen is reserved for the endoscopic or microscopic image.

CASE REPORTS
Middle Cranial Fossa

A 48-year-old Air Force pilot was referred with a 10-month history of tinnitus and progressive right-side hearing loss confirmed on audiogram. MRI revealed a 1.5-cm intracanalicular tumor on the right side (Fig 9, A). After reviewing all the options, the patient elected to undergo surgical excision by means of a middle cranial fossa approach with stereotactic guidance. The stereotactic probe assisted in the craniotomy by localizing the level of the floor of the middle cranial fossa. The dura propia was then elevated sharply, and the probe accurately identified Kawase's triangle in the petrous apex along the petrous ridge (Fig 9, B). Drilling was initiated in this area, and the probe

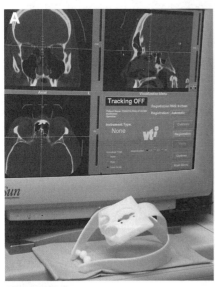
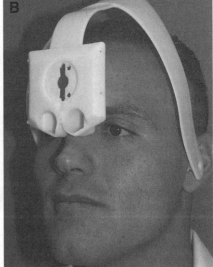

FIGURE 8.
A, Autoregistration headset with InstaTrak stereotactic system. B, Headset in place.

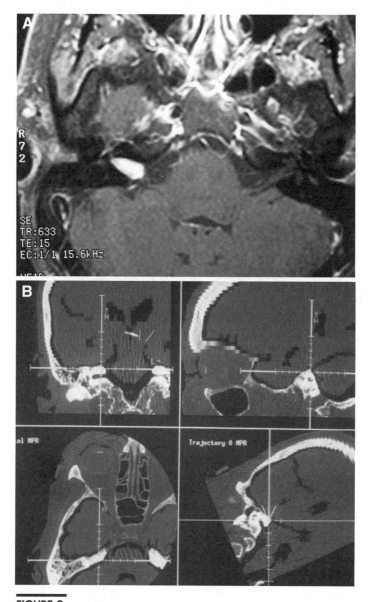

FIGURE 9.
Frameless stereotaxis case report 1: middle cranial fossa. **A,** IAC lesion.
B, Stereotactic view of the petrous apex.

(continued)

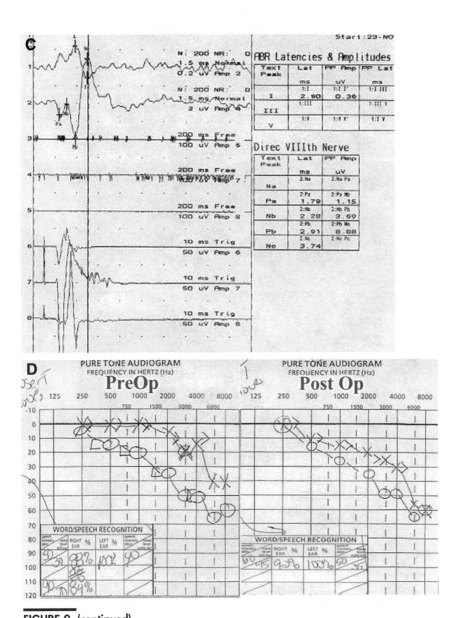

FIGURE 9. (continued)
C, Direct eighth nerve monitoring tracings throughout case. **D,** Preoperative **(left)** and postoperative **(right)** audiograms.

again was used to identify the IAC posteriorly. As the canal was unroofed, stereotaxy was used to help confirm the lateral extent of the canal. At this point, a platinum wire electrode was placed in the extradural space of the anterolateral bony IAC. A robust direct cochlear nerve potential was recorded throughout the case (Fig 9, C). The tumor was delicately removed under direct vision. The patient recovered without complication, and the postoperative audiogram showed preservation of his preoperative hearing thresholds (Fig 9, D). His facial nerve function remained a grade 1/6 postoperatively, and the patient returned to full duty.

Comments: Although it is not a prerequisite for this approach, use of the stereotactic probe enhanced the speed and accuracy with which the critical middle fossa landmarks were identified. The tolerances of current frameless stereotactic systems assist in navigation to large structures such as Kawase's triangle or the medial IAC but are of little use in the tight confines of the lateral IAC fundus. Here, traditional surgical landmarks such as the walls of the IAC provide the safest guidance to preserving the bony labyrinth.

Endoscopic Transphenoidal Surgery

During an evaluation for chronic migraine headaches, a 51-year-old woman was noted by MRI to have a 2-cm suprasellar mass that destroyed the dorsum sella, extended to the cavernous sinuses bilaterally, and lifted the optic chiasm and nerves bilaterally (Fig 10, A). The patient had multiple medical problems and was a Jehovah's Witness. An endocrine workup revealed an elevated serum prolactin level with normal adrenocorticotropic hormone and cortisol levels. After discussion of the available options, the patient elected to undergo surgical resection but declined to be transfused, a decision consistent with her religious beliefs. She agreed to enroll in a protocol for stereotactically guided endoscopic resection.

In the operating room (Fig 10, B and C), the sphenoid sinus was rapidly identified and confirmed by concomitant stereotactic localization. The inferior face of the sphenoid sinus was removed with a diamond drill upon stereotactic confirmation of locale (Fig 10, D). The posterior wall was identified and midline confirmed in the axial, coronal, and sagittal views. The posterior sphenoid sinus wall was penetrated without difficulty, and the tumor was debulked (Fig 10, E). Next, a 30° endoscope was placed within the capsule for further tumor removal. A clear identification of the

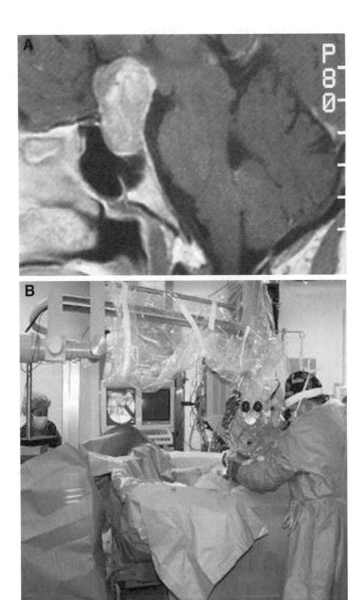

FIGURE 10.
Frameless stereotaxis case report 2: stereotactic endoscopic transsphenoidal surgery. **A,** MRI showing pituitary tumor. **B,** Traditional microsurgical approach: positioned for C-arm and microscope.

(continued)

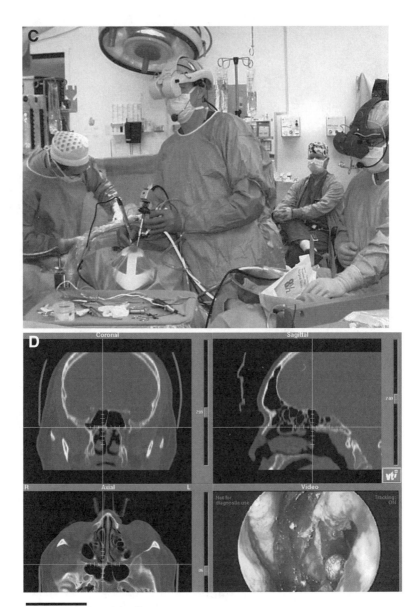

FIGURE 10. (continued)
C, Stereotactic endoscopic approach: no microscope, fluoroscope, or lead aprons. **D,** Head-mounted display view; drilling anterior wall of sphenoid sinus.

(continued)

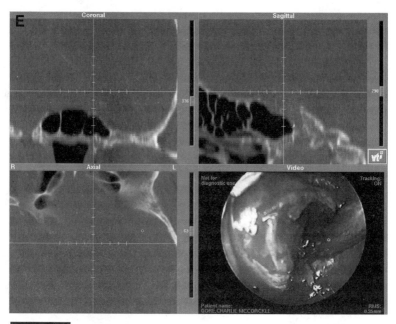

FIGURE 10. (continued)
E, Head-mounted display view; tumor removal.

optic chiasm and optic nerves were made, signaling adequate tumor removal. The sphenoid sinus was packed with autologous fascia, fat, and autologous platelet gel. Merocel (Merocel Corp, Mystic, Conn) packs were placed in the nostrils and removed at 6 hours without bleeding. Her postoperative course was unremarkable, and she noted a marked diminution of her "migraines" postoperatively.

Comments: This case best illustrates the enhancements offered by the stereotactic technology. From the patient's perspective, hemorrhage and dissection were markedly reduced by the direct approach compared with traditional sublabial or transnasal techniques. Accuracy and precision were improved by the three images offered in the stereotactic mode compared with the one lateral view provided by traditional fluoroscopy. Removal of the flouroscopy unit and the operating microscope further reduces operating time and, therefore, decreases costs. Tumor removal is improved by the addition of angled endoscopes within the tumor capsule once debulking has progressed satisfactorily. Finally, the elimination of prolonged nasal packing and mucosal flaps hastens and improves the recovery time. In the continually shrinking resources characterizing health care, only "enabling technologies" of this type can affordably be adopted.

DISCUSSION

Despite the benefits described in the widespread early use of the Viewing Wand,[25,26] it is somewhat bulky and unwieldy for delicate microsurgical procedures. Ultrasonic emitters are attractive conceptually but require further advances in the technology to literally "bring them up to speed" for the demands that moving instruments make on the longer time-of-flight sonic systems. Optical emitters offer a more rapid response but suffer from the requirement of direct visualization by the detectors, which requires multiple emitters attached to each instrument. Electromagnetic systems are susceptible to field artifact by large metal objects, but these were of little consequence, particularly when stationary (eg, operating table). A new crop of "hot" instruments, including powered sinus tools, can double as localizers. Perhaps the greatest feature of the magnetic system is the simple integration into surgery, adding the advantages of stereotactic guidance without increased time or complexity.

Although the current systems are useful in surgical procedures where inaccuracies up to several millimeters are tolerable, that clearly is not the situation in most ear surgery. Defining the IAC or Kawase's triangle is safer than relying on stereotaxy to find a semi-circular canal or facial nerve. To justify the expense of present systems, there must be a reduction in other costs accompanied by an improved patient outcome. The analogy of facial nerve monitoring holds here in many aspects. Originally intended as an adjunct in microsurgery for skull base tumors and acoustic neuromas, many otologists and otolaryngologists now use a facial nerve monitor routinely in chronic ear disease, rather than leaving it unplugged in the storage area. The frameless stereotactic system, procured because it reduced operating time and morbidity while removing the need for a microscope and fluoroscope in transphenoidal surgery, may be well deployed on a different day for a case of revision functional endoscopic sinus surgery. In the digital world, costs drop as the technology matures, and it is not too far-fetched to consider stereotactic systems evolving to become an integral part of many of our standard operations, performed to our patient's benefit with endoscopes through minimally invasive portals. With drill bits acting as localizers and coupled to intraoperative physiologic monitoring, we may eventually see systems beneficial even to the microsurgical domain of otology.

FUTURE STEREOTACTIC DEVELOPMENTS

The key design goals for future stereotactic systems include:

- Increased accuracy and precision below the 1-mm threshold
- Improved ergonomics
- Seamless integration into the operating room environment
- Reduced cost of ownership

Predicting the future in a field where the power doubles on an annual basis opens up the possibility for the most creative imaginations looking 20 years ahead. Instead, a 5- to 10-year view is more realistic, with many of the developments to be discussed already selectively deployed or in the advanced testing phases.

HARDWARE

Improved scanning techniques will greatly enrich the stereotactic environment. MR spectroscopy and angiography are in the early phases of development and hold great potential. PET scanners, using a variety of tissue-specific radioisotopes, offer a pathophysiologic correlate to the specific anatomical areas identified by more traditional imaging techniques. Functional stereotactic brain maps open up an array of new surgical approaches and may augment intraoperative physiologic measures for the accurate placement of various neural prostheses, such as the auditory brainstem implant. Beyond navigation, the integration of PET scan data may offer dramatic improvements in both SRS and functional stereotactic surgery. Whereas the original PET scan centers were determined by proximity to cyclotrons capable of generating the short-lived isotopes, new longer-lasting isotopes have made this technology available to many regional hospitals, greatly expanding the applications.

In addition to preoperative imaging techniques, many intraoperative technologies can be readily mapped to stereotactic coordinates and may be of assistance in updating the field as surgery is underway. Intraoperative ultrasound is perhaps the most promising, with significant 3-D rendering advances and several small contact probes for intraoperative use.[27] Doppler probes provide positional information on vascular structures. Additional information from nerve stimulators, evoked potentials, electromyography, and dye tracers can all be used to enhance the intraoperative localization of key structures.

Dedicated surgical CT scanners[28] and "open" MRI units[29] provide the ultimate real-time feedback throughout the procedure. Dramatic decreases in image access times and ongoing improvements in resolution have occurred since the introduction of this technology. At present, these systems are extremely costly, requiring an entire suite of specialized anesthetic and surgical equipment, and have many ergonomic constraints to be worked out.

Looking further down the road, advancing robotic technologies hold great promise. At least two microscope systems have been developed with active stereotactic robotics.[30,31] Safety issues have been addressed,[32] and industrial robotics adapted to the operating room have conducted successful human surgeries, but at present they remain ergonomically unacceptable because of their bulk.[33] Early robots may simply be added to a component of the surgery, such as a drill system designed to uncover the IAC once the petrous ridge has been identified. Ongoing support in this direction is a high priority for the Advanced Research Program Agency of the Department of Defense. Once developed, however, the entire field of remote robotic "telesurgery" opens up a host of intriguing possibilities.

SOFTWARE

The greatest future software advance lies in the maturation of surface-mapping registration techniques, which will expand stereotactic capabilities beyond the confines of the head. Extracranial stereotactic navigation can be readily applied to the endocrine aspects of head and neck surgery where excellent localizing technologies already exist. Image fusion technology is another software innovation that allows the simultaneous registration of multiple volumetric data sets. Currently, it is possible to switch rapidly between CT and MRI data sets, combining the bone window advantages of CT with the superior soft tissue resolution of MRI. In addition, the better spatial fidelity of CT can be used to correct for errors from magnetic field distortions. Future software will likely integrate multiple systems, including the intraoperative technologies discussed above.

Detailed stereotactic atlases are in development, accurately mapping intracranial routes in both anatomical and functional terms. Application of neural network style logic algorithms might be available to the surgeon at different points in the operation. Voice recognition software is already used in the accessories to stereotactic surgical guidance.

ACCESSORIES

Display technologies are emerging to manage the increase in information available to the stereotactic surgeon. We have been working with a Head Mounted Display (HMD) (Vista Medical

Technologies, Carlsbad, Calif), which provides a true stereoscopic image and multiple picture-in-picture displays similar to a computer screen (Fig 11). Voice recognition software allows the surgeon to control the type and location of images. Although the HMD can be used with any traditional microscope, its greatest utility comes when coupled to one of several new 3-D stereoendoscopes (Fig 12). Although the current VGA resolution is just below that of video monitors, it will soon reach SVGA resolution, which will likely be better than the most expensive 2-D monitors.

CONCLUSION

In summary, stereotactic systems have progressed beyond the research setting and into the operating room. Coupled with the digital technology "juggernaut," advances will rapidly influence many areas of medicine. Framed stereotactic systems open the door for noninvasive procedures through the precise application of radiation therapy. Frameless stereotactic surgery provides neural navigation with precision and accuracy within a few millimeters. Future stereotactic developments will allow the surgeon to

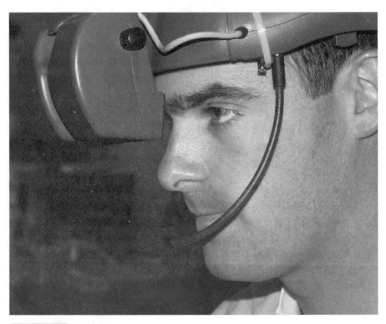

FIGURE 11.
Vista head-mounted display with voice controls.

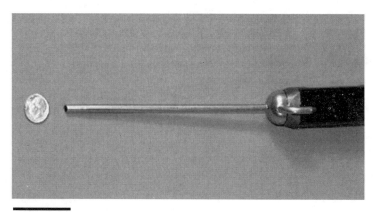

FIGURE 12.
Vista stereoendoscope.

accomplish even more, through a smaller view, to the patient's benefit.

ACKNOWLEDGMENTS
I acknowledge my neurosurgical colleagues Drs Mark E. Linskey and Catalano Dureza for their contributions in framed and frameless stereotaxy, respectively.

REFERENCES

1. Dittmar C: Ueber die lage des sogenannten gefaesszentrums in der medulla oblongata [German]. *Bersaechs Ges Wiss Leipzig (Math Phys).* 25:449-469, 1873.
2. Zernov DN: Encephalometer: A device for determination of the location of brain parts of living humans. *Proc Soc Physicomed Moscow Univ* 2:70-86, 1889.
3. Horsley V, Clarke RH: The structure and functions of the cerebellum examined by a new method. *Brain* 31:45-125, 1908.
4. Spiegel EA, Wycis HT, Marks M, et al: Stereotaxic apparatus for operations on the human brain. *Science* 106:349-350, 1947.
5. Spiegel EA, Wycis HT: Pallido-thalamotomy in chorea. *Arch Neurol Psychiatr* 64:495-496, 1950.
6. Spiegel EA, Wycis HT, Baird HW: Pallidotomy and pallidoamygdalotomy in certain types of convulsive disorders. *Arch Neurol* 80:714-728, 1958.
7. Spiegel EA, Wycis HT: Mesencephalotomy in the treatment of "intractable" facial pain. *Arch Neurol* 69:1-13, 1953.
8. Brown RA: A computerized tomography–computer graphics approach to stereotaxic localization. *J Neurosurg* 50:715-720, 1979.

9. Friets EM, Strohbehn JW, Roberts DW: Curvature-based nonfiducial registration for the frameless stereotactic operating microscope. *IEEE Trans Biomed Eng* 42:867-878, 1995.

10. Bragg WH, Kleeman RD: On the ionization curves of radium. *Philsoph Mag* 8:726-738, 1904.

11. Linskey ME, Flickinger JC, Lunsford D, et al: Cranial nerve length predicts the risk of delayed facial and trigeminal neuropathies after acoustic tumor stereotactic radiosurgery. *Int J Radiat Oncol Biol Phys* 27:397-401, 1993.

12. Bederson JB, von Ammon K, Wichmann WW, et al: Conservative treatment of patients with acoustic tumors. *Neurosurgery* 28:646-651, 1991.

13. Linskey ME, Lunsford LD, Flickinger JC: Neuroimaging of acoustic nerve sheath tumors after stereotaxic radiosurgery. *AJNR Am J Neuroradiol* 12:1165-1175, 1991.

14. Pasquier B, Gasnier F, Pasquier D, et al: Papillary meningioma: Clinicopathologic study of seven cases and review of the literature. *Cancer* 58:299-305, 1986.

15. Linskey ME, Martinez AJ, Kondziolka D, et al: The radiobiology of human acoustic schwannoma xenografts after stereotactic radiosurgery evaluated in the subrenal capsule of athymic mice. *J Neurosurg* 78:645-653, 1993.

16. Kondziolka D, Lunsford LD, McLaughlin MR, et al: Long-term outcomes after radiosurgery for acoustic neuromas. *N Engl J Med* 339:1426-1433, 1998.

17. House JW, Brackmann DE: Facial nerve grading system. *Otolaryngol Head Neck Surg* 93:146-147, 1985.

18. Gardner G, Robertson JH: Hearing preservation in unilateral acoustic neuroma surgery. *Ann Otol Rhinol Laryngol* 97:55-66, 1988.

19. Noren G, Hirsch A, Mosskin M: Long-term efficacy of gamma knife radiosurgery in vestibular schwannomas. *Acta Neurochir (Wien)* :122-164, 1993.

20. Slattery WE, Brackmann DE: Results of surgery following stereotactic irradiation for acoustic neuromas. *Am J Otol* 18:596-601, 1995.

21. Leggett W, Greenberg M, Gannon W: The viewing wand: A new system for three-dimensional CT correlated intraoperative localization. *Curr Surg* 48:674-678, 1991.

22. Zinreich S, Dekel D, Leggett B, et al: Three-dimensional CT interactive "Surgical Localizer" for endoscopic sinus surgery and neurosurgery. *Radiology* 177:217S, 1991.

23. Bucholz RD, Smith KR: A comparison of sonic digitizers versus light emitting diode-based localization, in Maciunas RJ (ed): *Interactive Image-Guided Neurosurgery*. Park Ridge, Ill, American Association of Neurosurgeons, 1993, pp 179-200.

24. Fried MP, Kleefield J, Gopal H, et al: Image-guided endoscopic surgery: Results of accuracy and performance in a multicenter clinical study using an electromagnetic tracking system. *Laryngoscope* 107:594-601, 1997.

25. Sipos EP, Tebo SA, Zinreich SJ, et al: In vivo accuracy testing and clinical experience with the ISG Viewing Wand. *Neurosurgery* 39:194-204, 1996.
26. Carrau RL, Snyderman CH, Curtin HD, et al: Computer-assisted intraoperative navigation during skull base surgery. *Am J Otolaryngol* 17:95-101, 1996.
27. Koivukangas J, Louhisalmi Y, Alakuijala J, et al: Ultrasound-controlled neuronavigator-guided brain surgery. *J Neurosurg* 79:36-42, 1993.
28. Kondziolka D, Lunsford LD: Results and expectations with image-integrated brainstem stereotactic biopsy. *Surg Neurol* 43:558-562, 1995.
29. Lee MH, Lufkin RB, Borges A, et al: MR-guided procedures using contemporaneous imaging frameless stereotaxis in an open-configuration system. *J Comput Assist Tomogr* 22:998-1005, 1998.
30. Roberts DW: Stereotactic guidance with the operating microscope: Surgiscope, in Alexander EMR (ed): *Advanced Neurosurgical Navigation.* New York, Thieme, 1999, pp 333-338.
31. Pillay PK: Image-guided stereotactic neurosurgery with the MKM microscope. *Surg Neurol* 47:171-176, 1997.
32. Cain P, Kazanzides P, Zuhars J, et al: Safety concerns in a surgical robot. *Biomed Sci Instrum* 29:291-294, 1993.
33. Drake JM, Joy M, Goldenberg A, et al: Computer-and-robot-assisted resection of thalamic astrocytomas in children. *Neurosurgery* 29:27-33, 1991.

Glossary

Accuracy: the measure of error in reaching any point in the entire volume

Cartesian coordinate system: named after the 17th century mathematician, René Descartes, who noted that three unique coordinates along perpendicular planes could define any point in space

Fiducial: an external prosthetic device, superficial or fixed

Frameless stereotactic surgery: a "catch-all" heading for a variety of emerging interactive computer technologies linking anatomical space and image space without the need for an intervening frame

Functional stereotactic surgery: the treatment of functional neurologic disorders (pain, movement, psychiatric) by ablation or stimulation of precise anatomical areas pinpointed by stereotactic guidance

Gamma knife: a stereotactic radiosurgery unit designed by Lars Leksell using 201 cobalt 60 sources focused by variable-sized collimators on a discrete intracranial target

Gamma rays: photons emitted during the radioactive decay of excited nuclei, as from the excited nickel nuclei produced by the decay of cobalt 60

Isocenter: the focus area of a single exposure to gamma knife irradiation. Dose-planning software can predict the isodose lines of up to 28 interacting isocenters in a single treatment plan for tumors with irregular shapes.

Isodose line: a line around a tumor target defined in terms of a percentage of the total dose applied within the line

LINAC: a linear accelerator generates high-energy x rays resulting from the collision of a focused electron beam aimed at a high-density metal target

Moore's Law: the doubling of transistor density on a manufactured die every year. This observation by Gordon Moore in 1965 correlates with an exponential yearly growth in computer power that is expected to continue through 2020.

PET scanner: positron emission tomography visualizes positron-emitting radiotracers, each of which reflects the physiology or pathophysiology of a discrete anatomical area

Pixel: a point in 2-D space defined by unique x and y coordinates

Polar coordinate systems: an arc-based, stereotactic system in which the target is always the center of the arc and can be described by a unique angle and distance

Precision: the repeatability of returning to a single point in the volume

Proton: charged particles produced by a cyclotron which travel a finite distance before depositing the majority of their energy over a short distance described as the Bragg peak

Registration: in stereotactic surgery, refers to the process of linking the volume of physical, anatomical space to the image space

Stereotactic radiosurgery (SRS): the single-fraction application of ionizing radiation to precise anatomical areas defined through framed stereotactic guidance

Stereotactic radiotherapy (SRT): the delivery of fractionated radiation focused stereotactically, as with a dedicated LINAC system

Voxel: a point in 3-D space defined by unique x, y, and z coordinates

CHAPTER 8

Office Treatment of the Draining Ear

Jed A. Kwartler, MD
Clinical Associate Professor, Division of Otolaryngology–Head and Neck Surgery, UMDNJ–New Jersey Medical School, Newark, NJ; Ear Specialty Group, Springfield, NJ

Clough Shelton, MD
Professor, Division of Otolaryngology–Head and Neck Surgery, University of Utah School of Medicine, Salt Lake City

Office treatment of the patient with a chronically draining ear can be quite frustrating for both patient and physician. A number of factors can interfere with treatment, including the physician's lack of recognition of underlying disease (such as cholesteatoma, immunodeficiency states, or ciliary immotility) as well as poor drainage of inflammatory exudates, lack of patient compliance with treatment, mucosal changes with subepithelial scarring and devascularization, and pathologic synergy between aerobic and anaerobic bacteria that promotes inhibition of phagocytosis. Because of the high rate of relapse associated with this condition, some authors have concluded that the goal of office management is not a completely dry ear but, rather, to achieve the best condition possible before definitive surgical treatment is undertaken.[1-3]

Office treatment can be successful, however, if it is approached systematically and if all those areas within the physician's control are addressed. Broadly, 4 categories of draining ears can be identified: (1) ears with perforations, (2) ears with mastoid cavities, 3) ears with ventilation tubes, and (4) ears with problems limited to the ear canal. These categories are useful because specific cleaning techniques vary, drug delivery systems can be modified for each category, and the bacteriology of each condition may be different (leading to different drug choices).

PATIENT HISTORY

Initial evaluation should include a thorough patient history designed to uncover causative or exacerbating factors that the physician can then change, treat, or eliminate. Some of the issues to be addressed at this stage are outlined below.

- What is the quality and pattern of the drainage? Is it serous, mucoid, mucopurulent, or bloody? Is it intermittent or constant? Is there any relationship between the drainage and recent upper respiratory infections or water contamination? (The latter are often seen in patients with perforation or ventilation tubes.)[4-6]
- Is there pain associated with the drainage? Pain is most often indicative of an external canal infection but may also be related to an underlying osteitis that might portend a potentially serious neurotologic complication.
- Does the patient have any underlying problems, such as anemia, malnutrition, long-term steroid use, or diabetes mellitus, that would compromise normal immune response?
- Does the patient have any chronic dermatologic conditions, such as seborrhea or eczema?
- Ear canal skin is quite thin and easily injured by manipulation. The use of a cotton swab (Q-Tip) is usually acknowledged by patients, but more persistent questioning is needed to determine whether bobby pins, paper clips, or similar objects were used to clean the ear.
- Does the patient exhibit any skin sensitivity to hairsprays, shampoos, or haircoloring? Have drops containing neomycin been used? These may cause contact dermatitis (easily treated by eliminating the offending chemical irritant).

EXAMINATION AND CLEANING

Ears of all patients with drainage are examined under the microscope. The microscope facilitates safer and more comfortable cleaning of the ear and provides appropriate lighting and magnification for determining the extent of the disease. A mental checklist of critical structural details is used, and the physician should be able to answer the following questions by the end of the examination:

1. Is the auricle normal in appearance? Is the underlying cartilage skeleton thickened or edematous? Is there irritation in the conchal bowl?

2. What is the shape and size of the ear canal? Is there any granulation tissue noted at the cartilage-bony junction? Is there erosion of the canal? Does pain result from manipulation of the canal?
3. What does the tympanic membrane look like? Is it retracted or atelectatic? Does it move with insufflation or Valsalva? Is there tympanosclerotic plaque?
4. Is a ventilation tube present? Is there peritubal granulation? Has squamous epithelium migrated into the middle ear cleft around the tube? Is there an occult or submucous cleft palate?
5. Is there a perforation? Is it a central or marginal perforation? What is the status of the middle ear mucosa? Is it normal, edematous, or covered with squamous epithelium?
6. Can the ossicular chain be seen? Is the malleus handle of normal length or eroded? Is the lenticular process of the incus seen, and is it attached to the stapes head?
7. Is there erosion of the scutum or canal wall?
8. If the patient has had a canal-wall-down mastoidectomy, is the cavity well saucerized and rounded? Is the facial ridge/posterior canal wall lowered to the level of the mastoid segment of the facial nerve creating a shallow transition between the middle ear and mastoid? Is the floor of the ear canal level with the floor of the mastoid bowl? Is the meatus large enough that a complete view of the cavity is possible?

The answers to these questions will help the physician separate out those patients who can respond to office-based management from those who will require some type of surgery. One example of a condition necessitating surgery is a mastoid cavity created with a high facial ridge and a small meatus relative to the size of the cavity. It is highly unlikely that a dry ear can be achieved with this set of structural problems. By identifying the underlying structural problem, the physician can avoid the time and expense to the patient of trying to medically treat such a condition.

Cleaning is the cornerstone of successful treatment of the draining ear. A variety of suctions, curettes, applicators, and hooks are needed to adequately (and with the least amount of pain) clean the ear. A long hook is particularly useful for cleaning the fenestration cavity in the rare case in which debris is trapped deep in the mastoid tip. A variety of curved and blunt suctions and probes are available for use in conjunction with oto-endoscopes for cleaning epitympanic pockets. Granulation tissue and areas of epithelitis can be cauterized with 5% or 10% solutions of silver nitrate. Care must be taken when working around the area of the facial nerve with silver nitrate, particularly when the canal wall has been removed, because silver nitrate can cause severe injury to an exposed nerve.

Cleaning the ear should not be limited to the office setting; rather, patients should mechanically clear any canal debris before using topical preparations. If this is not done, drops will not penetrate the mucoid layer of debris and will have essentially no effectiveness. Patients are instructed in the use of cotton-wire applicators to wick away any canal secretions. Another very effective way to mechanically dèbride the canal, middle ear or mastoid cavity is with half-strength vinegar irrigations. A solution of equal parts white vinegar and saline is warmed to body temperature (failure to do this leads to a caloric response) and "swished" back and forth in the ear with a bulb syringe or large medicine dropper.

BACTERIOLOGY

Knowledge of the most common pathogenic organisms, rather than routine cultures of the draining ear, should guide the initial treatment choice. The reason for this is 2-fold. Primary physicians have usually treated patients with a variety of topical or systemic antibiotics, which may lead to confusing isolates. More important, recovery of pathogenic organisms (particularly anaerobes) is poor when the sample is not plated immediately, when duration of incubation is too short, or when the aspirate is obtained from a swab of the ear canal, rather than from the middle ear.[7,8] If cultures are taken, the ear canal must be completely cleaned before culturing. Patients who do warrant cultures include immunocompromised patients, neonates, and those who are recidivists/nonresponders despite seemingly appropriate therapy.

Organisms most commonly cultured in chronic otitis media without cholesteatoma include *Pseudomonas aeruginosa, Escherichia coli, Enterobacter* species, *Proteus mirabilis, Staphylococcus aureus* and *Staphylococcus pyogenes*.[9,10] Anaerobes recovered include *Peptostreptococcus* species, pigmented *Prevotella* and *Porphyromonas*, and *Fusobacterium* species.[11,12]

Otorrhea from tympanostomy tubes is not uncommon, occurring in as many as 25% of patients.[13] It has been suggested that different organisms are responsible for the drainage, depending on the age of the patient and the season that the infection occurs in.[6,14] *Streptococcus pneumoniae, Haemophilus influenzae, Moraxella catarrhalis*, and *S pyogenes*, pathogens typical of acute otitis media, are seen in younger children (less than 6 years of age) and more commonly during the winter months. *P aeruginosa* and

Reservation Card for Advances

Yes! I would like my own copy of *Advances in Otolaryngology–Head and Neck Surgery*®, *Volume 14* (ISSN 0087-6916) at the price of **$94.00** (**$100.00** outside the U.S.) plus sales tax, postage, and handling. Please begin my subscription with the current edition according to the terms described below.* I understand that I will have 30 days to examine each annual edition.

Name _____

Address _____

City _____ State_____ ZIP _____

Method of Payment

❑ Check (in U.S. dollars, drawn on a U.S. bank, payable to **Mosby**)

❑ VISA　　❑ MasterCard　　❑ AmEx　　❑ Bill me

Card number _____　Exp. date _____

Signature _____

Prices are subject to change without notice.

MO141/D51532

Subscribe to the related journal in your field!

Yes! Begin my one-year subscription to *Otolaryngology–Head and Neck Surgery* (Volumes 122-123, 2000, 12 issues, ISSN 0194-5998).

Name _____

Institution _____

Address _____

City _____ State_____

ZIP/PC _____ Country _____

E-mail _____

Subscription prices

	USA	Int'l
Individuals ❑	$181.00	$219.00
Institutions ❑	307.00	345.00
Students/residents† ❑	89.00	127.00

Method of payment

❑ Check (in U.S. dollars, drawn on a U.S. bank, and payable to *Mosby*).

❑ VISA　　　❑ MasterCard

❑ AmEx　　❑ Bill me　Exp. date_____

Card #_____

Signature _____

†Please supply, on institution letterhead, your name, dates of study/residency, and signature of program coordinator. Orders will be billed at the individual rate until proof of status is received.

Airmail rates available upon request. Prices subject to change without notice.

MO141/D51540

---

*Your Advances service guarantee:

When you subscribe to *Advances*, you will receive advance notice of future annual volumes about two months before publication. To receive the new edition, you need do nothing—we'll send you the new volume as soon as it is available. If you want to discontinue, the advance notice allows you time to notify us of your decision. If you are not completely satisfied, you have 30 days to return any *Advances*.

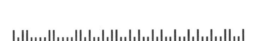

Want to speed up the process?

**To order a *Year Book* or *Advances*,
or to subscribe to a journal today,
call toll-free in the U.S.:
1-800-453-4351
Or fax 314-432-1158
Outside the U.S., call: 314-453-4351**
Visit us at: *www.mosby.com/periodicals*

Mosby
Subscription Services
11830 Westline Industrial Drive
St. Louis, MO   63146 U.S.A.

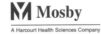

A Harcourt Health Sciences Company

S aureus are seen in older children (more than 6 years old) and more commonly in the summer months. More recently, it has been shown that the predominant organisms are similar to those isolated in chronic suppurative otitis media, such as *P aeruginosa, S aureus, Peptostreptococcus* species, *Prevotella* species and *Fusobacterium* species without regard to season or age.[15,16]

Otitis externa is caused predominantly by *P aeruginosa and S aureus* but may be complicated by fungal infections *(Aspergillus niger, Aspergillus fumigatus, Candida albicans)* and anaerobes.[17,18]

OTOTOPICAL THERAPY

After persistent mechanical cleansing, the mainstay of outpatient treatment of the draining ear is the use of topical antibiotic preparations. Advantages of this type of therapy, compared with the use of systemic antibiotics, include minimal side effects, direct delivery of medication to the affected area, and low rates of drug-resistant organisms developing in patients.[19]

Otic preparations (Table 1) usually are a combination of an antibiotic (choices are limited to neomycin, polymyxin B sulfate, polymyxin E, and chloramphenicol), a steroid, an acidifying agent, and an antiseptic. The pH of these preparations varies from 3.0 to 5.0.[20] Acidifying these preparations is recommended because drainage-causing organisms, particularly *P aeruginosa,* are killed in an acid environment.[21,22] Restoring the ear canal to its physiologic pH is also important in controlling drainage. The disadvantage of these drug choices is their lack of effectiveness against the common pathogens causing otorrhea. Neomycin and chloramphenicol have little activity against *P aeruginosa,* and the polymyxins are not active against gram-positive organisms and anaerobes. Acidifying the drops has 2 distinct disadvantages. Most apparent (for the patient) is the pain caused when the drops come in contact with middle ear mucosa. This is a common problem encountered when treating children, and it probably leads to failures in completing therapy or delivering drops appropriately. Second, the minimal inhibitory concentrations of neomycin are elevated, decreasing the effectiveness of an already marginally effective drug choice.

Ophthalmic drops (Table 2) and the newer ototopical preparations (Table 3) offer distinct advantages over the standard otic drops. There is a wider range of nonototoxic and lesser-ototoxic antibiotic choices that allow more specific and effective single-drug therapy. When steroid is added as an anti-inflammatory, it is

Text continues on page 175

TABLE 1.
Standard Otic Preparations

Product	Antimicrobial	Anti-inflammatory	Acidifying agent	Antiseptic	Other
Chloromycetin Otic Drops	Chloramphenicol				Propylene Glycol
Coly-Mycin S Otic Drops w/ Neomycin and Hydrocortisone	Colistin sulfate	Hydrocortisone 1%	Acetic acid	Thimerosal	Thonzium
	Neomycin sulfate				Polysorbate 80
					Sodium acetate
Cortisporin Otic Solution Sterile	Polymyxin B sulfate	Hydrocortisone 1%	Hydrochloric acid		Glycerin
	Neomycin sulfate				Propylene glycol
Cortisporin Otic Suspension	Polymyxin B sulfate	Hydrocortisone 1%	Sulfuric	Alcohol	Propylene glycol
	Neomycin sulfate				Polysorbate 80
LazerSporin-C Solution	Polymyxin B sulfate Neomycin sulfate	Hydrocortisone 1%		Thimerosal	
Domeboro Otic			Acetic acid		Aluminum sulfate

Product	Antibiotic	Steroid	Acid	Other ingredients
Otobiotic Otic Solution	Polymyxin B sulfate	Hydrocortisone 0.5%	Boric acid	Calcium carbonate; Propylene glycol
Pediotic	Polymyxin B sulfate	Hydrocortisone 1%	Sulfuric acid	Alcohol; Thimersol; Glycerin; Glyceryl monostearate; Mineral Oil; Polyoxyl 40 stearate; Propylene glycol
Pyocidin-Otic Solution	Polymyxin B sulfate	Hydrocortisone 0.5%	Hydrochloric acid	Propylene glycol
Star-Otic			Acetic acid; Boric acid	Propylene glycol
Tridesilon Otic		Desonide 0.05%	Acetic acid; Citric acid	Propylene glycol; Sodium acetate
VoSoL Otic solution			Acetic acid	Propylene glycol; Benzethonium chloride
VoSoL HC Otic Solution		Hydrocortisone 1%	Acetic acid	Propylene glycol; Benzethonium chloride

TABLE 2.
Ophthalmic Preparations

Product	Antimicrobial	Anti-inflammatory	Acidifying Agent	Antiseptic	Other
Chloromycetin	Chloramphenicol		Boric acid		Buffer
Chloromycetin/ Hydrocortisone	Chloramphenicol	Hydrocortisone 2.5%	Boric acid		Buffer Methylcellulose Benzethonium chloride
Ciloxan	Ciprofloxacin		Acetic acid		Benzethonium chloride
Cortisporin Opthalmic Suspension	Polymyxin B sulfate Neomycin sulfate	Hydrocortisone 1%	Hydrochloric acid Sulfuric acid	Cetyl alcohol	Mineral oil
Gantrisin	Sulfisoxazole				Propylene glycol Polyoxyl 40 Stearate Glyceryl mono- stearate Phenylmercuric nitrate

Product	Active ingredients	Steroid	Acid	Preservative	Other components
Garamycin	Gentamicin sulfate				Disodium phosphate, Monosodium phosphate, Benzalkonium chloride
Metimyd Opthalmic suspension	Sulfacetamide	Prednisolone acetate		Thiosulfate, Alcohol	Tyloxapol, Edetate disodium, Benzalkonium chloride
Neosporin Opthalmic Solution, Sterile	Polymyxin B sulfate, Neomycin sulfate			Alcohol, Thimerosal	Propylene glycol, Polyoxyethylene-polyoxypropylene
Polytrim	Gramicidin, Trimethoprim		Sulfuric acid		
Sodium Sulamyd Opthalmic Solution	Polymyxin B, Sulfacetamide sulfate			Thiosulfate	Benzalkonium chloride, Sodium hydroxide, Methylcellulose
Terra-Cortil	Oxytetracycline	Hydrocortisone 1.5%			Methylparaben, Propylparaben, Mineral oil

(continued)

TABLE 2. (continued)

Product	Antimicrobial	Anti-inflammatory	Acidifying Agent	Antiseptic	Other
TobraDex	Tobramycin	Dexamethasone	Sulfuric acid		Aluminum tristearate Benzalkonium chloride Tyloxapol Edetate disodium Hydroxyl cellulose
Tobrex	Tobramycin		Boric acid Sulfuric acid		Benzalkonium chloride Sodium sulfate Tyloxapol

typically at a greater concentration. These preparations are buffered to a near neutral pH that leads to fewer patients experiencing discomfort. Lastly, they have low viscosity, which allows better penetrations when ear wicks are used.

Several studies have documented the safety and effectiveness of the newer otic fluoroquinolone agents in both adult and pediatric populations.[23-28] Because of their effectiveness when compared with older ototopical therapies and because of the absence of ototoxicity with their use, these agents should be the ototopical treatment of choice.

Ototoxicity resulting from the use of ototopicals—particularly the older aminoglycoside agents that are still commonly used—is an area of controversy. Manufacturers usually advise against the use of these agents in patients with a perforated tympanic membrane. This recommendation is supported by animal studies that have shown the round window membrane is permeable with resultant inner ear injury.[29-32] It is unclear, however, what the actual incidence of ototoxicity is in human subjects. This issue is complicated by the fact that otitis media may be a cause of sensorineural hearing loss.[33,34] A survey of otolaryngologists suggests that the incidence of irreversible inner ear toxicity from the use of aminoglycoside ototopicals is fairly low (3.4%).[35] Others have demonstrated a similar lack of clinically significant inner ear toxicity.[36,37] Despite this apparent lack of strong clinical evidence for ototoxicity in patients with otitis media, aminoglycosides are used routinely to ablate inner ear function in Meniere's disease. It therefore follows that aminoglycoside drops should be used with caution in patients with tympanic membrane perforations, particularly as there now are nonototoxic topical medications.

Ototopical medications can also be delivered in powder form. This often works better in mastoid cavities where large surface areas need to be covered. The powders are packaged into capsules and delivered with an insufflator.[38] A variety of medications can be packaged as powders (Table 4).

Otomycotic infections are often the consequence of overgrowth resulting from the use of steroid-containing ototopicals. The mainstay of treatment is the discontinuation of the causative medication and thorough and frequent cleaning. A variety of antifungal medications are available (Table 5). Many of these medications are available in liquid or ointment/cream formulations. The latter are often highly effective because the ointment/cream can be applied so to fill the ear canal at the time of cleaning. Otic solutions (VoSoL, Cresylate), gentian violet, and thimerosal should not be used in the

TABLE 3.
New Otic Preparations

Product	Antimicrobial	Anti-inflammatory	Acidifying Agent	Antiseptic	Other
Ciloxan	Ciprofloxacin HCI	Hydrocortisone 1%	Hydrochloric acid	Benzyl alcohol	Sodium hydroxide
					Sodium acetate
				Polyvinyl alcohol	
Cortisporin TC	Polymyxin B sulfate	Hydrocortisone 1%	Acetic acid	Thimerosal	Thonzium bromide
	Neomycin sulfate				
Floxin Otic Solution	Ofloxacin		Hydrochloric acid		Sodium hydroxide
					Benzalkonium chloride
					Sodium chloride

TABLE 4.
Powder Preparations

CSF	CSF-H	CF	CF-H	BA
Chloromy-cetin 50 mg	Chloromy-cetin 50 mg	Chloromy-cetin 50 mg	Chloromy-cetin 50 mg	Boric acid 10% in talcum
Sulfanila-mide 50 mg	Sulfanila-mide 50 mg			
Fungizone 5 mg	Fungizone 5 mg	Fungizone 5 mg	Fungizone 5 mg	
	Hydrocortis-one 1 mg		Hydrocortis-one 1 mg	

presence of a tympanic membrane perforation. Systemic antifungal medication is rarely needed but may be a useful adjunct in refractory cases, particularly when *C albicans* is present.[39]

SYSTEMIC THERAPY

Is there any advantage to adding systemic therapy, either as oral or IV antibiotics, to the treatment of patients with draining ears? Several authors have advocated the use of IV antibiotics in chronic suppurative otitis media without cholesteatoma, with control of drainage being achieved in 90% of patients.[40-42] A limitation of these studies is that patients underwent daily cleaning of their ears in a clinic, so it remains unclear whether it was the IV antibiotics or the daily cleaning with appropriate placement of ototopical medication that led to the resolution of the drainage. Another drawback of IV antibiotics is the expense and morbidity associated with inpatient or at-home therapy. Similarly, it has not been clearly shown that oral antibiotics combined with ototopical therapy improve the cure rate of patients with draining ears. One large study compared the use of penicillin (Augmentin) alone with the use of ofloxacin in patients with otorrhea through a tympanostomy tube.[43] Treatment with topical ofloxacin resulted in a 76% cure rate, compared with 68% with penicillin. The American Academy of Otolaryngology-Head and Neck Surgery recently issued an expert panel consensus statement[44] recommending that, in the absence of systemic infection or serious underlying disease, oral or IV antibiotics should be avoided in chronic suppurative otitis media, infected tympanostomy tubes, and otitis externa. Further, they suggest that nonototoxic drops should be used as a first-line

TABLE 5.
Agents Used in Otomycosis

Product	Antifungal Agent	Other
Domeboro Otic	Acetic acid 2%	Aluminum sulfate
		Boric acid
VoSoL Otic	Acetic acid 2%	Propylene glycol 3%
Solution		
		Benzethonium chlo-
		ride
VoSoL HC Otic	Acetic acid 2%	Hydrocortisone 1%
Solution		Propylene glycol 3%
		Benzethonium chloride
Fungizone	Amphotericin B 3%	Propylene glycol
	Thimerosal	
Lotrimin	Clotrimazole	Polyethylene glycol
Mycelex	Clotrimazole	Polyethylene glycol
Cresylate	m-Cresyl acetate 24%	Propylene glycol
		Isopropanol 25%
Gentian violet	Gentian violet 1%	Ethanol 10%
Merthiolate	Thimerosal 1:1000	
Monistat-Derm	Miconazole	Pegoxol 7 stearate
Lotion		
		Mineral oil
		Benzoic acid
Nystatin	Nystatin, 100,000	
	units/mL	

treatment and that aminoglycoside drops should be added for treatment failures when cultures demonstrate sensitive organisms.

SUMMARY

Office treatment of the draining ear is a challenge, but one that can be met with an understanding of the factors contributing to the problem. Meticulous and repeated cleaning, which takes time and patience, is the mainstay of therapy to control the drainage. Another critical factor is the involvement of the patient in home care—appropriate instructions should be given for cleaning the ear and for the use of ototopical medications. Lastly, the timely use of ototopical antibiotics and anti-inflammatory agents should lead to a high rate of cure in most cases.

REFERENCES

1. Browning GG, Picozzi GL, Calder IT, et al: Controlled trial of medical treatment of active chronic otitis media. *BMJ* 287:1024, 1983.
2. Browning GG, Gatehouse S, Calder IT: Medical management of active chronic otitis media: A controlled study. *J Laryngol Otol* 102:491-495, 1988.
3. Hussain S: Conservative treatment in the management of inflammatory aural polyp. *J Laryngol Otol* 106:313-315, 1992.
4. Balkany T, Barkin RM, Suzuki BH, et al: A prospective study of infection following tympanostomy tube insertion. *Am J Otol* 4:288-291, 1983.
5. Gates GA, Avery C, Prihoda TJ, et al: Delayed onset post-tympanostomy otorrhea. *Otolaryngol Head Neck Surg* 98:111-115, 1988.
6. Schneider M: Bacteriology of otorrhea from tympanostomy tubes. *Arch Otolaryngol Head Neck Surg* 115:1225-1226, 1989.
7. Raju K, Unnykrishnan P, Nayar RC, et al: Reliability of conventional ear swabs in tubotympanic CSOM. *J Laryngol Otol* 102:460-462, 1990.
8. Brook I: Chronic otitis media in children. *Am J Dis Child* 134:564-566, 1980.
9. Brook I: Prevalence of beta-lactamase producing bacteria in chronic suppurative otitis media. *Am J Dis Child* 139:280-293, 1985.
10. Fliss D, Dagan R, Meidan N, et al: Aerobic bacteriology of chronic suppurative otitis media without cholesteatoma in children. *Ann Otol Rhinol Laryngol* 101:866-869, 1992.
11. Brook I: Otitis media: Microbiology and management. *J Otolaryngology* 23:269-275, 1994.
12. Sugita R, Kawamura S, Ichikawa G, et al: Studies of anaerobic bacteria in chronic otitis media. *Laryngoscope* 9:816-821, 1981.
13. Gates GA, Avery CA, Cooper JC, et al: Chronic secretory otitis media: Effects of surgical management. *Ann Otol Laryngol* 38:2S-32S, 1989.
14. Mandel E, Casselbrant ML, Kurs-Lasky M: Acute otorrhea: Bacteriology of a common complication of tympanostomy tubes. *Ann Otol Rhinol Laryngol* 103:713-718, 1994.
15. Brook I, Yocum P, Shah K: Aerobic and anaerobic bacteriology of otorrhea associated with tympanostomy tubes in children. *Acta Otolaryngol (Stockh)* 118:206-210, 1998.
16. Dohar J, Garner ET, Nielsen RW: Topical ofloxacin treatment of otorrhea in children with tympanostomy tube. *Arch Otolaryngol Head Neck Surg* 125:537-545, 1999.
17. Clark W, Brook I, Bianki D, et al: Microbiology of otitis externa. *Otolaryngol Head Neck Surg* 116:23-25, 1997.
18. Brook I, Frazier EH, Thompson DH: Aerobic and anaerobic microbiology of external otitis. *Clin Infect Dis* 15:955-958, 1992.
19. Dohar JE, Kenna MA, Wadowsky RM: In vitro susceptibility of aural isolates of *P aeruginosa* to commonly used ototopical antibiotics. *Am J Otol* 17:207-209, 1996.

20. Hoffman RA, Goldofsky E: Topical ophthalmologics in otology. *Ear Nose Throat J* 70:201-205, 1991.

21. Thorp MA, Kruger J, Oliver S, et al: The antibacterial activity of acetic acid and Burow's Solution as topical otologic preparations. *J Laryngol Otol* 112:925-928, 1998.

22. Aminifarshidemehr N: The management of chronic suppurative otitis media with acid media solution. *Am J Otol* 17:24-25, 1996.

23. Wintermeyer SM, Hart MC, Nahat MC: Efficacy of ototopical ciprofloxacin in pediatric patients with otorrhea. *Otolargngol Head Neck Surg* 114:450-453, 1997.

24. Fombeur JP, Barrault S, Koubbi G, et al: Study of the efficacy and safety of ciprofloxacin in the treatment of chronic otitis. *Chemotherapy* 40:29S-34S, 1994.

25. Kiris M, Berktas M, Egeli E, et al: The efficacy of topical ciprofloxacin in the treatment of chronic suppurative otitis media. *Ear Nose Throat J* 77:904-909, 1998.

26. Altunas A, Aslan A, Eren N, et al: Susceptibility of microorganisms isolated from chronic suppurative otitis media to ciprofloxacin. *Eur Arch Otorhinolaryngol* 253:364-366, 1996.

27. Agro AS, Garner ET, Wright JW, et al: Clinical trial of ototopical ofloxacin for treatment of chronic suppurative otitis media. *Clin Ther* 20:744-759, 1998.

28. Tong MC, Woo JK, van Hasselt CA: A double-blind comparative study of ofloxacin otic drops versus neomycin-polymyxin B-hydrocortisone otic drops in the medical treatment of chronic suppurative otitis media. *J Laryngol Otol* 110:309-314, 1996.

29. Brummet RE, Harris RF, Lindgren JA. Detection of ototoxicity from drugs applied topically to the middle ear space. *Laryngoscope* 86:1177-1187, 1976.

30. Meyerhoff WL, Morizono T, Wright CG, et al: Tympanostomy tubes and otic drops. *Laryngoscope* 93:1022-1027,1996.

31. Morizono T: Toxicity of ototopical drugs: animal modeling. *Ann Otol Rhinol Laryngol* 99:42-45, 1990.

32. Barlow DK, Duckert LG, Kreig CS et al: Ototoxicity of topical antimicrobial agents. *Acta Otolaryngol (Stockh)* 115:231-235, 1994.

33. Hunter LL, Marogolis RH, Rykken JR et al: High frequency hearing loss associated with otitis media. *Ear Hear* 17:1-11, 1996.

34. Paparella MM, Hiraide F, Oda H, et al: Pathology of sensorineural hearing loss in otitis media. *Ann Otol Rhinol Laryngol* 81:632-647, 1972.

35. Lundy LB, Graham MD: Ototoxicity and ototopical medications: A survey of otolaryngologists. *Am J Otol* 14:141-146, 1993.

36. Merifeld D, et al: Therapeutic management of chronic suppurativeotitis media with otic drops. *Otolaryngol Head Neck Surg* 109:77-82, 1993.

37. Ozagar A, Koc A, Ciprut A, et al: Effects of topical otic preparations on hearing in chronic otitis media. *Otolaryngol Head Neck Surg* 117:405-408, 1997.

38. House JW, Sheehy JL: Powder insufflator for the ear. *Otolaryngol Head Neck Surg* 91:461-462, 1983.
39. Cohen SR, Thompson JW: Otitic candidiasis in children: An evaluation of the problem and effectiveness of ketoconazole in 10 children. *Ann Otol Rhinol Laryngol* 99:427-431, 1990.
40. Kenna MA, Bluestone CD, Reilly JS, et al: Medical management of chronic suppurative otitis media without cholesteatoma in children. *Laryngoscope* 96:146-151, 1986.
41. Kenna MA, Rosane BA, Bluestone CD: Medical management of chronic suppurative otitis media without cholesteatoma in children-update. *Am J Otol* 14:469-473, 1993.
42. Lieberman A, Fliss DM, Dagan R: Medical treatment of chronic suppurative otitis media without cholesteatoma in children—A two-year follow-up. *Int J Pediatr Otorhinolaryngol* 24:25-33, 1992.
43. Goldblatt EL, Dohar JE, Nozza RJ, et al: Topical ofloxacin versus systemic amoxicillin/clavulanate in purulent otorrhea in children with tympanostomy tubes. *Int J Pediatr Otorhinolaryngol* 15:91-101, 1998.
44. *American Academy of Otolarygology–Head and Neck Surgery Bulletin*, June, 1999, p 9.

C HAPTER 9

Recent Advances in Molecular Genetics of Hereditary Hearing Loss

Xiaoyan Cindy Li, MD, PhD
Senior Research Associate, House Ear Institute, Los Angeles

Rick A. Friedman, MD, PhD
Associate, House Ear Clinic; Section Chief, Hereditary Disorders of the Ear, House Ear Institute, University of Southern California, Los Angeles

For the last decade, mammalian genetics has enjoyed tremendous progress. Advances in molecular methodologies, the identification of genetic markers and the development of high resolution genetic maps, the sequencing of the human genome, and the establishment of expressed sequence tag databases have resulted in the mapping and cloning of human disease genes at a rapid rate. Because of the extreme genetic heterogeneity of hereditary hearing loss and the difficulty of studying the molecular components of the cochlea, the study of hereditary hearing loss only recently has begun to bear fruit. The first autosomal gene responsible for nonsyndromic hearing impairment was mapped to chromosome 5q31 in 1992,[1] and the first autosomal nonsyndromic deafness gene, Connexin 26, was identified in May 1997.[2] Since then, more than 50 nonsyndromic deafness loci have been identified by linkage analysis, and 12 autosomal nonsyndromic deafness genes have been cloned.[3] The identification of genes involved in inner ear development and function is opening the door to a broader understanding of inner ear developmental biology and to potential genetic therapies for hearing loss.

In this review, we first briefly introduce the basic concepts of human genetics and genetic diseases. We then discuss the molecular methodologies that have facilitated gene mapping and cloning. Finally, we review the recent advances in the molecular genetics of hereditary hearing impairment.

HUMAN CHROMOSOMES AND GENETIC DISEASES

Genetic information is normally stored in DNA molecules that are used as templates to synthesize RNA molecules. The RNA molecules then are used as a template for the synthesis of the polypeptides of proteins, which carry out the biological function of the living cells and organisms. In humans, DNA can be found in chromosomes of the nucleus as long, linear, double-stranded helices and in the mitochondria as a single, circular, double-stranded molecule. The human mitochondria genome is small, 16.6 kb, and contains only 37 genes. The human nuclear genome is approximately 3000 Mb and contains approximately 65,000 to 80,000 genes.

In human somatic cells, there are 23 pairs of homologous chromosomes. Of those 23 pairs, 22 are alike in males and females and are called autosomes. The remaining pair has the sex chromosomes: XX in the female and XY in the male. Each pair of chromosomes carries almost identical genetic information, that is, each has the same gene loci in the same sequence. However, at any specific locus, pairs may have either identical or slightly different forms known as alleles. One member of each pair of chromosomes (homologues) is inherited from the father, the other from the mother. In females, the sex chromosomes are two indistinguishable X chromosomes. In males, the sex chromosomes differ. One is an X, identical to the Xs of the female, inherited by a male from his mother and transmitted to his daughters; the other, the Y chromosome, is inherited from his father and transmitted to his sons. When there are 2 identical alleles at a locus, a person is homozygous; when the alleles are different, the person is heterozygous. When there is only a single copy of a gene, such as X and Y in males, the situation is referred to as hemizygous.

Each species has a characteristic chromosome complement (karyotype) in terms of the number and morphology of its chromosomes. The human karyogram and the chromosomal locations of syndromic and nonsyndromic deafness genes are shown in Fig 1. The genes are in linear order along the chromosomes, each gene having a precise position or locus. The chromosomal location of each gene also is characteristic for each species and is believed to be the same in all individuals within a species. The relative position of some genes appears to have been highly conserved in

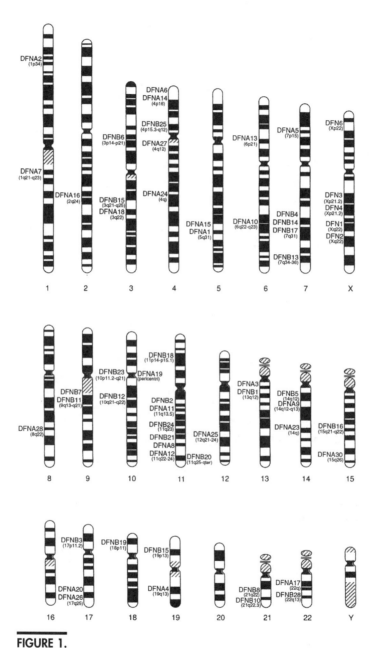

FIGURE 1.

Chromosomal locations of genes for hereditary hearing loss on a human male karyotype.

recent evolution, even among species as diverse as man and mouse. Thus, animals are a particularly valuable tool with which to identify human disease genes and study the function of the genes.

Genetic disease, a very broad term, includes disorders in which the genetic defects are entirely responsible for the pathology, as well as those in which genetic factors are only partially involved. The spectrum of genetic diseases is divided into 3 major categories: single-gene disorders, chromosome disorders, and multifactorial disorders. Single-gene disorders, also referred to as Mendelian disorders, are caused by a mutant allele or a pair of mutant alleles at a single genetic locus. They may be either inherited or the result of new mutations. When inherited, such disorders usually exhibit obvious and characteristic transmission patterns. Almost all forms of nonsyndromic and some forms of syndromic hereditary hearing loss are single-gene disorders. Chromosome disorders are caused by the loss, gain, or abnormal arrangement of 1 or more of the 46 chromosomes. The majority of chromosome disorders are de novo events arising from major mutations in the parents' germ cells. Some examples of inherited chromosomal aberrations show modified patterns of Mendelian transmission. Multifactorial disorders include many common disorders of adulthood, as well as the majority of developmental disorders that result in congenital malformations. These arise when mutations in more than one gene contribute to the disease, a combination of small variations that together can produce or predispose to a serious defect. In multifactorial disorders, environmental factors often contribute to the disease. These disorders tend to recur in families but do not show the characteristic inheritance patterns of Mendelian traits. Presbyacusis is an example of a multifactorial genetic disorder.

There are 5 basic pedigree patterns for single-gene inheritance: autosomal-dominant, autosomal-recessive, X-linked dominant, X-linked recessive, and mitochondrial inheritance. Classic pedigree patterns are shown in Fig 2. Rarely, Y-linked disorders, caused by mutations in the few genes carried on the Y chromosome, have been reported.

The genes for autosomal-dominant disorders are carried on the autosomes. Only a single copy of the mutant gene is needed to cause the disease (Fig 2, A). Dominant characters are the phenotypes expressed in both heterozygotes and homozygotes. They are typically more severe in homozygotes than in heterozygotes; however, so far only one such disorder, Huntington's disease, is known to be equally severe in both genotypes. Dominant traits often are

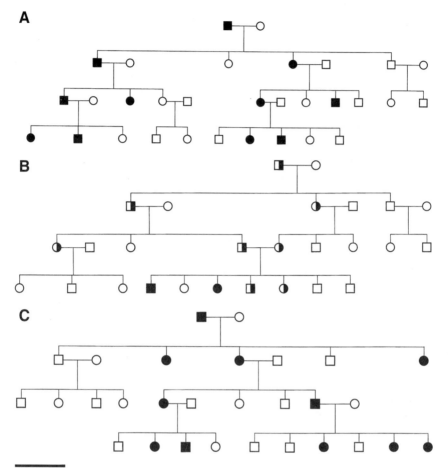

FIGURE 2.

Pedigree patterns of basic single-gene inheritance. **A,** Autosomal-dominant inheritance with nonpenetrance in individual III-6. **B,** Autosomal-recessive inheritance. **C,** X-linked dominant inheritance.

(continued)

observed with late-onset and variable expression. A common finding in dominant conditions is that a dominant character is not expressed in every individual who carries the gene. This is called reduced penetrance.

Autosomal recessive disorders are expressed only in homozygotes— affected individuals who inherited 2 mutant alleles, 1 from each parent (Fig 2, B). Heterozygotes with one mutant gene are usually unaffected and are called carriers. Both parents of an affected person are heterozygotes and are obligate carriers.

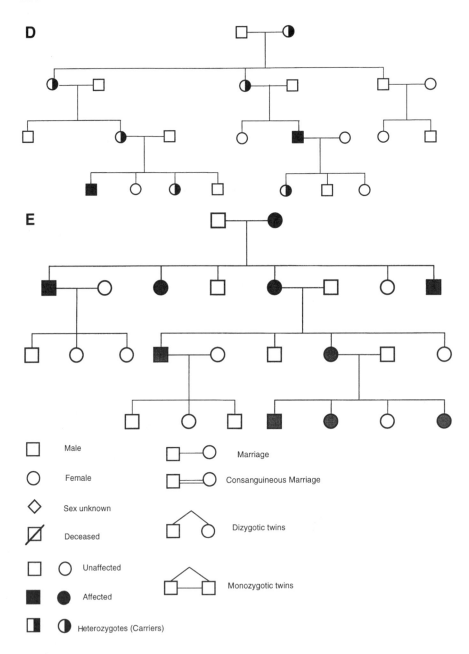

Symbols commonly used in pedigrees.

FIGURE 2. (continued)
D, X-linked recessive inheritance. E, Mitochondrial inheritance.

X-linked disorders are caused by mutations in genes present on the X chromosome. The characteristic feature of X-linked disorders is that male-to-male transmission never occurs. X-linked disorders can be either dominant or recessive. The dominant conditions affect either sex, whereas the recessive conditions affect males almost exclusively, because males are hemizygous for the genes on the X and Y chromosomes (Fig 2, C and Fig 2, D). Y-linked disorders are rare. They only affect males, and all sons of an affected male are affected.

Mitochondrial disorders arise from mutations in genes in the mitochondrial genome, which is distinct from the genes carried on the nuclear chromosomes. A unique feature of mitochondrial disorders is maternal inheritance. Although these diseases can affect both sexes, they are only passed on by affected mothers (Fig 2, E), because the egg, not the sperm, contributes nearly all the mitochondria to the developing offspring. Therefore, male transmission is not seen with mitochondrial disorders.

METHODS OF IDENTIFYING HEARING LOSS GENES

The identification of genes responsible for inherited disorders has been helped by recent advances in molecular methodologies. There are 4 general approaches to gene identification: functional cloning, positional cloning, position-independent candidate gene cloning, and positional candidate gene cloning. Functional cloning is used when the biochemical basis of an inherited disease is known, the gene product can be purified, and the amino acid sequence of the protein is determined. By reverse genetic coding, a DNA probe is designed to identify the gene encoding this protein. However, this approach has very limited utility, because the biochemical bases for most human diseases are unknown. Positional cloning is used to identify a disease gene when nothing is known about the pathogenesis or biochemical basis of the disease except its subchromosomal location.

The general approach is to construct genetic and physical maps of the targeted chromosomal region, refine the subchromosomal location, and then identify genes in the region to investigate as disease gene candidates. Strategies for gene identification include direct cDNA selection, exon trapping, and CpG island selection, among others. Positional cloning is a powerful, yet arduous method. The positional-independent candidate gene approaches can be used when a human disease phenotype resembles another phenotype in an animal or human for which the gene is known. Also, if the molecular pathogenesis suggests that the gene may be a member of a gene family, the gene can be directly tested as the candidate gene without its chromosomal location being known. However, this method has only rarely been successful. In positional candidate gene approaches, once a disease gene has been mapped, candidate genes will be identified for mutation analysis through database search.* With more and more human genes being mapped to specific subchromosomal regions, the positional candidate gene approach has become the most-used strategy.

In both positional cloning and positional candidate gene approaches, the first step toward identifying the gene underlying a clinical phenotype is to map the gene into a chromosomal region. This can be achieved either by identification of chromosomal rearrangements or by genetic linkage analysis. Genetic linkage analysis is one of the most powerful approaches in medical genetics because it alone allows mapping of genes that are detectable only as phenotypic traits. The majority of genes that underlie genetic disease fall into this category. Genetic linkage mapping also could be used to diagnose genetic disease even in the absence of any concrete information about the biochemical or molecular nature of the disorder.

Genetic linkage is a method of mapping genes by virtue of their cosegregation on a chromosome through meiosis. In humans, there are 2 types of cell divisions: mitosis and meiosis. Mitosis is the normal process of somatic cell division by which the body grows, differentiates, and effects repair. Mitotic division results in 2 daughter cells, each with chromosomes and genes identical to those of the parent cell. Meiosis is a specialized form of cell division by which the diploid cells of the germline give rise to haploid gametes. This results in the formation of reproductive cells, each of which contains 23 chromosomes: one each of the autosomes and either an X or Y chromosome. In the distribution of homologous chromosomes, the selection of either the paternally or maternally derived chromosome of each pair in a specific daughter cell is random (Mendel's first law of random assortment). When a sperm fertilizes an egg, the 2 haploid chromosome sets are combined, making a new zygote containing 2 copies of each chromosome (diploid chromosome set). This diploid cell then develops into a whole new organism whose every cell contains an identical full diploid set of chromosomes.

---

*The Human GeneMap (www.ncbi.nlm.nih.gov/genemap/) and Human Cochlear cDNA Library and EST Database (http://hearing.bwh.harvard.edu/cochlearcdnalibrary.htm) and many other useful databases are available on the Internet.

During meiosis, the pairs of homologous chromosomes line up side by side and undergo a process called "crossing over," resulting in the exchange of genetic material between homologous chromosomes. This physical phenomenon also is referred to as recombination (Fig 3). Recombinations occur frequently, and it appears that at least one crossover must occur on each chromosome arm (or chromosome) in each meiosis. Recombination can occur between loci on the same chromosome if they are far enough apart. However, loci that are physically close together on the same chromosome tend to be inherited together through meiosis as the chromosome is transmitted to the next generation. The chance that a crossover will occur between 2 loci is proportional to the distance between them. Hence, the probability of a recombination event occurring between the 2 loci, referred to as the recombination fraction denoted by (θ), can be used to measure the genetic distance between 2 loci. The formal unit for recombination fractions is the centimorgan (cM), with 1 cM equal to 0.01, or 1% frequency of recombination. There is a rough correlation between genetic distance and physical distance, with 1 cM measuring approximately 1000 kb or 1 megabase (Mb) of genomic DNA. However, this relationship is not completely linear because of regional variations in recombination rate and differences in recombination frequency in male and female meioses.

The entire basis of linkage analysis is that recombination events occur between 2 genetic loci (genes, DNA makers, chromosomal aberrations) at a rate related to the distance between them on the same chromosome. The first step in gene localization is to detect that there is reduced recombination between the gene and a specific marker so that its exact chromosomal position is already known. The known locus or marker may be another gene or sequence of DNA of unknown function. Currently, the most-used DNA markers for linkage mappings are a type of DNA polymorphism called "microsatellites." They belong to a group of short regions of repetitive DNA sequences with variable-number tandem repeats. These types of DNA marker are abundant throughout the genome, highly informative, and easy to use. Through linkage analysis, the transmission of the disease phenotype and the marker are compared to see if recombination between them is reduced.

To distinguish between coincidence and significance, formal mathematics was used in linkage analysis. The probability of a set of observations representing true linkage is expressed as the logarithm (base 10) of the odds, or lod score (Z). Lod scores are

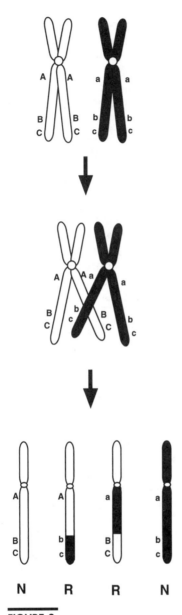

FIGURE 3.
Recombination (crossing over) between homologous chromosomes in meiosis. The white chromosome carries A, B, and C alleles at 3 loci, while the black chromosome carries a, b, and c alleles (*N*, Nonrecombinant; *R*, recombinant). This illustrates the principle that recombination is likely occur to between two loci if they are physically far apart; and loci that are physically close together tend to cosegregate through meiosis.

calculated at various possible values of recombination fraction θ, ranging from θ = 0 (no recombination) to θ = 0.5 (random assortment), and represent the likelihood that 2 loci are linked at a given recombination fraction compared with the likelihood that they are not linked at all (θ = 0.5). Because the logs are used, the lod scores can be summed between families. The recombination fraction giving the highest lod score is taken as the best estimate of the distance between the loci. Positive values of Z suggest that 2 loci are linked, whereas negative values suggest that 2 loci are not linked (at the given value of θ). By convention, a lod score equal to or greater than 3 is the threshold for accepting linkage, which represents 1000:1 odds that 2 loci are linked. Linkage can be rejected if Z < −2.[5,6]

Once a disease gene is localized into a subchromosomal region, the next step is to identify the disease gene within the target chromosomal region, using the strategies described earlier. Linkage analyses usually result in a large candidate region that is seldom smaller than several million base pairs. Although the traditional positional cloning approach is straightforward, it is extremely laborious and time consuming. In such cases, the positional candidate gene approach is the most appropriate cloning strategy.

Animal models, especially mouse models, have proven to be a valuable tool for the study of human diseases.[7,8] A major advantage of using the mouse for identification of disease genes is the ease of obtaining large numbers of informative progeny. The adult mouse cochlea is structurally and functionally similar to the human cochlea, and each shares similar developmental processes. Furthermore, some hereditary disorders of the inner ear are similar in the 2 species.[9] The modeling of human genetic disorders in the mouse is facilitated further by the high degree of homology between the human and mouse genomes, with regions of each demonstrating highly conserved gene content, as well as by the numbers of mouse mutations with hearing impairment.[10]

The analysis of inner ear mutations in mice is invaluable in the identification of genes involved in human hereditary hearing loss. A good example is the identification of the *MYO7A* gene. Mice homozygous for the shaker-1 mutation *(sh1)* demonstrated a waltzing phenotype consisting of head-bobbing, hyperactivity, circling, and deafness secondary to a neuroepithelial defect in the inner ear. Positional cloning identified a mutation in an unconventional myosin gene, *Myo7A*, as causative in this mouse.[11] The homologous gene in humans, *MYO7A,* has subsequently been implicated in 2 forms of nonsyndromic hearing loss (DFNA11 and DFNB2) and in 1 form of syndromic hearing loss, Usher syndrome 1B (USH1B).[12-14]

RECENT PROGRESS IN HEREDITARY HEARING LOSS

Hearing loss is the most common sensory disorder in humans. It can lead to alterations in language, speech and cognitive and psychosocial development. About 1 in every 1000 children is affected by severe deafness, either at birth or during early childhood. A further 1 in 1000 children becomes deaf before adulthood. More than 50% of all cases are linked to a genetic cause.[15,16] This number is even higher in the developed countries.[17] Finally, nearly half the population is affected by age 80.[15]

Hearing loss can be classified in many ways, such as prelingual versus postlingual, conductive versus sensorineural, syndromic versus nonsyndromic, and genetic versus acquired. The 3 general categories, conductive, neurosensory, and mixed, are based on the site of the physiologic defect. Conductive hearing loss is the result of outer or middle ear dysfunction; neurosensory hearing loss is caused by malfunction of the cochlea, the auditory nervous system, or both; mixed hearing loss results from a combination of the two. Hereditary hearing loss is usually classified into syndromic and nonsyndromic forms. Nonsyndromic hearing loss occurs in isolation, whereas syndromic hearing loss is associated with abnormalities in other systems, such as pigmentation or renal dysfunction. Syndromic hearing loss accounts for 30% of deafness in children, and the deafness is, in most cases, conductive or mixed. Nonsyndromic hearing loss accounts for approximately 70% of hereditary hearing loss. It is almost exclusively monogenic with extremely high genetic heterogeneity. It is estimated that several hundred different genes are involved in inherited deafness.[15] Approximately 80% of the genes are autosomal recessive, 18% are autosomal dominant, and 2% are X-linked or mitochondrial. In some cases, defects in multiple genes appear to account for the pattern of inheritance. Genetic factors also are highly likely to play a role in susceptibility to hearing loss later in life.

NONSYNDROMIC HEARING LOSS

The nonsyndromic forms of hearing loss are collectively referred to as DFNA for the autosomal dominant forms, DFNB for the autosomal recessive forms, and DFN for the X-linked forms. The autosomal recessive forms of hearing loss often are the most severe and account for the vast majority of congenital deafness. These forms are almost exclusively sensorineural. Autosomal-dominant and mitochondrial forms of hearing loss are frequently postlingual, with the age of onset varying from the first to the third decades. Postlingual forms also seem to be mainly sensorineural and progressive. However, 3 DFNA loci with congenital profound deafness have been described.[18-21]

The extreme genetic heterogeneity of nonsyndromic deafness combined with the absence of unambiguous phenotypic criteria that would allow differentiation of the inner ear defects caused by various genes has hampered progress in the genetic mapping of nonsyndromic deafness genes. This genetic complexity is even greater in large, outbred populations, such as in the United States, where large numbers of different genes causing deafness are expected to be found. Recently, these impediments have been overcome by successfully using different approaches to map the genes responsible for nonsyndromic recessive deafness, including selecting geographically isolated populations, homozygosity mapping using small but consanguineous families, and disequilibrium mapping.[22] These strategies, along with advances in gene cloning methods, have led to an exponential increase in the number of deafness genes that have been mapped and cloned. To date, more than 40 nonsyndromic hearing loss loci have been mapped by genetic linkage analysis, 14 DFNA (Table 1), 20 DFNB (Table 2), and 4 DFN (Table 3). Fifteen genes responsible for nonsyndromic deafness have been cloned, and all of the autosomal deafness genes were identified within the last 2 years.[3] The names of the cloned nonsyndromic deafness genes, their encoded protein, and their designation are listed in Table 4. Included in this list are 3 different genes in the mitochondrial genome associated with maternally inherited nonsyndromic deafness. These nonsyndromic deafness genes encode proteins of diverse functions, from transcription factors, cytoskeletal and extracelluar matrix components to membrane components of ion channel.

In the category of genes encoding membrane components, Connexin 26 (also called *GJB2*) is the first identified nonsyndromic autosomal deafness gene. It causes hearing loss in patients of both recessive DFNB1[2] and dominant DFNA3.[23] *Cx26* is a gap junction protein that forms intercellular channels, allowing ion and small molecule exchange between adjacent cells. *Cx26* is expressed in the supporting cells and fibrocytes in and around the organ of Corti, the spiral limbus, and the spiral ligament.[24] This supports the notion that *Cx26* is involved in the recycling of K^+ back to the endolymph of the cochlear duct after auditory stimulation.[25] *Cx26* is a small gene with a single exon, which makes

TABLE 1.
Nonsyndromic Autosomal Dominant Hearing-Impairment Loci

DFNA Locus	Chromosomal Location	Gene	References*
DFNA1	5q31	HDIA1	1, 2
DFNA2	1p34	GJB3/KCNQ4	3, 4, 5
DFNA3	13q12	GJB2/GJB6	6, 7, 8
DFNA4	19q13		9
DFNA5	7p15	DFNA5	10, 11
DFNA6	4p16.3		12
DFNA7	1q21-q23		13
DFNA8/A12†	11q22-q24	TECTA	14, 15, 16
DFNA9	14q12-q13	COCH	17, 18
DFNA10	6q22-q23		19
DFNA11	11q12.3-q21	MYO7A	20, 21
DFNA13	6q21		22
DFNA14	4p16		23
DFNA15	5q31	POU4F3	24
DFNA16	2q24		25
DFNA17	22q		26
DFNA18	3q22		27
DFNA19	10 (pericentromeric)		28
DFNA20‡	17q25		29
DFNA21	Reserved		
DFNA22	Reserved		
DFNA23	14q		30
DFNA24	4q		31
DFNA25	12q21-24		32
DFNA26‡	17q25		33
DFNA27	4q12		34
DFNA28	8q22		35
DFNA29	9p		36
DFNA30	15q26		37
DFNA31	Reserved		
DFNA32	11p		38

*References available by request from the authors.
†The original linkage of DFNA8 to 15q15-21 was retracted later, and a linkege to DFNA12 locus was reported in the same family.
‡DFNA20 and DFNA26 are overlapped.

TABLE 2.
Nonsyndromic Autosomal Recessive Hearing-Impairment Loci

DFNB Locus	Chromosomal Location	Gene	References*
DFNB1	13q12	GJB2	1, 2
DFNB2	11q13.5	MYO7A	3, 4, 5
DFNB3	17p11.2	MYO15	6, 7
DFNB4	7q31	PDS	8†, 9
DFNB5	14q12		10
DFNB6	3p14-p21		11
DFNB7/B11‡	9q13-q21		12
DFNB8	21q22		13
DFNB9	2p22-p23	OTOF	14, 15
DFNB10	21q22.3		16
DFNB11	9q13-q21		17
DFNB12	10q21-q22		18
DFNB13	7q34-36		19
DFNB14	7q31		20
DFNB15†	3q21-q25/19p13		21
DFNB16	15q21-q22		22
DFNB17	7q31		23
DFNB18	11p14-p15		24
DFNB19	18p11		25
DFNB20	11q25-qter		26
DFNB21	11q22-q24	TECTA	27
DFNB22	Reserved		
DFNB23	10p11-q21		28
DFNB24	11q23		29
DFNB25	4p15-q12		30
DFNB26†	4q2/1q22-23		31
DFNB27	Reserved		
DFNB28	22q13		32

*References available by request from the authors.
†This family was later found to have Pendred syndrome.
‡DFNB7 and DFNB11 are mapped to the same region; DFNB15 is linked to both chromosome 3 and 19; DFNB26 is mapped to 4q and a modifier gene is mapped to 1q in the same family.

TABLE 3.

Nonsyndromic X-linked Hearing-Impairment Loci

DFN	Chromosomal	Gene	References*
DFN1	Xq22	DDP	1, 2
DFN2	Xq22		3
DFN3	Xq22	POU3F4	4
DFN4	Xq21.1		5
DFN5	withdrawn		
DFN6	Xp22		6
DFN7	Withdrawn		
DFN8	Reserved		

*References available on request from the authors.

mutation screening relatively easy. Population studies have shown that mutations in *Cx26* are responsible for more than 50% of all recessive deafness.[26] One particular mutation, *30delG,* was the most common mutation in the populations studied and accounted for approximately 70% of all *Cx26* mutations.[23] In Mediterranean Europeans, the *30delG* is responsible for more than 80% of all cases of nonsyndromic recessive deafness. These findings make prenatal diagnosis, genetic counseling, and even genetic therapy an approachable goal. Recently, a second gap junction protein, connexin 31 (*GJB3*), has been reported to cause DFNA2.[27] Interestingly, another deafness gene, *KCNQ4*, which encodes a novel potassium channel protein, has been identified in the same DFNA2 locus.[28] Studies in mice and in Xenopus oocytes showed that *KCNQ4* is unique to outer hair cells and it likely plays a role in the removal of potassium ions from out hair cells.[28] Another gene encoding a membrane component is *PDS*. Mutations in *PDS* are reported to cause both nonsyndromic deafness (DFNB4)[29] and syndromic deafness (Pendred syndrome).[30] The *PDS*-encoded protein, pendrin, functions as a chloride-iodide transporter.[31]

Several molecules encoding cytoskeletal components have been identified as causing hereditary hearing loss. It was first demonstrated in *sh1* mice and Usher syndrome type IB patients that myosin7A is important for hearing.[11,14] Mutations in *MYO7A* genes have been shown to cause nonsyndromic deafness DFNA11[12] and DFNB2.[13] Recently, mutations in *MYO15/Myo15* have been implicated as causing deafness in nonsyndromic recessive DFNB3 patients and *sh2* mice.[32,33] *MYO7A* and *MYO15* belong to a group of unconventional myosins that are motor molecules involved in the movement of actin

TABLE 4.
Cloned Nonsyndromic Hearing Impairment Genes

Category	Encoded Gene	Protein	Locus	Reference*
Extracellular matrix components				
	TECTA	Tectorin	DFNA8/12, DFNB21	1,2
	COCH	COCH	DFNA9	3
	OTOF	otoferlin	DFNB9	4
Transcription factors				
	POU3F4	POU3F4	DFN3	5
	POU4F3	POU3F4	DFNA15	6
Cytoskeletal components				
Motor molecule	MYO7A	Myosin VIIA	DFNA11, DFNB2	7, 8, 9
Motor molecule	MYO15	Myosin XV	DFNB3	10
	HDIA1	Diaphanous 1	DFNA1	11
Membrane components				
Gap junction	GJB2	connexin 26	DFNA3, DFNB1	12
Gap junction	GJB6	connexin 30	DFNA3	13
Gap junction	GJB3	connexin 31	DFNA2	14
K channel	KCNQ4	KCNQ4	DFNA2	15
Ion transporter	PDS	Pendrin	DFNB4	16
Novel				
	DFNA5	DFNA5	DFNA5	17
Mitochrondrial genes				
	12s rRNA	12s rRNA		18
	tRNAser (UCN)	tRNAser(UCN)		19

*References available on request from the authors.

filaments. There are 3 rows of precisely arranged actin-packed stereocilia in each hair cell of the organ of Corti. These stereocilia are connected by lateral crosslinks. Myosin VIIA has a potential role in the formation of lateral crosslinks.[34] Mutations in *HDIA1* gene have been identified in patients with DFNA1.[35] Diaphanous, a human homologue of *Drosophila diaphanous*, is thought to regulate the polymerization of actin and maintain the actin cytoskeleton of the hair cell.

Among the transcription factors, *POU4F3* has been identified as causative in patients with a late-onset, dominant progressive deafness (DFNA15).[36] Its encoded protein is required for hair cell maturation, maintenance, survival.[37]

In several instances, mutations in the same genes cause both syndromic and nonsyndromic, autosomal-dominant and autosomal-recessive hearing loss. For example, mutations in *TECTA* are responsible for dominant DFNA8, DFNA12, as well as DFNB21.[38,39] The protein, α-Tectorin, is an extracellular matrix component of the tectorial membrane and the only protein known to be cochlear specific. Mutations in the unconventional *MYO7A* have been reported as causing DFNA11, DFNB2, as well as the syndromic hearing loss Usher syndrome type IB.[12-14]

Finally, among the late-onset forms of nonsyndromic deafness that appear in young adulthood, otosclerosis is the most common. Otosclerosis affects bone homeostasis of the labyrinthine capsule, resulting in abnormal resorption and redeposition of bone. It usually presents as unilateral or bilateral (70%) mixed hearing loss often accompanied with low-pitched tinnitus[40] This disorder has an autosomal-dominant mode of transmission with incomplete penetrance and variable expression.[41] It is thought to be genetically heterogeneous, with involvement of modifying genes and environmental factors. The first otosclerosis locus recently was localized to 15q25 -q26 by genetic linkage mapping.[42]

SYNDROMIC HEARING LOSS

It has been estimated that 30% of hereditary hearing loss is syndromic. Syndromic hearing loss can have many modes of transmission, including mitochondrial inheritance. For example, Waardenburg syndrome (WS), Treacher Collins' syndrome, and Stickler and Branchio-oto-renal (BOR) syndrome are transmitted as autosomal-dominant traits. Usher syndrome, Pendred syndrome, and Jervelle and Lange-Nielsen syndrome are autosomal-recessive disorders. Alport syndrome, Hunter syndrome, and Norrie syndrome are the examples for X-linked syndromic deafness.[42a] The hearing loss may be conductive, sensorineural, or mixed; however, the majority are conductive or mixed and are associated with malformations of the outer and middle ear. In this review, we only focus on a few forms of syndromic hereditary hearing loss whose molecular bases have been elucidated recently. A list of syndromic deafness genes and their encoded molecules are shown in Table 5.

Pendred Syndrome

Pendred syndrome is the most prevalent form of syndromic hearing loss, accounting for about 10% of all hereditary hearing loss.[43] Pendred syndrome is an autosomal recessive disorder characterized by congenital sensorineural deafness and thyroid goiter. Variable interfamilial and intrafamilial expression has been noted, particularly with respect to goiter, which may appear congenitally or in mid-childhood, but is often postpubertal.[44] The delay in the onset of goiter can make accurate diagnosis difficult. A positive perchlorate discharge test is suggested for early diagnosis of this disorder.

The hearing loss in Pendred syndrome is usually profound, but it can be progressive. It is often associated with radiologically detectable malformations of the inner ear.[45] The classic type of defect in Pendred syndrome is a Mondini malformation, which reflects an arrest of development at approximately 8 weeks of gestation. Features of Mondini malformation include a reduced number of cochlear turns and an enlarged vestibular aqueduct. Partial and complete forms of Mondini malformation have been reported in patients with Pendred syndrome. The basis for the abnormal perchlorate discharge test in Pendred syndrome suggests a fundamental defect in the ability to organify iodide in the thyroid.

The Pendred syndrome gene (*PDS*) was localized to a broad region on chromosome 7q22.3-q31.1 by linkage analysis.[46,47] Pendred syndrome has been linked to a single locus in more than 19 families from different geographic areas and ethnic backgrounds, suggesting locus homogeneity for this disorder.[48] Using a positional cloning strategy, Everett et al[49] identified and isolated the *PDS* gene, which was found to contain 21 exons and an open reading frame of 2343 bp. Mutations in *PDS* also cause a recessive nonsyndromic deafness, DFNB4.[29] Recent studies have shown that the *PDS*-encoded protein, pendrin, functions as a chloride-iodide transporter.[31] The expression of mouse orthologue (*Pds*) was detected in several regions thought to be important for endolymphatic fluid resorption in the inner ear, consistent with the putative function of pendrin as an anion transporter.[49]

An intriguing aspect of Pendred syndrome is the fact that defects in a single gene and its encoded protein can lead to such divergent pathology as deafness associated with a malformed inner ear and thyroid disease in the form of goiter. A better appreciation of these findings requires characterizing the role of pendrin in the developing inner ear and thyroid.

TABLE 5.
Cloned Syndromic Hearing-Impairment Genes

Category	Encoded Gene	Protein	Chromosomal Syndrome	Location	Reference*
Extracellular matrix components					
	COL4A3, COL4A4	Type VI collagen	Alport, AR	2q35-37	1
	COL4A5	Type VI collagen	Alport, X-linked	Xq22	2
	COL2A1	Type II collagen	Stickler, AD	12q13.1-13.3	3
	COL11A2	Type XI collagen	Stickler, AD	6p21.3	4
	COL11A1	Type XI collagen	Stickler, type II	1p21	5
	NDP	Norrin	Norrie	Xp11.3	6, 7
	USH2A	USH2A	Usher Type 2A	1q41	8
Transcription factors					
	PAX3	PAX3	Waardenburg type I/III	2q36	9, 10
	MITF	MITF	Waardenburg type II	3p12.3-p14.1	11
	SOX10	SOX10	Waardenburg type VI	22q13	12
	EYA1	EYA1	Branchi-Oto-Renal	8q13.3	13
	SALLI	SALLI	Townes-Brocks	16q12.1	14

Cytoskeletal components				
	MYO7A	Myosin VIIA	Usher Type 1B	11q13.5	15
	NF2	Merlin	Neurofibromatosis type II	22q12	16
Membrane component				
Receptor	EDNRB receptor	endothelin-B	Waardenburg type VI	13q22	17
Receptor ligand	EDN3	Endothelin-3	Waardenburg type VI	20q13.2-q13.3	18
Ion transporter	PDS	Pendin	Pendred	7q31	19
K channel	KCNQ1/KVLQT1	KCNQ1/KVLQT1	Jervell and Lange-Nielson	11p15.5	20
K channel	KCNE1/IsK	minK/IsK	Jervell and Lange-Nielson	21q22	21, 22
Neucleolar phosphater	TCOF1	Treacle	Treacher Collins	5q32-q33.1	23
Mitochrondrial genes				
	tRNA(leu)(UUR)	tRNA(leu)(UUR)	NIDDM, MELAS	Mitochondrial	24
	tRNA(lys)	tRNA(lys)	MERRF, MERRF/MELAS	Mitochondrial	25

*References available on request from the authors.

Usher Syndrome

Usher syndrome is an autosomal-recessive disorder character-ized by hearing loss and retinitis pigmentosa (RP). The preva-lence of Usher syndrome in the United States is estimated between 3 to 5 per 100,000.[50] Usher syndrome can be classified into 3 subtypes on the basis of clinical findings. Type I is the most severe form, characterized by congenital profound hearing loss, absent vestibular responses, and early-onset RP. It is also the most prevalent among the 3 subtypes, which comprise about 90% of all Usher syndromes. Type II is characterized by con-genital hearing loss with normal vestibular responses and the onset of RP in the first or second decade. Type III includes pro-gressive hearing loss with variable vestibular responses and variable onset of RP.

Usher syndrome is extremely heterogeneous. To date, 6 type I loci (USH1A to USH1F), 2 type II loci (USH2A and USH2B), and one type III locus (USH3) have been localized to different chromo-somal locations.[3] Two Usher syndrome-causing genes have been cloned. USH1B is caused by mutations in an unconventional myosin, MYO7A.[14] MYOVIIA is also responsible for 2 forms of nonsyndromic deafness: the recessive DFNB2 and the dominant DFNA11.[12,13] The expression studies in humans and mice showed that deafness in Usher1B is caused by a sensory hair cell defect, and RP is possibly the result of a primary cone and rod defect.[51,52] The second gene, USH2A, encodes a novel tissue-specific extra-celluar matrix protein.[53]

Jervell Lange-Nielsen Syndrome

Jervell Lange-Nielsen syndrome, also referred to as cardio-audito-ry syndrome, is an autosomal-recessive disorder characterized by congenital, severe to profound hearing loss with prolonged QT interval on electrocardiogram. Episodes of arrhythmia can result in dizziness, fainting, and even sudden death.

Recently, 2 potassium channel genes, KCNQ1 and KCNE1, have been identified in individuals with Jervell Lange-Nielsen syn-drome.[54-56] The KCNQ1 (or KVLQT1) encodes an atypical voltage-gated potassium channel protein with 6 transmembrane domains.[54] The KCNE1 gene (or IsK) encodes a potassium channel protein with a single transmembrane domain. This protein interacts with KVLQT1 to form a functional channel.[56,57] In the inner ear, the IsK and KVLQT1 are coexpressed in vestibular dark cells and in the marginal cells of the stria vascularis.[56] This suggests that IsK/KVLQT1 is involved in endolymph homeostasis.

Waardenburg Syndrome

WS is an auditory-pigmentary syndrome characterized by hearing loss with various combinations of dystopia canthorum, pigmentary abnormalities such as white forelock, heterochromia irises, and white skin patches. The prevalence of WS is 1 in 4000 live births. WS is classified into 4 types on the basis of clinical findings: WSI (with dystopia canthorum), WSII (without dystopia canthorum), WSIII (WSI and upper limb abnormalities, also called Klein-Waardenburg syndrome), and WSIV (WSII with autosomal-recessive inheritance and megacolon, also called Waardenburg-Shah syndrome).

Five genes underlying Waardenburg syndrome have been cloned. WSI and WSIII are caused by mutations in *PAX3* gene.[58,59] WSII is caused by mutations in MITF (microphthalmia-associated transcription factor).[60] Three genes, *Sox10*,[61] 1998), *EDNRB*,[62] 1995), and *EDN3*[63] have been identified as causing WSVI. *PAX3* belongs to a family of transcription factors that contain 2 putative DNA-binding domains (a paired box domain and homeobox domain).[64] *MITF* encodes a transcription factor of the basic-helix-loop-helix-zipper family.[65] *SOX10* is also a transcription factor that contains a domain similar to the high-mobility group DNA-binding motif present in the mammalian sex-determining protein *SRY*. *EDNRB* and *EDN3* encode peptide hormone endothelin B receptor and its ligand, endothelin-3. Both *PAX3* and *SOX10* are expressed in the dorsal neural tube from which neural crest cells originated.[64,66] *MITF* is expressed in cells that represent migrating neural crest-derived melanocyte precursors.[67] These results suggest that these genes play roles in the early development of neural crest-derived melanocytes. It has been shown recently that *PAX3* can directly transactivate *MITF* promoter.[68] *SOX10* also enhances the transcriptional activity.[69] These genes may function in the common pathway controlling the differentiation of neural crest cells into melanocytes. *EDNRB* and *EDN-3* are thought to be involved in an autocrine signal pathway necessary to maintain migration and tissue colonization by neural crest-derived melanocytes.[70]

Branchio-Oto-Renal Syndrome

Although the association of branchial arch anomalies and hearing loss has been recognized for nearly a century, it has only been in the last 25 years that BOR syndrome has been defined. In 1976, Melnick et al[71] reported a father and 3 of his 6 children with mixed hearing loss, abnormally cupped pinnae, preauricular pits, branchial cleft fistulae, and renal anomalies. BOR syndrome is an autosomal-dominant disorder with incomplete penetrance and variable expressivity. Several reports in the literature detail families with affected members demonstrating variability in both affected organs and degree of affectation, particularly with regard to anomalies of the renal system, including normal kidneys (BO syndrome) to total renal agenesis.[71a]

Despite these factors, a few salient features of the syndrome, including cup-shaped pinnae, preauricular pits, branchial fistulae, and renal anomalies are notable. Other less common features include lacrimal duct stenosis, anomalies of the maxilla, and palate and preauricular tags.[72,73] In a thorough study of more than 100 affected individuals, Fraser et al[73] demonstrated that the most commonly affected organ in patients with BOR was the ear, with 89% of those affected exhibiting some degree of hearing loss. The authors identified preauricular pits in 77%, branchial cleft fistulae or sinuses in 63%, and renal anomalies in 13%.

A better understanding of the molecular defect underlying BOR syndrome came in 1989 when Haan et al[74] described a family with a rearrangement of chromosome 8q, dir ins (8) (q24.11;q13.3;q21.13) and BO syndrome, and tricho-rhino-phalangeal syndrome.[74] This provided the first genetic map of this syndrome to chromosome 8q13.3 or 8q21.13. The causative gene, *EYA1,* was subsequently identified.[75] We recently described a mouse mutant at the *Eya1* locus.[76] This will provide a model system for the study of this syndrome.

Neurofibromatosis Type II

Neurofibromatosis type II(NF2) is a dominantly inherited disorder. It predisposes affected individuals to the development of a variety of intracranial and intraspinal neoplasms, most commonly bilateral vestibular schwannomas. NF2 occurs in about 1 in every 40,000 live births and from 1 in 20,000 to 1 in 1 million adults. Hearing loss, which is a result of vestibular schwannomas and is progressive, occurs in 45% of NF2 patients.

The responsible gene was localized to chromosome 22q12 by chromosomal abnormalities and linkage studies.[77,78] No evidence of genetic heterogeneity has been found. The gene encodes a membrane protein called merlin,[79] or schwanomin.[80]

MITOCHONDRIAL HEARING IMPAIRMENT

Mutations in the mitochondrial genome cause both nonsyndromic and syndromic deafness. Two mitochondrial genes have been identified as causing nonsyndromic hearing loss.[81,82] A mutation at position 1555 (A → G) in 12S rRNA gene was the first mito-chondrial mutation identified as causing nonsyndromic deaf-ness.[81] Later studies have shown that this mutation also influences susceptibility to aminoglycoside ototoxicity. Some of the syn-dromic hearing impairments caused by mutations in mitochondrial genes include lactic acidosis, encephalopathy, myopathy, diabetes mellitus, ophthalmoplegia, ataxia, and optic atrophy.

CONCLUSIONS

Like many areas of medicine, the rapid advances in genetics and molecular biology are revolutionizing our understanding of hear-ing and balance disorders. It is hoped that with a sound molecular foundation, some of these disorders may be diagnosed and treated at the genetic level.

REFERENCES

1. Leon PE, Raventos H, Lynch E, et al: The gene for an inherited form of deafness maps to chromosome 5q31. *Proc Natl Acad Sci USA* 89:5181-5184, 1992.
2. Kelsell DP, Dunlop J, Stevens HP, et al: Connexin 26 mutations in hered-itary non-syndromic sensorineural deafness. *Nature* 387:80-83, 1997.
3. Hereditary Hearing Loss Homepage, http://dnalab-www.uia.ac.be/dnal-ab/hhh/.
4. Reference withdrawn.
5. Terwilliger JD, Ott J: *Handbook of Human Genetic Linkage*. Baltimore: Johns Hopkins University Press, 1994.
6. Ott J: *Analysis of Human Genetic Linkage*. Baltimore: Johns Hopkins University Press, 1991.
7. Brown SD, Steel KP: Genetic deafness: Progress with mouse models. *Hum Mol Genet* 3:1453-1456, 1994.
8. Steel KP, Brown SD: Genetic deafness. *Curr Opin Neurobiol* 6:520-525, 1996.
9. Steel KP: Similarities between mice and human with hereditary deaf-ness. *Ann N Y Acad Sci* 630:68-79, 1991.
10. Steel KP: Inherited hearing defects in mice. *Annu Rev Genet* 29:675-701, 1995.
11. Gibson F, Walsh J, Mburu P, et al: A type VII myosin encoded by the mouse deafness gene shaker-1. *Nature* 374:62-64, 1995.
12. Liu XZ, Walsh J, Mburu P, et al: Mutations in the myosin VIIA gene cause non-syndromic recessive deafness. *Nat Genet* 16:188-190,1997a.
13. Liu XZ, Walsh J, Tamagawa Y, et al: Autosomal dominant non-syn-dromic deafness caused by a mutation in the myosin VIIA gene. *Nat Genet* 17:268-269, 1997b.
14. Weil D, Blanchard S, Kaplan J, et al: Defective myosin VIIA gene responsible for Usher syndrome type 1B. *Nature* 374:60-61, 1995.

15. Morton ME: Genetic epidemiology of hearing impairment. *Ann N Y Acad Sci* 630:16-31, 1991.
16. Reardon W: Genetic deafness. *J Med Genet* 29:521-526, 1992.
17. Marazita ML, Ploughman LM, Rawlings B, et al: Genetic epidemiological studies of early onset deafness in the U.S. school-age population. *Am J Med Genet* 46:486-491, 1993.
18. Chaib H, Lina-Granade G, Guilford P, et al: A gene responsible for a dominant form of neurosensory non-syndromic deafness maps to the NSRD1 recessive deafness gene interval. *Hum Mol Genet* 3:2219-2222, 1994.
19. Kirschhofer K, Kenyon JB, Hoover DM, et al: Autosomal dominant, prelingual, nonprogressive sensorineural hearing loss: Localization of the gene (DFNA8) to chromosome 11q by linkage in an Austrian family. *Cytogenet Cell Genet* 82:126-130, 1998.
20. Verhoeven K, Van Camp G, Govaerts PJ, et al: A gene for autosomal dominant nonsyndromic hearing loss (DFNA12) maps to chromosome 11q22-24. *Am J Hum Genet* 60:1168-1173, 1997.
21. Brown MR, Tomek MS, Van Laer L, et al: A novel locus for autosomal dominant nonsyndromic hearing loss, DFNA13, maps to chromosome 6p. *Am J Hum Genet* 61:924-927, 1997.
22. Petit C: Genes responsible for human hereditary deafness: Symphony of thousands. *Nat Genet* 14:385-391, 1996.
23. Denoyelle F, Lina-Granade G, Plauchu H, et al: Connexin 26 gene linked to a dominant deafness. *Nature* 393:319-320, 1998.
24. Kikuchi T, Kimura RS, Paul DL, et al: Gap junctions in the rat cochlea: Immunohistochemical and ultrastructural analysis. *Anat Embryol (Berl)* 191:101-118, 1995.
25. Spicer SS, Schulter BA: Evidence for a medial K^+ recycling pathway from inner hair cells. *Hear Res* 118:1-12, 1998.
26. Zelante L, Gasparini P, Estivill X, et al: Connexin 26 mutations associated with the most common form of non-syndromic neurosensory autosomal recessive deafness (DFNB1) in Mediterraneans. *Hum Mol Genet* 6:1605-1609, 1997.
26a. Denoyelle F, Weil D, Maw MA, et al: Prelingual deafness: High prevalence of a 30 del G mutation in the connexin 26 gene. *Hum Mol Genet* 6:2173-2177, 1997.
27. Xia JH, Liu CY, Tang BS, et al: Mutations in the gene encoding gap junction protein beta-3 associated with autosomal dominant hearing impairment. *Nat Genet* 20:370-373, 1998.
28. Kubisch C, Schroeder BC, Friedrich T, et al: KCNQ4, a novel potassium channel expressed in sensory outer hair cells, is mutated in dominant deafness. *Cell* 96:437-446, 1999.
29. Li XC, Everett LA, Lalwani AK, et al: A mutation in PDS causes non-syndromic recessive deafness. *Nat Genet* 18:215-217, 1998.
30. Everett LA, Glaser B, Beck JC, et al: Pendred syndrome is caused by mutations in a putative sulphate transporter gene (PDS). *Nat Genet* 17:411-422, 1997.

31. Scott DA, Wang R, Kreman TM, et al: The Pendred syndrome gene encodes a chloride-iodide transport protein. *Nat Genet* 21:440-443, 1999.
32. Wang A, Liang Y, Fridell RA, et al: Association of unconventional myosin MYO15 mutations with human nonsyndromic deafness DFNB3. *Science* 280:1447-1451, 1998.
33. Probst FJ, Fridell RA, Raphael Y, et al: Correction of deafness in shaker-2 mice by an unconventional myosin in a BAC transgene. *Science* 280:1444-1447, 1998.
34. Hasson T, Mooseker MS: The growing family of myosine motors and their role in neurons and sensory cells. *Curr Opin Neurobiol* 7:615-623, 1997.
35. Lynch ED, Lee MK, Morrow JE, et al: Non-syndromic deafness DFNA1 associated with mutation of the human homolog HDIA1 of the *Drosophila diaphanous* gene. *Science* 278:1315-1318, 1997.
36. Vahava O, Morell R, Lynch ED, et al: Mutation in transcription factor POU4F3 associated with inherited progressive hearing loss in humans. *Science* 279:1950-1954, 1998.
37. Erkman L, McEvilly RJ, Luo L, et al: Role of transcription factors Brn-3.1 and Brn-3.2 in auditory and visual system development. *Nature* 381:603-606, 1996.
38. Verhoeven K, Van Laer L, Kirschhofer K, et al: Mutations in the human alpha-tectorin cause autosomal dominant non-syndromic hearing impairment. *Nat Genet* 19:60-62, 1998.
39. Mustapha M, Weil D, Chardenoux S, et al: An alpha-tectorin gene defect causes a newly identified autosomal recessive form of sensorineural pre-lingual non-syndromic deafness, DFNB21. *Hum Mol Genet* 8:409-12, 1999.
40. Larson A: Otosclerosis, a genetic and clinical study. *Acta Otolaryngol* 154:1S-86S, 1960.
41. Ben Arab S, Bonaiti-Pellie C, Belkahia A: A genetic study of otosclerosis in a population living in the north of Tunisia. *Ann Genet* 36:111-116, 1993.
42. Tomek MS, Brown MR, Mani SR, et al: Localization of a gene for otosclerosis to chromosome 15q25-q26. *Hum Mol Genet* 7:285-290, 1998.
42a. Holmes LB: Norrie's disease—An X-linked syndrome of retinal malformation, mental retardation and deafness. *N Engl J Med* 284:367-368, 1971.
43. Batsakis JG, Nishiyama RH: Deafness with sporidic goiter: Pendred syndrome. *Arch Otolaryngol Head Neck Surg* 76:401-406, 1962.
44. Reardon W, Trembath, RC: Pendred syndrome. *J Med Genet* 33:1037-1040, 1996.
45. Johnsen T, Sorensen MS, Feldt-Rasmussen, et al: CT-scanning of the cochlear in Pendred's syndrome, Clin Otolaryngol 14:389-393, 1989.
46. Sheffield VC, Kraiem Z, Beck JC, et al: Pendred syndrome maps to chromosome 7q21-34 and is caused by an intrinsic defect in thyroid iodine organification. *Nat Genet* 12:424-426, 1996.

47. Coyel B, Coffey R, Armour JA, et al: Pendred syndrome (goiter and sensorineural hearing loss) maps to chromosome 7 in the region containing the nonsyndromic deafness gene DFNB4. *Nat Genet* 12:421-423, 1996.

48. Gausden E, Coyle B, Armour JA, et al: Pendred syndrome: Evidence for genetic homogeneity. *J Med Genet* 34:126-129, 1997.

49. Everett LA, Morsli H, Wu D, et al: Expression pattern of the mouse ortholog of the Pendred's syndrome gene (Pds) suggests a key role for pendrin in the inner ear. *Proc Natl Acad Sci U S A* 96:9727-9732, 1999.

50. Grondahl J, Mjoen S: Usher syndrome in four Norwegian countries. *Clin Genet* 30:14-28, 1986.

51. Hasson T, Heintzelman MB, Santos-Sacchi J, et al: expression in cochlear and retina of myosin VIIa, the gene product defective in Usher syndrome type 1B. *Proc Natl Acad Sci U S A* 92:9815-9819, 1995.

52. El-Amraoui A, et al: Human Usher 1B/mouse shaker-1: The retinal phenotype discrepancy explained by the presence/absence of myosin VIIA in the photoreceptor cells. *Hum Mol Genet* 5:1171-1178, 1996.

53. Eudy JD, Weston MD, Yao S, et al: Mutation of a gene encoding a protein with extracelluar matrix motif in Usher syndrome type IIa. *Science* 280:1753-1757, 1998.

54. Neyround N, Tesson F, Denjoy I, et al: A novel mutation I the potassium channel gene KVLQT1 causes the Jervell and Lange-Nielsen cardioauditory syndrome. *Nat Genet* 15:186-189, 1997.

55. Tyson J, Tranebjaerg L, Bellman S, et al: IsK and KvLQT1: Mutations in either of the two subunits of the slow component of the delayed recitifier potassium channel can cause Jervell and Lange-Nielsen syndrome. *Hum Mol Genet* 6:2179-2185, 1997.

56. Schulze-Bahr E, Wang Q, Wedekind H, et al: KCNE1 mutations cause Jervell and Lange-Nielsen syndrome. *Nat Genet* 17:267-268, 1997.

57. Sanguinetti MC, Curran ME, Zou A, et al: Coassembly of K(V)LQT1 and minK (IsK) proteins to form cardiac I(Ks) potassium channel. *Nature* 384:80-83, 1996.

58. Tassabehji M, Read AP, Newton VE, et al: Waardenburg's syndrome patients have mutations in the human homologue of the Pax-3 paired box gene. *Nature* 355:635-636, 1992.

59. Hoth CF, Milunsky A, Lipsky N, et al: Mutations in the paired domain of the human PAX3 gene cause Klein-Waardanburg syndrome (WSIII) as well as Waardenburg syndrome type I (WSI). *Am J Hum Genet* 52:455-462, 1993.

60. Tassabehji M, Newton VE, Read AP: Waardenburg syndrome type 2 caused by mutations I the human microphthalmia (MITF) gene. *Nat Genet* 8:251-255, 1994.

61. Pingault V, Bondurant N, Kuhlbrodt K, et al: SOX10 mutations in patients with Waardenburg-Hirschsprung disease. *Nat Genet* 18:171-173, 1998.

62. Attie T, Till M, Pelet A, et al: Mutation of the endothelin-receptor B gene in Waardenburg-Hirschsprung disease. *Hum Mol Genet* 4:2407-2409, 1995.

63. Edery P, Attie T, Amiel J, et al: Mutation of the endothelin-3 gene in the Waardenburg-Hirschsprung disease (Shah-Waardenburg syndrome). *Nat Genet* 12:442-444, 1996.

64. Goulding NJ, et al: Pax-3, a novel murine DNA binding protein expressed during early neurogenesis. *EMBO J* 10:1135-1147, 1991.

65. Hodgkinson CA, et al: Mutations at the mouse microphthalmia locus are associated with defects in a gene encoding a novel basic-helix-loop-helix-zipper protein. *Cell* 74:395-404, 1993.

66. Southard-Smith EM, et al: SOX10 mutation disrupts neural crest development in Dom Hirschsprung mouse model. *Nat Genet* 18:60-64, 1998.

67. Nakayama A, Nguyen M, Chen CC, et al: Mutations in microphthalmia, the mouse homolog of the human deafness gene MITF, affect neurepithelial and neural crest-derived melanocytes differently. *Mech Dev* 70:155-166, 1998.

68. Watanabe A, Tekeda K, Ploplis B, et al: Epistatic relationship between Waardenburg syndrome genes MITF and PAX3. *Nat Genet* 18:283-286, 1998.

69. Herbarth B, et al: mutations of the Sry-related Sox10 in dominant megacolon, a mouse model for human Hirschsprung disease. *Proc Natl Acad Sci U S A* 95:5161-5165, 1998.

70. Greenstein-Baynash A, Hosoda K, Giaid A, et al: Interaction of endothelin-3 with endothelin-B receptor is essential for development of epidermal melanocytes and enteric neurons. *Cell* 79:1277-1285, 1994.

71. Melnick M, Bixler D, Nance WE, et al: Familial branchio-oto-renal dysplasia: A new addition to the branchial arch syndromes. *Clin Genet* 9:25-34, 1976.

71a. Heimler A, Lieber E: Branchio-oto-renal syndrome: Reduced penetrance and variable expressivity in four generations of a large kindred. *Am J Med Genet* 25:15-27, 1986.

72. Cremers CWRJ, Fikkers-van Noord M: The earpits-deafness syndrome: Clinical and genetic aspects. *Int J Pediatr Otorhinolaryngol* 2:309-322, 1980.

73. Fraser FC, Ling D, Cbogg D, et al: Genetic aspects of the BOR syndrome: Branchial fistulas, ear pits, hearing loss, and renal abnormalities. *Med Genet* 2:241-252, 1978.

74. Haan EA, Hull YJ, White S, et al: Thricho-rhino-phalangeal and branchio-oto syndromes in a family with an inherited rearrangement of chromosome 8q. *Am J Med Genet* 32:490-494, 1989.

75. Abdelhak S, Kalatzis V, Heilig R, et al: A human homologue of the drosophila eyes absent gene underlies branchio-oto-renal (BOR) syndrome and identifies a novel gene family. *Nat Genet* 15:157-164, 1997.

76. Johnson KR, Cook SA, Erway LC, et al: Inner ear and kidney anomalies caused by IAP insertion in an intron of Eya 1 gene in a mouse model of BOR syndrome. *Hum Mol Genet* 8:645-653, 1999.

77. Seizinger BR, Martuza RL, Gusella JF: Loss of gene on chromosome 22 in tumorigenesis of human acoustic neuroma. *Nature* 322:644-647, 1986.

78. Rouleau GA, Wertelecki W, Hanine JL, et al: Genetic linkage of bilateral acoustic neurofibromatosis to a DNA marker on chromosome 22. *Nature* 329:246-248, 1987.

79. Trofatter JA, MacCollin MM, Rutter JL, et al: A novel moesin-, ezrin-, radixin-like gene is a candidate for the neurofibromatosis 2 tumor suppressor. *Cell* 72:791-800, 1993.

80. Rouleau GA, Merel P, Lutchman M, et al: Alteration in a new gene encoding a putative membrane-organizing protein causes neuro-fibromatosis type 2. *Nature* 363:515-521, 1993.

81. Prezant TR, Agapian JV, Bohlman MC, et al: Mitochondrial ribosomal RNA mutation associated with both antibiotic-induced and non-syndromic deafness. *Nat Genet* 4:289-294, 1993.

82. Reid FM, Vernham GA, Jacobs HT: A novel mitochondrial point mutation in a maternal pedigree with sensorineural deafness. *Hum Mutat* 3:243-247, 1994.

83. Sue CM, Tanji K, Hadjigeorgiou G, et al: Maternally inherited hearing loss in a large kindred with a novel T7511C mutation in the mitochondrial DNA tRNA(Ser(UCN)) gene. *Neurology* 52:1905-1908, 1999.

CHAPTER 10

Advances in the Treatment of Epistaxis

Carl H. Snyderman, MD
Associate Professor, Department of Otolaryngology, University of
Pittsburgh Medical Center, Pittsburgh, Pa

Ricardo L. Carrau, MD
Associate Professor, Department of Otolaryngology, University of
Pittsburgh Medical Center, Pittsburgh, Pa

Patients with epistaxis are frequently encountered in the practice of otolaryngology–head and neck surgery. Most episodes are minor in severity and duration and are managed adequately with the use of simple techniques in the outpatient setting. The majority of nosebleeds take place in the anterior nasal septum near Kiesselbach's area. Bleeding from this area may be effectively controlled with direct external pressure, topical vasoconstrictive agents, chemical cautery, electrocautery, or anterior nasal packing. Recurrent epistaxis may necessitate more extensive cautery or correction of a septal deformity.

Severe epistaxis usually originates from branches of the anterior ethmoid and sphenopalatine arteries. There are a number of treatment options, including anterior and posterior nasal packing, endoscopic electrocautery, surgical arterial ligation, and angiographic embolization. Considerable controversy remains regarding the optimal management of patients with epistaxis when considering factors of efficacy, cost, and morbidity. Additional issues to be considered include the identification of risk factors for epistaxis and effective prevention for high-risk patients.

RISK FACTORS

For many patients, specific risk factors for the development of epistaxis can be identified, including nasal trauma, desiccation of mucosa, use of anticoagulants and antiplatelet drugs, congenital or acquired coagulation disorders, and mucosal lesions (tumors, telangiectasias). More often, however, a specific precipitating cause is not identified. It is commonly believed, despite a lack of convincing data, that hypertension is a contributing factor. A recent study by Neto et al[1] of 323 adults with hypertension did not find any association between a history of adult epistaxis and blood pressure. However, there was a positive trend associating the duration of hypertension and left ventricular hypertrophy with epistaxis, suggesting that "epistaxis might be a consequence of long-lasting hypertension." Patient age was not a risk factor in this study population.

NONSURGICAL TREATMENT

Nonoperative management of patients with severe epistaxis usually involves some form of tamponade with the use of gauze packing, balloon catheters, or absorbable sponges. One overlooked therapy, hot water irrigation, is at least 100 years old. Stangerup et al[2,3] randomly assigned 122 patients hospitalized for treatment of posterior epistaxis to receive either hot water irrigation or tamponade treatment. A specially designed balloon catheter was used to prevent aspiration, and the nasal cavity was irrigated with 500 mL of 50°C water. Compared with tamponade, hot water irrigation was as effective, less traumatic to nasal tissues, less painful, and resulted in a shorter hospitalization. Based on a prior experimental study of rabbits, they have proposed that the hemostatic effect of hot water irrigation is caused by (1) edema and narrowing of the intranasal lumen, (2) vasodilation of the mucosal vessels resulting in decreased flow and intraluminal blood pressure, (3) cleaning of blood clots from the nose, and (4) possibly an increased speed of the clotting cascade.[4]

Angiography and embolization have been successfully used to treat patients with posterior epistaxis. Angiographic embolization yields results that are comparable to tamponade and surgery. Cost, availability, and risks that range widely among different institutions often limit the use of this technique. In addition, patients whose epistaxis arises from the anterior ethmoidal arteries cannot be managed with embolization because of the high risk that the embolization material could produce a stroke.

SURGICAL TREATMENT

If the site of bleeding can be located, the vessel can be ligated or the bleeding point can be cauterized. If the bleeding is profuse or the site of bleeding cannot be located, both the anterior ethmoid artery and the sphenopalatine artery (SPA) are ligated. The anterior ethmoid artery is ligated with the use of an external approach along the frontoethmoid suture. The internal maxillary artery and its branches (including the SPA) can be ligated with the use of buccal, transantral, or intranasal approaches. Transantral ligation of the internal maxillary artery has historically been the most widely used approach. Although a high success rate of 80% to 95% has been reported, transantral ligation of the internal maxillary artery is associated with significant morbidity. Additionally, because the terminal branches of the IMA may not all be ligated, there is a risk of failure due to collateral blood flow. Investigation of nasal blood flow in a swine model demonstrated a longer reduction in nasal blood flow with more distal occlusion of vessels.[5] To address the shortcomings of the transantral approach, researchers have introduced a number of transnasal techniques.

Microsurgical ligation of the SPA was first introduced by Prades[6] in the 1970s. Simpson et al[7] demonstrated that the SPA may be selectively ligated at the sphenopalatine foramen using a transantral approach without dissection of the pterygopalatine space. A transnasal microsurgical approach for the treatment of posterior epistaxis was described by Stamm,[8] in 1982, and by Stamm et al,[9] in 1985. For 145 patients undergoing this procedure, the immediate and delayed failure rate was 6.1%. A similar experience with this technique was reported in 1987 by Sulsenti et al.[10]

The most significant advance in the treatment of epistaxis in recent years has been the use of endoscopic techniques with selective ligation of the SPA at the sphenopalatine foramen. In 1992, Budrovich and Saetti[11] were the first to report endoscopic ligation of the SPA. They successfully applied this technique to 3 patients with epistaxis under local anesthesia. Since that time, multiple authors have described their experiences with endoscopic ligation of the SPA, with slight variations in the surgical technique. We have previously reported our technique[12] and clinical experience[13] with endoscopic SPA ligation.

SURGICAL TECHNIQUE

Surgery is preferably performed with the patient under general anesthesia to ensure the patient's comfort and to minimize risk of aspiration. After the induction of general anesthesia, nasal packing or balloon catheters are removed and replaced with cottonoids soaked in 0.05% oxymetazoline solution. After several minutes, the cottonoids are removed and the nasal cavity is inspected with

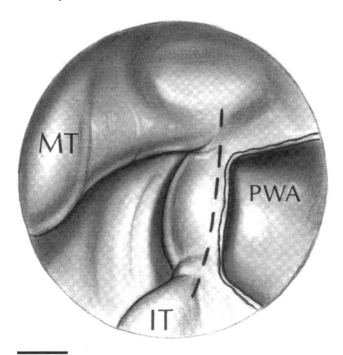

FIGURE 1.

A large middle meatal antrostomy is created. The mucosa is elevated in a subperiosteal plane at the posterior margin of the antrostomy *(dotted line)*. *Abbreviations: MT,* Middle turbinate; *IT,* inferior turbinate; *PWA,* posterior wall of antrum. (Adapted from Snyderman CH, Carrau RL: Endoscopic ligation of the sphenopalatine artery for epistaxis. *Operative Techniques in Otolaryngology–Head and Neck Surgery* 8:85-89, 1997. Used with permission.)

the use of a nasal endoscope. If a bleeding site is readily apparent, suction or bipolar electrocautery of the site is performed. More often, there is no visible bleeding site and surgical ligation proceeds. In rare cases, profuse bleeding may necessitate an ethmoidectomy to expose the bleeding site for control by direct electrocautery.

If access to the middle meatus is limited, a septoplasty or partial resection of the middle turbinate may be necessary. The inferior half of the uncinate process is removed and the opening into the maxillary sinus is enlarged posteriorly so that the opening is flush with the posterior wall of the maxillary sinus. At the posterior margin of the antrostomy, a Cottle elevator or a small Frazier suction tip is used to elevate the mucosa of the lateral nasal wall in a subperiosteal plane (Fig 1). It is easier to start the dissection inferiorly and sweep the instrument superiorly toward the sphenopalatine foramen. The SPA is easily identified where it exits the foramen posterosuperior to the maxillary antrostomy (Fig 2). On exiting the foramen, the SPA diverges into lateral nasal and posterior (septal) branches. To have enough room to place a hemoclip on the main trunk of the SPA, surgeons have found it is occasionally helpful to open the sphenopalatine foramen with a fine-tip Kerrison rongeur (Fig 3). Although seldom necessary, additional bone may be removed from the posterior wall of the maxillary sinus to expose the entire course of the SPA and other branches of the internal maxillary artery (Fig 4). The branches of the SPA and IMA may be carefully dissected with a blunt hook and a suction tip. Experienced endoscopic surgeons may forgo the opening of an

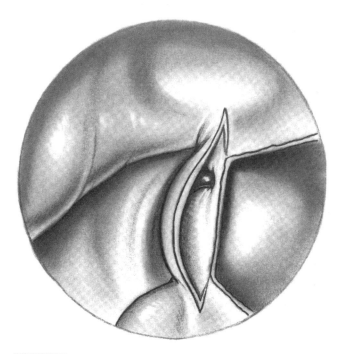

FIGURE 2.
The sphenopalatine foramen is located posterior to the antrostomy near the superomedial corner of the maxillary sinus. (Adapted from Snyderman CH, Carrau RL: Endoscopic ligation of the sphenopalatine artery for epistaxis. *Operative Techniques in Otolaryngology–Head and Neck Surgery* 8:85-89, 1997. Used with permission.)

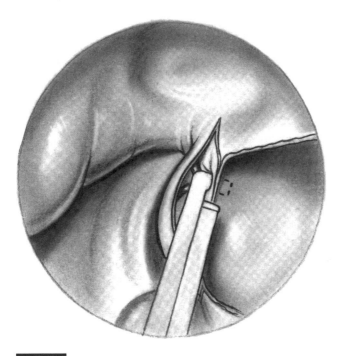

FIGURE 3.
Once the sphenopalatine artery is identified where it exits the foramen, a fine-tip rongeur is used to trace the artery laterally into the pterygopalatine fossa. (Adapted from Snyderman CH, Carrau RL: Endoscopic ligation of the sphenopalatine artery for epistaxis. *Operative Techniques in Otolaryngology–Head and Neck Surgery* 8:85-89, 1997. Used with permission.)

antral window and vertically incise the mucosa of the middle meatus at the posterior fontanelle. The identification and dissection of the SPA proceeds as described. Under direct endoscopic guidance, hemoclips are applied to the main trunk of the SPA and its major branches (Fig 5, *A*). Some hemoclip appliers may be too large for transnasal application. We have had better success using a flat-handled rather than a barrel-shaped instrument. More room for surgical manipulation may also be provided by performing a puncture antrostomy of the anterior wall of the maxillary sinus and passing the endoscope through the trocar (Fig 5, *B*). A piece of absorbable gelatin sponge is placed over the exposed vessels after clipping. Nasal packing is usually not necessary, although silicone splints may be used to prevent intranasal synechiae between the turbinates and the nasal septum, especially for patients who have had multiple packings or prior surgical procedures aimed at controlling the epistaxis.

Patients are discharged the day of surgery or the following day, depending on medical comorbidities and social factors. Saline spray is used postoperatively to minimize crusting, and silicone splints are removed after 4 to 7 days. Serial endoscopic examinations, with gentle removal of blood clots and crusts, are performed over the next month. Mucosalization of the surgical site with coverage of the clips and vessels is observed during this time.

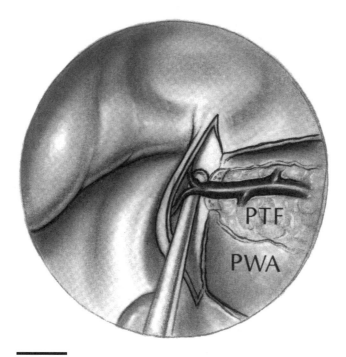

FIGURE 4.
After removal of bone from the posterior wall of the antrum, the course of the sphenopalatine artery in the pterygopalatine fossa can be observed. The distal portion of the vessel is carefully dissected free from the adipose tissue using a blunt hook and suction. *Abbreviations: PWA,* Posterior wall of the antrum; *PTF,* pterygopalatine fossa. (Adapted from Snyderman CH, Carrau RL: Endoscopic ligation of the sphenopalatine artery for epistaxis. *Operative Techniques in Otolaryngology–Head and Neck Surgery* 8:85-89, 1997. Used with permission.)

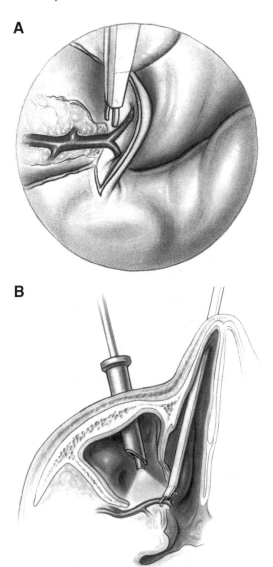

FIGURE 5.

A, If there is adequate space for instrumentation, hemoclips may be applied
to the sphenopalatine artery under endoscopic guidance through the middle
meatus. **B,** If there is too much bleeding or insufficient space, it is helpful to
use a transantral approach for the endoscope. This allows the introduction of
a hook or suction intranasally in addition to the hemoclip applier. (Adapted
from Snyderman CH, Carrau RL: Endoscopic ligation of the sphenopalatine
artery for epistaxis. *Operative Techniques in Otolaryngology–Head and Neck
Surgery* 8:85-89, 1997. Used with permission.)

CLINICAL EXPERIENCE

Recently, we reviewed our experience with endoscopic SPA ligation for the treatment of posterior epistaxis.[13] Five of 38 patients (13%) had recurrent epistaxis develop during follow-up, necessitating further treatment. Two of these patients had coagulopathies that contributed to the recurrence. When a coagulopathy was not present, endoscopic SPA ligation was effective for 92% of the patients. Ligation of the anterior ethmoid artery was performed concurrently in 25 patients; it was not a predictor of recurrent bleeding.

None of the patients experienced major complications related to their procedure. Minor nasal crusting occurred in 13 patients (34%) and was similar in nature to the crusting noted after endoscopic sinus surgery. Five patients (13%) complained of transient numbness of the teeth, palate, or upper lip. This may have resulted from trauma to the greater palatine nerve. One patient had a septal perforation develop after bilateral SPA ligation, but the causal relationship is unclear because multiple attempts failed to control the epistaxis by nasal cautery and packing. Four other patients underwent bilateral SPA ligation without adverse sequelae.

The median hospital stay was 3 days (range, 1-10 days). Most patients were discharged the day after surgery. We have recently been discharging patients on the day of surgery if there is no significant postoperative bleeding and they have adequate access to emergency medical care. The shortened hospital stay with endoscopic SPA ligation has the potential for significant cost savings in comparison with other therapies. Additional cost savings may accrue with a shorter operative time compared with transantral internal maxillary artery ligation. At our institution, endoscopic SPA ligation is more cost-effective than internal maxillary artery ligation, embolization, or posterior packing (unpublished data).

HEREDITARY HEMORRHAGIC TELANGIECTASIA

The treatment of patients with hereditary hemorrhagic telangiectasia, also known as Osler-Weber-Rendu disease, is frustrating. The number of therapies described in the medical literature is an indication of the inadequacy of treatment. Treatments include hormone therapy, antifibrinolytic agents, embolization, brachytherapy, cautery, injection of sclerosing agents, septal dermoplasty, and surgical closure of the nasal cavity. Laser photocoagulation has been investigated in recent years. Argon, KTP, and Nd:YAG lasers have been used with variable success.[14,15] The Nd:YAG laser is most commonly used because of its availability and better coagulative properties.

Argon plasma coagulation has been used successfully in the nasal cavity for the treatment of telangiectasias. Argon plasma coagulation is based on high-frequency electric energy transmitted through ionized argon gas to the tissue without direct contact. Its major advantage is limited tissue penetration (1-2 mm) with decreased tissue damage. Lennox et al[16] treated 19 patients and found it to be beneficial for patients with mild or moderate epistaxis. Bergler et al[17] studied 12 patients and found that the frequency and intensity of bleeding were significantly reduced. All of the patients felt that the results were superior to previous therapies. Further experience is needed with argon plasma coagulation to determine its relative advantages and disadvantages compared with other techniques in the treatment of this condition.

SUMMARY

The treatment of epistaxis continues to evolve. Outcomes analyses are needed to determine the most effective and least costly therapies for the treatment of patients with anterior and posterior epistaxis. For patients with severe posterior epistaxis, endoscopic SPA ligation appears to be more cost-effective than other treatment approaches and potentially causes less morbidity.

REFERENCES

1. Lubianca JF, Fuchs FD, Facco SR, et al: Is epistaxis evidence of end-organ damage in patients with hypertension? *Laryngoscope* 109:1111-1115, 1999.
2. Stangerup SE, Dommerby H, Sim C, et al: New modification of hot-water irrigation in the treatment of posterior epistaxis. *Arch Otolaryngol Head Neck Surg* 125:686-690, 1999.
3. Stangerup SE, Dommerby H, Lau T: Hot-water irrigation as a treatment of posterior epistasis. *Rhinology* 34:18-20, 1996.
4. Stangerup SE, Thomsen HK: Histological changes in the nasal mucosa after "hot-water-irrigation": An animal study. *Rhinology* 34:14-17, 1996.
5. Weaver EM, Chaloupka JC, Putman CM: Effect of internal maxillary arterial occlusion on nasal blood flow in swine. *Laryngoscope* 109:8-14, 1999.
6. Prades J: Abord endonasal de la fosse pterygo-maxillaire. LXXII Cong Franc Compt Rendus Seanc 290-296, 1976.
7. Simpson GT, Janfaza P, Becker GD : Transantral sphenopalatine artery ligation. *Laryngoscope* 92:1001-1005, 1982.
8. Stamm WK: Eine mikrochirurgische Methode zur Koagulation der A spheno-palatina als Therapie der hinteren Epistaxis. *Aktuelle Probleme ORL* 55:265, 1982.

9. Stamm AC, Pinto JA, Neto AF, et al: Microsurgery in severe posterior epistaxis. *Rhinology* 23:321-325, 1985.
10. Sulsenti G, Yanez C, Kadiri M: Recurrent epistaxis: Microscopic endonasal clipping of the sphenopalatine artery. *Rhinology* 25:141-142, 1987.
11. Budrovich R, Saetti R: Microscopic and endoscopic ligature of the sphenopalatine artery. *Laryngoscope* 102:1390-1394, 1992.
12. Snyderman CH, Carrau RL: Endoscopic ligation of the sphenopalatine artery for epistaxis. *Operative Techniques in Otolaryngology–Head and Neck Surgery* 8:85-89, 1997.
13. Snyderman CH, Goldman SA, Carrau RL, et al: Endoscopic sphenopalatine artery ligation is an effective method of treatment for posterior epistaxis. *Am J Rhinol* 13:137-140, 1999.
14. Werner JA, Geisthoff UW, Lippert BM, et al: Treatment of recurrent epistaxis in Rendu-Osler-Weber disease. *HNO* 45:673-681, 1997.
15. Velegrakis GA, Prokopakis EP, Papadakis, CE, et al: Nd:YAG laser treatment of recurrent epistaxis in heredity hemorrhagic telangiectasia. *J Otolaryngol* 26:384-386, 1997.
16. Lennox PA, Harries M, Lund VJ, et al: A retrospective study of the role of the argon laser in the management of epistaxis secondary to hereditary haemorrhagic telangiectasia. *J Laryngol Otol* 111:34-37, 1997.
17. Bergler W, Gotte K, Riedel F, et al: Argon plasma coagulation in treatment of hereditary hemorrhagic telangiectasia of the nasal mucosa. *HNO* 46:228-232, 1998.

CHAPTER 11

Contemporary Management of Chronic Facial Paralysis

Eugene L. Alford, MD
Clinical Assistant Professor, Baylor College of Medicine; Director, Texas Center for Facial Plastic and Reconstructive Surgery, Houston

Chronic, unilateral facial paralysis is a devastating condition that affects more than 5000 people each year. The etiology of facial paralysis is varied, ranging from viral neuropathy to surgical sacrifice of the seventh nerve. Chronic facial paralysis can encompass a wide spectrum of effects but is most often seen as a flaccid, unilateral, hemifacial paralysis. Management of this serious and debilitating problem has evolved dramatically during the last 30 years. At one time, patients were told that nothing could be done; now, there are many surgical and nonsurgical ways to help restore the vital functions and physical appearance lost as a result of chronic facial paralysis. As our methods for reanimation of the paralyzed face have improved, so have our goals and definitions of success in facial reanimation changed. Just 10 years ago, most surgeons would have accepted restoration of bilateral facial symmetry at rest as a successful outcome. Today's specialists in the treatment of chronic facial paralysis would not find this to be an acceptable result by itself. Results once thought to be unattainable are now the expected standards in all cases of chronic facial paralysis. The primary goals of facial reanimation—restoration and protection of vital functions such as vision, speech, and swallowing—have remained the same, whereas the secondary goals have changed dramatically. These secondary goals are now defined as: (1) superior outcome: restoration of bilateral, symmetric, emotional facial motion; (2) excellent outcome: restoration of bilateral, symmetric, volitional facial motion; (3) fair outcome: restoration of bilateral facial symmetry at rest. The ability to achieve these secondary goals and outcomes is what distinguishes the contemporary surgeon from his predecessors with regard to management of chronic facial paralysis.

The ultimate achievement in chronic facial paralysis surgery is the restoration of bilateral, symmetric facial movement in response to emotion. Emotional facial movements are those subtle facial movements that occur without conscious thought or effort as the result of deep-seated emotions, thoughts, or feelings. Emotional facial expressions are the small facial movements that communicate to others, without words, feelings such as happiness, sadness, joy, pain, and contentment. Restoration of emotional facial movement can be achieved most consistently through methods of facial reanimation that provide neural input from the ipsilateral facial nerve, central facial nucleus, and higher processing centers of the brain to all the ipsilateral facial muscles in a coordinated and non-synkinetic fashion. Achieving this result is a formidable task that requires that the surgeon possess exemplary surgical skills and talent. It is also important for the patient to be motivated and willing to dedicate the time necessary for rehabilitation and retraining to "learn" how to use the restored facial nerve.

Although restoration of emotional facial movement cannot always be achieved, the goal of bilateral, symmetric, volitional facial movement can be attained in the vast majority of patients. Bilateral, volitional facial movement and symmetry occur as a result of conscious effort to move the once-paralyzed side of the face. This goal may be achieved through a variety of methods, typically involving muscle transfers such as the temporalis or masseter regional muscle transfer, or the use of microvascular free tissue transfer. Each of these procedures uses a cranial nerve other than the seventh nerve—usually the fifth or twelfth nerve—to provide motor input to the new contractile unit of the face. Stimulation of the cranial nerve other than the seventh nerve requires a conscious effort to achieve and is thus volitional. In highly motivated patients, usually younger patients in whom restoration of neural input to the face occurs soon after the onset of facial paralysis, this volitional effort may begin to occur without conscious effort. Therefore, bilateral, emotional facial motion may be restored in a small percentage of patients without neural input from the ipsilateral facial nerve processing centers. It is important to note that this is the exception, not the rule, with regard to the use of muscle transfers in facial paralysis surgery.

Restoration of facial symmetry at rest, without symmetry of motion, was once considered the best one could achieve in any patient with chronic facial paralysis. Today, this result is considered only fair and can usually be achieved in almost every patient with chronic facial paralysis, regardless of the patient's age, duration of paralysis, or comorbidity factors. A variety of surgical procedures, including those listed above, as well as traditional cosmetic surgical procedures such as facelift, browlift, soft tissue implants, blepharoplasty, or muscle transpositions, can be used to obtain symmetry at rest.

Restoration of facial motion and symmetry is a delicate and arduous process. In no case of facial paralysis can results such as those outlined above be achieved with a single surgical procedure or even multiple surgical procedures in a single operative setting. To achieve a superior result, contemporary management of chronic facial nerve paralysis requires at least 2, and often 3 to 5 separate surgical steps, each from 2 months to 2 years apart. Every surgical step should build upon the results of the preceding step or steps. No procedure should occur until the maximum benefit of therapy, rehabilitation, and retraining has been realized after each step.

Contemporary management of facial nerve paralysis, attempting to achieve bilateral, symmetric, emotional facial movement, can occur only in healthy, highly motivated patients who are willing to undergo rehabilitation, therapy, and retraining after each phase of restoration. Surgical procedures performed on patients with facial nerve paralysis of long-standing duration who lack motivation, have multiple comorbidities, are older or unable to comply with postoperative rehabilitation training and therapy generally do not achieve restoration of emotional facial movement.

Early restoration of neural input to the facial nerve is the key factor in achieving return of emotional, bilateral, symmetric facial motion; however, precipitous decisions to undertake surgical restoration of neural input can be more harmful than helpful, depending on the circumstances. The only scenario that would allow the physician to undertake a surgical plan to restore neural input to the facial nerve within days of onset of paralysis would require that the physician know there is no chance of spontaneous facial nerve recovery. This situation usually occurs in those patients in whom a fully functional facial nerve is sacrificed as part of a surgical procedure, as in the treatment of posterior or middle fossa tumors, skull base surgery, acoustic neuroma surgery, or parotid surgery.[1] Early restoration of neural input to the facial nerve is best achieved through a primary end-to-end facial nerve repair at the time of injury. When possible, a primary end-to-end, tension-free anastomosis of the facial nerve will provide the best chance of facial nerve recovery.[2] This type of repair is only possible in a small percentage of cases. Far more commonly, grafting of the seventh nerve is required. When facial nerve grafting is necessary, the nerve graft should be of the same diameter as the native facial nerve and should be sutured end to end, without tension, using epineural sutures. Primary facial nerve grafting, however, is not without certain deficiencies. Standard facial nerve grafting techniques use 2 anastomoses and, thus, 2 sites of scarring to impede neural growth and input. Additionally, in some cases a donor graft of the same or similar size may not be available and size mismatch may be a problem. In many cases of skull base surgery, primary facial nerve grafting is not technically possible, especially in those patients requiring intratemporal sacrifice of the seventh nerve. Although primary facial nerve grafting has for years been the standard of care to achieve the best facial nerve reanimation results, newer techniques recently published in the literature are showing promise of better results.

The twelfth to seventh nerve side-to-end anastomosis procedure, illustrated with patient results by Jung et al,[3] avoids 2 anastomoses and eliminates the problem of facial nerve graft size mismatch. This procedure is also feasible in patients requiring intratemporal sacrifice of the seventh nerve. Although the twelfth to seventh nerve side-to-end procedure does not restore input from the ipsilateral facial nerve nucleus to the facial nerve, its advantages far outweigh its disadvantages. Recovery of facial muscle tone and motion that resulted from this procedure in 8 patients was clinically equivalent or superior to results from primary facial nerve grafting techniques. Use of the twelfth to seventh nerve side-to-end procedure for facial reanimation may allow an earlier return of facial muscle tone (usually within 6 weeks), earlier return of facial nerve volitional motion (usually within 3 months), and less synkinesis than with primary seventh nerve grafts.

The twelfth to seventh nerve side-to-end procedure calls for a complete decompression and rerouting of the seventh nerve, distal to the transection, from the geniculate ganglion down to the mastoid tip and through the stylomastoid foramen. The posterior belly of the digastric muscle is divided and the seventh nerve is rotated down to lie immediately against the ipsilateral twelfth nerve. A site along the seventh nerve is chosen to allow a tension-free, side-to-end anastomosis between the distal stump of the seventh nerve and the side of the twelfth nerve. A neurotomy is made one third to one half the width of the twelfth nerve at an angle of

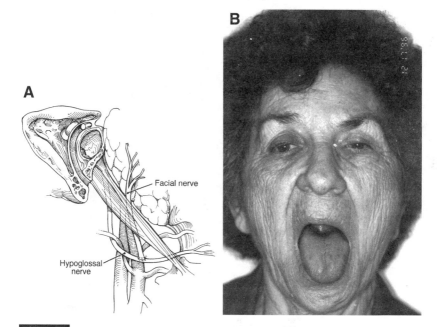

FIGURE 1.
A, A schematic drawing of the XII to VII side-to-end anastomosis for facial rean-imation. **B,** Patient 1 year after XII to VII side-to-end anastomosis.

(continued)

30 degrees to 45 degrees. The distal end of the seventh nerve is inserted into the neurotomy and sutured to the twelfth nerve with 8×0 perineural suture. Rehabilitation and retraining of facial nerve function begins as soon as possible after surgery. Highly motivated, healthy young patients have achieved some restoration of emotional facial motion with the twelfth to seventh nerve procedure. All patients in the paper by Jung et al have had restoration of ipsilateral, volitional facial motion and facial symmetry with excellent resting tone and symmetry (Fig 1, A–F).

Another neural procedure that has had good results in the restoration of volitional facial muscle movement and tone is the twelfth to seventh interposition nerve graft, as first described by Dr. Mark May.[4] This procedure has a long history of success and, in many cases, gives excellent results with separate volitional facial muscle control, restoration of resting tone, and excellent symmetry. Only rarely does this procedure provide emotional facial motion. Recovery of facial nerve function does not occur as quickly as with the twelfth to seventh nerve side-to-end proce-

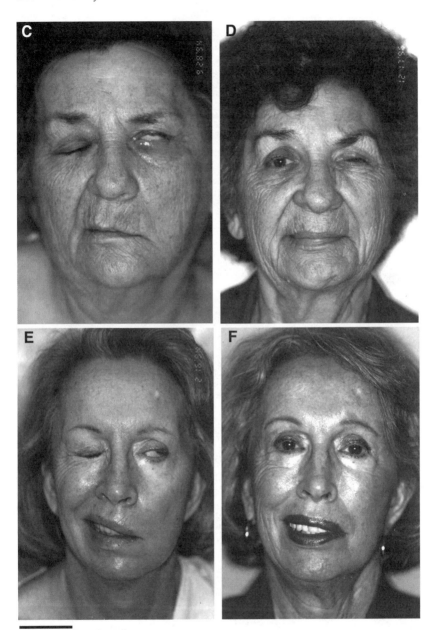

FIGURE 1. (continued)
C, Preoperative photo. D, Patient 1 year postoperative demonstrating volitional symmetry of smile with preservation of normal tongue function. E, Preoperative appearance. F, Eight months after XII to VII side-to-end procedure demonstrating flaccid left facial paralysis and postoperative spontaneous emotional smile without mass motion or synkinesis.

dure, as the twelfth to seventh interposition uses a nerve graft that requires 2 anastomoses. This procedure, however, does not cause ipsilateral twelfth nerve paralysis and, therefore, does not affect speech or swallowing (Fig 2, A and B).

The classic twelfth to seventh nerve end-to-end procedure has the longest history of success; however, 2 major problems are associated with its use.[2,5] This procedure guarantees loss of ipsilateral tongue function in all cases and, more importantly, can often result in overpowering facial muscle mass motion or facial twitching when patients talk or eat. These drawbacks suggest that this method be used only when there is no other choice of reanimation, and then only in those cases in which facial nerve paralysis has been apparent for more than 1 year. By allowing 1 year to pass between onset of paralysis and reanimation with a twelfth to seventh nerve end-to-end anastomosis, enough fibrosis of the affected facial nerve has occurred so that both involuntary twitching of the

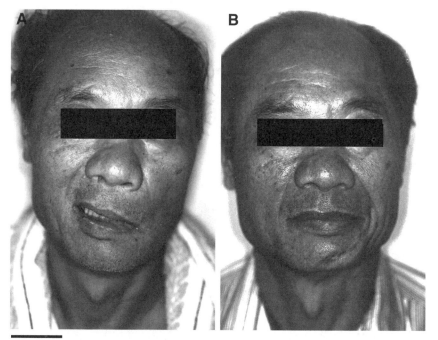

FIGURE 2.
A, B, Preoperative and 4 years postoperative photos of patient after XII to VII interpositional graft requiring sacrifice of VII nerve for removal of a 4-cm acoustic neuroma. (Note lack of synkinesis or mass motion of face.)

(continued)

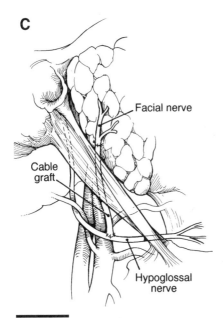

C

Facial nerve

Cable graft

Hypoglossal nerve

FIGURE 2. (continued)
C, A schematic drawing of the XII to VII interpositional nerve graft for facial reanimation. Compare to Figure 1A and note additional anastomosis necessary for successful completion of interpositional nerve graft.

face with eating and mass motion of the face with voluntary contraction may be avoided. The classic twelfth to seventh nerve end-to-end anastomosis may be indicated in cases of facial nerve paralysis of unknown etiology in which no evidence of spontaneous recovery has been observed even after long-term follow-up. However, the surgeon must not overlook or minimize the morbidity of the loss of ipsilateral tongue function and its effect on speech and swallowing.

Temporalis, masseter, or free muscle transfers have been used for more than 60 years to restore facial symmetry and movement. The primary limitation of all muscle transfer procedures is that they provide contraction and facial movement in only one vector. These procedures can never restore the limitless vectors of contraction in facial movement provided by the multiple muscles of facial expression. Therefore, muscle transfer procedures are used in contemporary management of facial paralysis primarily for elevation of the oral commissure to prevent drooling, improve speech and swallowing, and to allow for voluntary commissure elevation to mimic a smile. Temporalis or masseter muscle transfers for treatment of facial paralysis were first described by Edgerton[6] in 1932. These procedures have been used thousands of times by hundreds of surgeons for treatment of chronic facial paralysis. Limitations of vector movement and donor site morbidity can make these procedures less-than-perfect methods for facial reanimation; however, a surgeon, through careful planning and execution of these regional muscle transfer procedures, can overcome these shortfalls. By careful analysis of the contralateral vectors of facial motion, one can determine the best points of insertion for the distal temporalis or masseter muscle to provide matching elevation of the oral commissure to that of the nonparalyzed side. Although pull of the temporalis muscle is primarily superior and lateral, if the lower lip smile needs to move posteriorly and inferiorly, the masseter muscle can be used to provide this vector when necessary. Successful use of the temporalis muscle also demands that the oral commissure be overcorrected initially to allow for the temporalis muscle stretching that occurs after transfer. The donor site of the temporalis muscle also must be camouflaged by use of

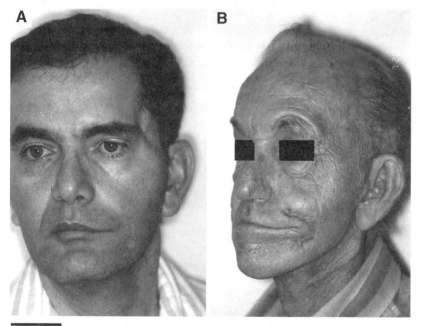

FIGURE 3.
Comparison of donor site morbidity after temporalis muscle transfer. **A,** A carved silicone block was used to fill the donor site. **B,** Photo demonstrates the use of a folded temporoparietal fascia flap and Gore-Tex strips for donor site camouflage.

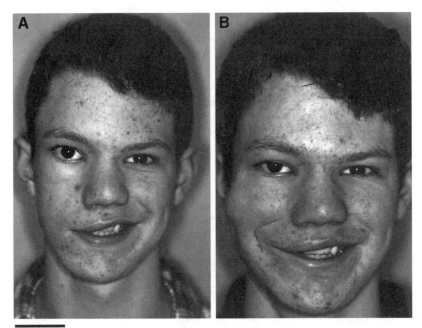

FIGURE 4.
A, Preoperative. **B,** Twelve weeks after surgery for free gracilis muscle transfer and end-to-side anastomosis between the motor branch of the gracilis and hypoglossal nerve in a 16-year-old male with right congenital facial paralysis. (Note early return of muscle contractility and commissure elevation.)

autologous materials such as a temporoparietal fascia flap or implants such as Gore-Tex or Alloderm (Fig 3, A and B). Bunching of the temporalis muscle over the zygomatic arch should be minimized by using the smallest width of muscle necessary to achieve elevation of the oral commissure. The zygomatic arch should never be taken down or removed, as this provides an important fulcrum for contraction of the temporalis muscle and elevation of the oral commissure.[7]

Free muscle transfers are used when all facial muscle contractility has been lost, such as in cases of long-standing facial paralysis in which muscle atrophy and loss of motor end-plate function has occurred or when surgical sacrifice of the muscles of facial expression is required. The same limitations of vector pull and commissure elevation apply in the use of both free muscle transfers and regional muscle transfers. Donor sites for free muscle transfer include the gracilis, pectoralis minor, latissimus dorsi, or rectus abdominus. The gracilis muscle is favored by most surgeons as it is the best match with existing facial muscle mass, and its harvest site is well hidden. Other donor sites have drawbacks related to their large bulk of muscle mass, which makes them less acceptable alternatives than the gracilis muscle transfer.[8]

Neural input to the free muscle transfer can be provided in a variety of ways. Whenever possible, the ipsilateral facial nerve should be anastomosed to the motor branch of the free muscle transfer. This is possible only in cases of traumatic or surgical tissue loss involving the muscles of facial expression. Cross-facial nerve grafting may be used to help provide symmetrical, emotional facial muscle contraction, but this result is rarely realized. Cross-facial nerve grafting usually does not supply adequate neural input and contractile power to the transferred muscle to achieve the desired result. The use of an end-to-side anastomosis between the motor nerve of the transferred muscle and the ipsilateral seventh nerve, as previously described for the seventh to twelfth nerve end-to-side procedure, followed by retraining and rehabilitation, usually leads to a far better aesthetic and functional outcome (Fig 4, A and B).

ANCILLARY PROCEDURES IN THE TREATMENT OF CHRONIC FACIAL PARALYSIS

Ancillary procedures enhance the aesthetic and functional results obtained with the procedures thus far described. They are essential to achieving superior surgical results. Ancillary procedures should be performed only after maximum benefit of the primary procedures has been achieved. They include brow lifting, rhytidectomy, the use of autologous and nonautologous implants, and Botox.[7,9,10]

In contemporary management of facial nerve paralysis, endoscopic brow lifting has replaced all other methods of forehead, brow, temporal, and midface rejuvenation and restoration of static symmetry. The advantages of the endoscopic subperiosteal dissection include its ability to lift the midface and malar fatpad with minimal potential for facial nerve damage while still achieving a long-lasting elevation of soft tissue, making it a superior way to achieve facial balance and symmetry. With the advent of resorbable screw fixation devices and long-acting, yet resorbable suture materials for fixation of the elevated brow, malar fatpad, and temporal area, the problem of achieving exact, long-lasting results with endoscopic facial plastic surgery has been reduced.

Deep-plane or tri-plane rhytidectomy with buccal fatpad repositioning to bring about further soft tissue symmetry between the affected and nonaffected side is the method of choice for restoring

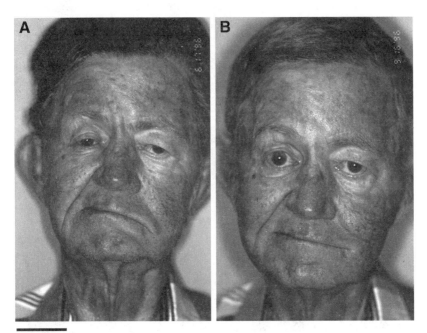

FIGURE 5.
A, Preoperative. B, Postoperative, showing results of ancillary procedures (deep-plane facelift, endoscopic browlift, and platysma plication) and temporalis muscle transfer in a 72-year-old male with a long-standing left facial paralysis.

static symmetry to the lower two thirds of the face. Deep-plane or tri-plane techniques of facelifting allow for removal of excessive wrinkled or lax skin on the paralyzed side of the face. They also permit repositioning of soft tissues that tend to sag further inferiorly and to a greater degree than do the tissues on the nonparalyzed side. The ability to reposition this soft tissue provides a long-lasting, natural appearance and symmetry of facial features (Fig 5, A and B).

Autologous and nonautologous implants such as fat injections, submalar implants, Gore-Tex, and Alloderm,[7] to fill in soft tissue losses and provide mechanical support of sagging, soft tissues are useful adjuncts in the management of long-term, chronic facial muscle atrophy. Autologous fat injections, when properly performed, are long lasting. There is little or no resorption, and they virtually eliminate small depressions caused by muscle and soft tissue atrophy that result from long-term facial paralysis. Nonautologous, nonresorbable implants such as solid silicone, rolled Gore-Tex, or Alloderm can be used to fill in larger, soft tissue losses in which the volume of fat required is too great and the risk of fat resorption is too high. Strips of Gore-Tex can also be used as static support of areas in which neural or muscle transfers have not provided the desired symmetry at rest. The key to successful use of Gore-Tex is placement of the implant at the same point of origin and insertion as the muscle whose effect is being recreated. The use of gold weights to provide upper eyelid closure and protection is the standard of care for all cases of incomplete eye closure associated with facial paralysis. Although some surgeons have noted success with upper eyelid springs, most authors report the extrusion rate and complications with this procedure to be extremely high. Botulinum toxin or limited myectomys, especially around the eye and platysmal muscle, can be used to manage the problems of synkinesis, twitching, or mass motion that commonly affect these areas. Botulinum toxin, although not a permanent solution, can usually render better overall appearance with fewer side effects and a higher degree of accuracy than myectomy.

In summary, contemporary management of facial nerve paralysis has evolved from a relatively small number of procedures with limited goals and success to a complex arena of procedures used either alone or in concert with others. When undertaken in conjunction with postoperative therapy, rehabilitation, and retraining, successful restoration of nearly normal facial nerve function can be the result. This is an opportunity for the otolaryngologist or facial plastic surgeon to have a dramatic impact on a significant group of patients. Although our surgical results have improved significantly in recent years, we can be confident that advancing knowledge and technology will allow even more dramatic outcomes in the future.

REFERENCES

1. Burkey B, Coleman JR: The selection of rehabilitation techniques and the timing of procedures in facial reanimation. *Facial Plast Surg Clin North Am* 5:279-285, 1997.
2. May M: Facial nerve grafting, in *Complications in Otolaryngology–Head and Neck Surgery. Volume 1: Ear and Skull Base.* Philadelphia: B.C. Decker, 1986, pp 87-89.
3. Jung TM, Alford EL, Telian SA, et al: An end-to-side cranial nerve VII to cranial nerve XII anastomosis. Presented at the American Neurotology Society, Palm Springs, California, May 8, 1996.
4. May M, Sobol SM, Mester SJ: Hypoglossal-facial nerve interpositional-jump graft for facial reanimation without tongue atrophy. *Otolaryngol Head Neck Surg* 104:818-825, 1991.
5. McKenna MJ, Cheney ML, Borodic G, et al: Management of facial paralysis after intracranial surgery. *Contemp Neurol* 13:159-165, 1991.

6. Edgerton MJ, Turek DB, Fischer JC: Surgical treatment of Mobius syndrome by platysma and temporalis muscle transfers. *Plast Reconstr Surg* 55:3305, 1975.

7. Alford EL: Temporalis and masseter muscle transfer for facial paralysis. *Facial Plast Surg Clin North Am* 5:241-245, 1997.

8. Fong B, Shindo M: Dynamic facial reanimation using free tissue transfer. *Facial Plast Surg Clin North Am* 5:247-255, 1997.

9. Alford EL: Eyelid reanimation procedures, in Bailey BJ, ed: *Atlas of Head and Neck Surgery–Otolaryngology.* Philadelphia, J. B. Lippincott Co, 1996, pp 374-375.

10. Biglan AW, May M, Bowers RA: Management of facial spasm with *Clostridium botulinum* toxin, type A (Oculinum). *Arch Otolaryngol Head Neck Surg* 114:1407-1412, 1998.

CHAPTER 12

Rhytidectomy in the Male Patient

Ira D. Papel, MD
Associate Professor, Division of Facial Plastic and Reconstructive
Surgery, Department of Otolaryngology—Head and Neck Surgery, The
Johns Hopkins Medical Institutions, Baltimore, Md

Daniel F. Jiannetto, MD
Fellow in Facial Plastic and Reconstructive Surgery, American Academy
of Facial Plastic and Reconstructive Surgery, Baltimore, Md

S trategies for rhytidectomy for the male patient are examined, with advances and trends discussed and analyzed. Differences in the procedure for males and females have been illustrated by examining the doctor-patient interaction and planning process, from initial consultation through the late postoperative period.

The concept of self-adornment in society is an old one. In Western society, women who seek cosmetic surgery are well accepted. Men do not commonly seek cosmetic surgery, although this prejudice seems to be fading. Western society places great emphasis on a youthful, energetic appearance for both men and women. Competition at work is high, and many middle-aged men who seek a competitive edge are turning to cosmetic surgery. The benefits of improved self-image extend beyond the workplace to social spheres. Men have long known to maintain their appearance with diet, exercise, and good grooming. They are beginning to view cosmetic surgery in the same positive light.

The number of men pursuing cosmetic facial surgery is increasing. Men accounted for approximately 10% of all patients requesting rhytidectomy in the early 1990s. In some practices, men may comprise 25% of rhytidectomy patients.[1-3] Therefore, it is prudent for the facial plastic surgeon to be familiar with the special considerations and techniques in rhytidectomy for men.

HISTORICAL REVIEW

To appreciate such considerations and techniques, a brief historical review is necessary. In 1916, Lexer[4] was one of the first to publish a detailed description of a subcutaneous rhytidectomy. This approach, with many modifications, was used extensively until the 1970s. Rhytidectomy is a procedure in evolution.

In 1974, Skoog[5] published descriptions of platysma elevation with the cutaneous flap. This approach emphasized improvement in the contour of the neck and jowl region but did not address the midface adequately. In a landmark article in 1976, Mitz and Peyronie[6] described the concept of the superficial musculoaponeurotic system (SMAS) in the midface. In this description, the SMAS envelops all the muscles of facial expression and is a distinct fascial layer superficial to the parotideomasseteric fascia. Appreciation of the surgical significance of this structure led to the development of rhytidectomy procedures that plicate or imbricate this layer for the purpose of obtaining better and longer-lasting facial rejuvenation. In the standard SMAS rhytidectomy, skin is first elevated superficial to the SMAS before it is modified. The overall results of the SMAS rhytidectomy were an improvement over those of subcutaneous rhytidectomy, especially in the jawline and neck. However, rejuvenation in the areas of the medial cheek and nasolabial folds was still lacking.[4]

In 1990, Hamra[7] described the deep-plane rhytidectomy. The goal of this technique is to address the medial cheek and nasolabial fold region. One highlight of this technique is minimal subcutaneous dissection, keeping the intimate relationships of the skin to SMAS and platysma. A thick musculocutaneous flap is developed by dissection in the preplatysmal plane below the jawline and the subplatysmal plane in the midface. The malar fat pad is included with the flap after separation from the underlying zygomaticus musculature. The orbicularis oculi muscle is deep to the plane of dissection. Dissection is carried medially and anterior to the parotid, where branches of the facial nerve become more superficial.

Hamra[8] described the composite rhytidectomy in 1992. To improve rejuvenation in the periorbital region, the orbicularis oculi muscle was raised with the musculocutaneous flap previously described in the deep-plane rhytidectomy. In experienced hands, complications have been comparable to the standard SMAS rhytidectomy. For selected patients, this technique may provide improved results in the midface and nasolabial region and is a safe alternative to standard SMAS rhytidectomy.[4]

Ramirez[9] in 1994 described the subperiosteal facelift. This technique frees the midface and periorbital regions by endoscopic dissection in the subperiosteal plane from both forehead and sublabial approaches. Repositioning of the resulting composite flap attempts to create a more harmonious result. This approach has been helpful for rejuvenation of the forehead and brow. Midface results have been mixed, and further analysis is required before any conclusions may be reached regarding the efficacy of this approach.[4]

Rhytidectomy will continue to evolve into the new millennium. Advances in technology, innovative approaches, and refinement of established methods will contribute to the process.

PREOPERATIVE CONSIDERATIONS

As with any cosmetic procedure, patient selection is extremely important. At the first meeting with the patient, psychological factors must be assessed along with physical attributes. The patient's goals and motivations for seeking surgery are ascertained. Patients with unrealistic expectations, those who display overly manipulative or aggressive behavior, or those suffering from psychiatric disorders such as depression are identified. These patients may not be psychologically fit to undergo surgery. It is up to the surgeon to decide whether to proceed. No specific preoperative test can screen for potential psychiatric problems.[4,10]

The male patient's concerns are centered more on the midface, nasolabial folds, and neck. Women, on the other hand, seem to place greater emphasis on the upper third of the face and eyes in addition to the midface and neck. The majority of men seeking rhytidectomy are middle-aged professionals or businessmen with busy and demanding lifestyles.[2,4,11] Men can be demanding with regard to expectations and services. Most do not wear makeup and, therefore, may accept scars less readily. In general, men do not change hairstyle or appearance as often as women do; therefore, it may be assumed that they will accept severe self-image changes poorly. It may be wise to consider staged procedures if extensive surgery is planned in addition to rhytidectomy. Because most men have few peers who have had rhytidectomy, unrealistic expectations may exist with regard to results and recovery times. These psychological differences between the sexes, along with physical constraints unique to men, mandate a thorough discussion of the entire surgical process from the first consultation through return to social and business activity.[2] Significant time must be expended by the surgeon on preoperative patient education.

There is no ideal age for facelift surgery. Patients who are well into their 80s can be good candidates, provided they are in good general health. A thorough medical history is taken. Particular attention is paid to eliciting a history of cardiovascular or pulmonary problems. Men have a higher incidence of these problems during the ages when rhytidectomy is usually sought.

Other areas of concern are a history of diabetes, hypothyroidism, connective tissue diseases, previous problems in healing, bruising, or bleeding, scarring, intolerance to previous local or general anesthesia, allergies to medications or iodine, present medications, and vitamins. Aspirin or anti-inflammatory drugs and smoking present special risks. Patients must discontinue use of aspirin and related products 2 weeks before surgery, and smoking should be stopped 4 weeks before surgery. Failure to do so greatly increases the chances of hematoma and flap necrosis.[12] Depending on the patient's age and medical history, appropriate laboratory, electrocardiography, chest radiographs, or other studies are ordered. Patients should have an independent medical evaluation by their family practitioner or internist before surgery.[4]

The physical examination during the consultation includes a complete head and neck evaluation with cranial nerve examination. Asymmetry is noted and signs of aging documented. Attention is paid to skin condition and characteristics of the facial skeleton. In a systematic fashion, the brow position, nasolabial folds, jowls, condition of the platysma, and neck are examined. For men, special attention is paid to the beard pattern and the position of the temporal and occipital hairline. Frontal hairline and male pattern baldness are noted, especially if the brow needs intervention.

The need for ancillary procedures to maximize facial harmony and rejuvenation also is assessed. Common procedures include browlift, blepharoplasty, mentoplasty, malarplasty. Indications for adjunct techniques, such as direct excision of nasolabial folds and midline neck, are noted.[13]

At this point, a surgical plan is formulated and discussed with the patient. Normal sequelae of male rhytidectomy, such as alterations in beard pattern and hairline and scar location, are reviewed. The patient must be told that bearded skin may be advanced behind the ear, which may require that this area be shaved. Transient periauricular hypoesthesia should be mentioned. Suggestions such as using an electric razor until normal sensation returns may be given. The incisions used in men attempt to preserve the natural contour of the temporal tuft of hair, the hairless area immediately in front and below the ear, and the postauricular hairline. It must be explained that resulting scars may be more apparent because of these constraints. Recommendations for any ancillary procedures are then made, if indicated. If a browlift is contemplated, potential alterations in the frontal hairline with standard techniques should be addressed. Patients exhibiting signs of male pattern baldness will benefit from an endoscopic approach to the brow, thereby avoiding large incisions, concomitant scarring, further alopecia, and significant alteration of the frontal hairline.[4]

A thorough discussion of risks versus benefits and possible common complications of the procedure then ensues. Complications to be outlined include bleeding, hematoma, infection, tissue necrosis, temporary or permanent hypoesthesia or anesthesia of the lateral face and earlobe, facial nerve injury, scarring, alopecia, deformity of the earlobe, and significant alteration of hairline and beard patterns.

The type of anesthesia is also agreed on. Local anesthesia with intravenous sedation or general anesthesia can be used safely. The patient and surgeon, in conjunction with the anesthesiologist or anesthetist, guide the choice. The senior author prefers general anesthesia. If deep plane lifting techniques are used, it is more difficult to get an adequate level of local anesthesia in the anterior midface region without affecting branches of the facial nerve. General anesthesia is more suited to patient comfort and airway control in lengthy cases. After all questions are answered, informed consent must be obtained.

Photographs are taken in multiple views. Standard views include frontal, profiles, three-quarter, and submental. If computer-imaging equipment is available, it may be used at this time. Computer imaging is of some value, especially in the profile view, for illustrating expected changes in the jawline and neck. However, it must be used with some caution because it can create expectations that are not easily attainable.[14] Showing previous patients' preoperative and postoperative photographs is also of some value. Photographs and imaging are an integral part of the planning process and are important for documentation and teaching purposes.

At the conclusion of the consultation, a decision is made about whether additional preoperative visits are required to answer all questions. Printed information and preoperative instructions are given for home review. Financial arrangements and scheduling are then discussed.[4]

INTRAOPERATIVE CONSIDERATIONS

On the day of surgery, the patient arrives early at the surgical facility. An operative gown is provided and the patient is brought to the preoperative area. With the patient in the seated position, all incisions are drawn on the skin (Fig 1). This reiterates the location of the final scars and takes into account the effects of gravity on the tissues when the patient assumes a supine position intraoperatively. The incisions drawn attempt to preserve the male characteristics of the hairline and beard. Superiorly, the incision follows the anterior edge of the temporal hair tuft extending slightly posterior to the superior aspect of the auricle. Sweeping anteriorly and inferiorly, the incision is located 1 cm anterior to the tragus to preserve the hairless strip of skin. This is continued inferior to the crease of the earlobe, then superiorly and posteriorly up onto the posterior auricular skin to the level of the superior ear canal. Crossing the crease with a W-plasty, the incision runs along the occipital hairline at its inferior edge, or it may extend inside the hair. Before sedation is administered, all questions are answered

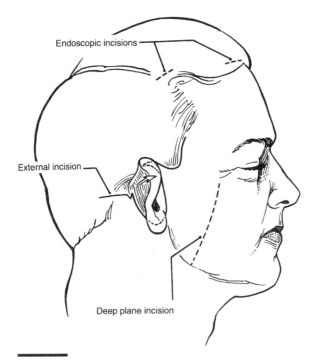

Endoscopic incisions

External incision

Deep plane incision

FIGURE 1.
Incisions used in rhytidectomy in men. (Courtesy of Papel ID, Lee EL: *Facial Plast Surg* 12:257-263, 1996.)

and the procedure is reviewed again. If informed consent has not been obtained, it should be done now.[11]

The patient is now brought to the operating suite. The senior author prefers general anesthesia for the reasons previously discussed. The endotracheal tube is secured to the upper central incisors with dental floss. The hair is stabilized clear of scalp incisions without shaving. Incisions on the face and scalp and areas designated for direct undermining or suction-assisted lipectomy are infiltrated with 1% lidocaine with 1:100,000 epinephrine. If an endoscopic browlift is planned, the superior bony orbital rims also are infiltrated. It is the senior author's preference to perform any scheduled browlift before blepharoplasty or rhytidectomy. This order allows better appreciation of the actual tissue laxity around the eyes and in the temporal hairline region. The face, neck, and scalp are then completely prepped and draped.

The deep-plane rhytidectomy technique for men is preferred by the senior author for several reasons. The presence of a beard is associated with an extensive subdermal plexus of blood vessels. This characteristic has been cited as a source of increased incidence of hematoma among men—about 6%, 2 to 3 times the incidence reported for women.[2] The deep-plane lift creates a myocutaneous flap with superior blood supply and less risk of bleeding from the subdermal plexus.[15] The deep-plane lift technique minimizes the actual subcutaneous dissection. This technique also addresses more directly the problem of laxity of the nasolabial folds that is common among men.[7]

Making skin incisions with a 15 blade on one side of the face begins the operation. The hairline incisions are beveled to promote hair growth through the scar. Cutaneous undermining to a limited, predetermined extent is carried out. The superior portion of the dissection adjacent to the temporal hair tuft is in a subcutaneous plane. If desired, an alternative incision may be curved superiorly and posteriorly into the hair, and then the plane becomes subgaleal. Immediately anterior to the ear, the dissection proceeds subcutaneously, approximately 2 to 3 cm. The subcutaneous line of dissection in the midface extends from the anterior zygoma along a line inferior to the angle of the mandible. The inferior dissection is carried subcutaneously anteriorly from the posterior auricular and occipital hairline incisions to the posterior border of the platysma below the mandible. A supraplatysmal plane is then developed and carried toward the midline to a variable degree, depending on the surgeon's preference. This plane is directly above the muscle and is deeper than the subcutaneous plane in an attempt to elevate all of the fat with the skin.

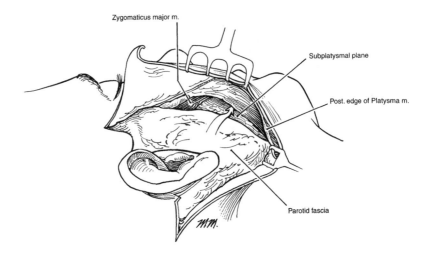

Zygomaticus major m.

Subplatysmal plane

Post. edge of Platysma m.

Parotid fascia

FIGURE 2.
Flap elevation for deep plane rhytidectomy. (Courtesy of Papel ID, Lee EL: *Facial Plast Surg* 12:257-263, 1996.)

The deep plane is now entered in the midface. Under direct vision with proper retraction, an incision is made in the thin SMAS/platysma layer, extending from the zygoma to the angle of the mandible. Dissection continues anteriorly toward the nasolabial fold region with blunt scissors. Superiorly, the zygomaticus major muscle is identified just below the orbicularis oculi muscle. The dissection proceeds inferiorly just superficial to the zygomaticus major to its confluence with the orbicularis oris muscle at the modiolus, which is preserved. This frees the malar fat pad from the deeper tissue, allowing it to be repositioned with the musculocutaneous flap. The proper level of dissection in the sub-SMAS/platysma plane is just above the parotideomasseteric fascia. Below this fascia lie the branches of the facial nerve as they exit the anterior border of the parotid, coursing superficially toward the undersurface of the muscles of facial expression (Fig 2).

Attention then turns to the left side of the face, and the identical dissection is performed. After this side is completed, but before the myocutaneous flaps are advanced and rotated, the anterior neck and platysma are addressed. A submental incision is made and fat is removed either directly or with suction-assisted lipectomy. Depending on the extent of the preplatysmal dissections laterally, the right and left dissections may be joined. The medial borders of the platysma are then plicated with 3.0 polyglactin 910, burying the knot in an interrupted fashion to the level of the hyoid. It is usually not necessary to transect the muscle at the hyoid; however, a partial incision may be done if needed to avoid a bowstring deformity.

Rotation-advancement of the musculocutaneous flap in a superioposterior direction is then accomplished starting on the right side of the face. The senior author prefers 3.0 permanent suture, such as silk or other material, for fixation. The posterior border of the platysma is sutured to the preauricular fascia near the lobule of the ear. Advancement and fixation of SMAS/platysma to preauricular parotid fascia in the superior portion of the upper face flap are then accomplished in a similar fashion. Inferior to the mandible, the posterior edge of the platysma is sutured to mastoid periosteum (Fig 3).

Skin closure is then performed in the standard fashion. Tacking sutures are placed anterosuperior and posterosuperior to the ear. The flap is tailored, and redundant skin is excised. The dog-ear that results in the temporal area is addressed by excising non–hair-bearing facial skin. Periauricular trimming, with attention to creating a natural earlobe, is accomplished. The posterior auricular W-plasty is carefully approximated. Incisions in the hair-bearing scalp are closed with staples. Cutaneous closure, including the

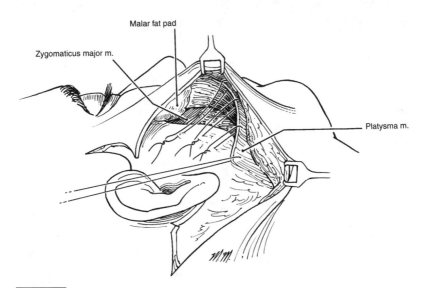

FIGURE 3.
Midface fixation sutures. (Courtesy of Papel ID, Lee EL: *Facial Plast Surg* 12:257-263, 1996.)

submental incision, is accomplished with running and interrupted 5.0 nylon suture. Drains usually are not necessary. A bulky compression dressing is then placed.[11]

POSTOPERATIVE CONSIDERATIONS

After the patient is stable in the recovery room, he may be discharged to a recovery facility or to the care of a family member who has received adequate postoperative instruction. The dressing is kept in place for 24 to 48 hours, depending on the surgeon's preference. During this time, adequate analgesia is maintained. The patient is instructed to sleep with the head of the bed elevated and to avoid straining or exertion. Instruction is given to report any severe pain or bleeding immediately, which may herald a hematoma. When the patient returns to the office, the bulky dressing is taken down. Incisions are examined and cleaned, and instructions are reinforced. A lighter compression dressing is applied and is to be worn for 1 week. The patient returns on postoperative day 7 to have all staples and sutures removed. Restriction of strenuous activity is encouraged for 2 weeks postoperatively, followed by a gradual return to the preoperative level of activity.

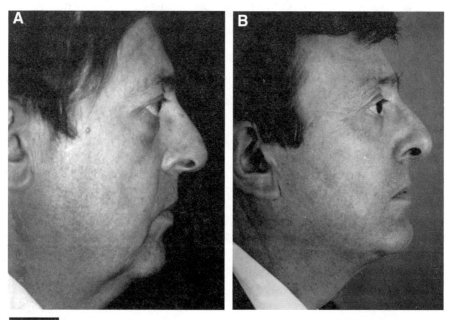

FIGURE 4.
A 60-year-old rhytidectomy patient. **A,** Preoperative. **B,** Postoperative.

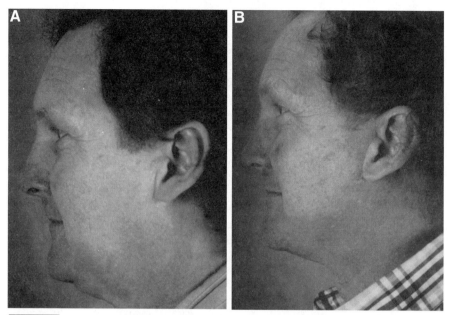

FIGURE 5.
A 55-year-old rhytidectomy patient. **A,** Preoperative. **B,** Postoperative.

Generally the patient may return to work as soon as the ecchymosis resolves, at about 2 weeks. Later postoperative visits are scheduled as needed to assess progress (Figs 4,*A* and *B* and 5,*A* and *B*).

In the immediate postoperative period, men are less likely to ask for pain medication. On the other hand, men tend to be more difficult to manage and are generally more impatient with regard to resolution of ecchymosis and swelling.

In the later postoperative period, men complain less about minor problems and tend to be pleased with the result. They request revision surgery less often and will seek a second facelift about half often as their female counterparts.[2,11]

Hematoma is the only complication that occurs with greater frequency among men. Management includes early recognition of the hematoma, with immediate evacuation and drainage. If concomitant tissue loss occurs, local wound care and débridement, along with reassurance, will minimize scarring. Healing by secondary intent is often adequate, and grafting is rarely needed. Minor alterations of beard pattern and hairline along with transient alopecia are to be expected, as discussed. Major alterations may be treated with hair grafting and flap transposition techniques.[4,16-19]

SUMMARY

Goals of male rhytidectomy address the concerns of the patient while attempting to preserve male characteristics and to avoid complications. Psychological and anatomical differences require modifications in management and technique. The combination of the deep-plane rhytidectomy technique with modified incisions and endoscopic brow intervention provides predictable results with minimal complications. For men, the rhytidectomy procedure offers some unique challenges. When handled appropriately, a satisfied patient with a good result can be expected.

REFERENCES

1. Vistnes L, Jobe R: Rhytidectomy, with emphasis on the differences between males and females, in Courtiss EH (ed): *Male Aesthetic Surgery.* St Louis, Mosby, 1982, pp 253-262.
2. Baker TJ: Face-lift, in Courtiss EH (ed): *Male Aesthetic Surgery,* ed 2. St Louis, Mosby, 1991, pp 347-364.
3. McCollough EG: Facelifting in the male patient. *Facial Plast Surg Clin North Am* 1:217-229, 1993.
4. Papel ID: Advances in rhytidectomy, in Gluckman JL (ed): *Renewal of Certification Study Guide in Otolaryngology—Head and Neck Surgery.* Dubuque, Kendall/Hunt, 1998, pp 586-590.
5. Skoog T: *Plastic surgery: New methods and refinements.* Philadelphia, WB Saunders, 1974.
6. Mitz V, Peyronie M: The superficial musculoaponeurotic system (SMAS) in the parotid and cheek area. *Plast Reconstr Surg* 58:80-88, 1976.
7. Hamra S: The deep-plane rhytidectomy. *Plast Reconstr Surg* 86:53-68, 1990.
8. Hamra S: Composite rhytidectomy. *Plast Reconstr Surg* 90:1-21, 1992.
9. Ramirez OM: Endoscopic techniques in facial rejuvenation: An overview. I. *Aesthetic Plast Surg* 18:141, 1994.
10. Goin J, Goin M: *Changing the body image: The psychological effects of plastic surgery.* Baltimore, Williams & Wilkins, 1981.
11. Papel ID, Lee EL: The male facelift: Considerations and techniques. Facial Plast Surg 12: 257-263, 1996.
12. Rees TD, Liverett DM, Guy CL: The effect of cigarette smoking on skin flap survival in the face lift patient. *Plast Reconstr Surg* 73:911-915, 1984.
13. Miller TA, Orringer JS: Excision of neck redundancy with single Z-plasty closure. *Plast Reconstr Surg* 97:219-221, 1996.
14. Papel ID, Schoenrock LD: Computer imaging, in Papel ID, Nachlas NE (eds): *Facial Plastic and Reconstructive Surgery.* St Louis, Mosby, 1992, pp 110-115.

15. Schuster RH, Gamble WB, Hamra ST: A comparison of flap vascular anatomy in three rhytidectomy techniques. *Plast Reconstr Surg* 90:683-690, 1992.

16. Barrera A: The use of micrografts and minigrafts for the correction of the postrhytidectomy lost sideburn. *Plast Reconstr Surg* 102:2237-2240, 1998.

17. Juri J: Sideburn reconstruction in secondary lifting. *Plast Reconstr Surg* 102:2241-2243, 1998.

18. Marten TJ: Hairline lowering during foreheadplasty. *Plast Reconstr Surg* 103:224-236, 1999.

19. Hamas RS, Rohrich RJ: Preventing hairline elevation in endoscopic browlifts. *Plast Reconstr Surg* 99:1018-1022, 1997.

SUGGESTED READING

Baker TJ: Face-lift, in Courtiss EH (ed): *Male Aesthetic Surgery*, ed 2. St Louis, Mosby, 1991, pp 347-364.

Hamra ST: *Composite rhytidectomy*. St Louis, Quality Medical, 1993.

McCollough EG: Facelifting in the male patient. *Facial Plast Surg Clin North Am* 1:217-229, 1993.

Mitz V, Peyronie M: The superficial musculoaponeurotic system (SMAS) in the parotid and cheek area. *Plast Reconstr Surg* 58:80-88, 1976.

Owsley JQ: *Aesthetic Facial Surgery*. Philadelphia, WB Saunders, 1994.

Rees TD: *Aesthetic Plastic Surgery*. Philadelphia, WB Saunders, 1980.

CHAPTER 13

Laser Hair Modification

W. Gregory Chernoff, MD, BSc, FRCS(C)

Clinical Assistant Professor, Indiana University, Indianapolis

Unwanted hair is an aesthetic problem that has plagued women and men alike for centuries. Hair has most commonly been removed by shaving or by mechanical epilation with waxes or epilating devices. Various epilating products have also appeared on the market. For decades, electrolysis was the only treatment considered to be a permanent solution for superfluous hair. The American Electrology Association was founded in 1958. This not-for-profit professional organization strives to maintain the highest of standards of education and professional practice, endeavoring to provide consistency in the state licensing and regulation of the electrology profession.

In the past 5 years tremendous strides have been made in the field of laser technology and its use in modifying hair growth. The focus of most research has been 2-fold: first, to more closely narrow the "ideal" wavelength, for the purposes of causing damage to the hair follicle, and second, to more closely identify which anatomical portion of the hair follicle is the best target for the laser.

Unwanted hair can be caused by hereditary, malignant, or endochronologic diseases such as hypertrichosis (ie, excess hair) and hirsutism (ie, androgen-influenced hair). Hirsutism in women, especially if it involves the face, can have a tremendously negative effect on self-esteem. Temporary hair removal has been a major component in the management of hirsute patients. Hair can be temporarily removed with the use of a number of techniques, including wax epilation, depilatory creams, and shaving, the most frequently used method. Careful plucking can be helpful, if tolerated; however, folliculitis, hyperpigmentation, and scarring have been associated with excessively aggressively plucking. Waxing and depilatory agents are used by less than 5% of patients on the face and by 20% on other parts of the body.

The physician should keep abreast with the rapid evolution of improved laser technology and have a good working knowledge about the choices of wavelengths available, their respective advantages, and potential disadvantages.

ANATOMY AND PHYSIOLOGY

It is critical that one understand the anatomy of the hair follicle and the associated physiology as it pertains to hair removal or modification. The histologic appearance of the hair follicle varies with the stage of hair growth in the region being examined.

Hair follicles develop embryologically through a complex series of interactions between the epidermis and the dermis. Anatomically, hair follicles consist of 3 distinct units: the hair bulb, the isthmus, and infundibulum. The hair bulb is the region that extends from the base of the follicle to the insertion site of the arrectores pilorum muscle. The isthmus encompasses the region between the arrectores pilorum insertion in the entrance of the sebaceous duct. The infundibulum includes the region from the sebaceous duct entrance to the hair follicle orifice. Several key elements also add to the composition of the hair follicle. These are the dermal papillae, the hair matrix, and the hair shaft. The cellular linings from interior to exterior include the cuticle, the inner root sheath, Huxley's layer, the outer root sheath, and the vitreous layer.

The histologic appearance of the hair follicle changes with the stage of hair growth in the region being examined. There are 3 distinct phases of growth: the anagen, or the active growth, phase; the telogen, or resting, phase; and the catagen, or the regression, phase. At any given time, in any given region of the body, different percentages of hairs are in the growth and resting phases. The length of time of the growth phase in each region of the body also differs, from an average of 6 months to 1 year. This becomes important when considering words such as *permanent, removal,* and *modification.* The anagen, or growth, phase yields to the catagen, or regression, phase. The telogen, or resting, phase follows just before the resumption of the anagen phase. The anagen phase is variable and can last up to 3 years. The catagen phase is relatively constant and lasts usually 3 weeks. Telogen usually lasts for 3 months. In any region of the body, the majority of hair follicles are in anagen, while the remaining follicles are in either the catagen or the telogen phase.

Hair follicle sensation occurs by the terminal arborization of nonmyelinated fibers that terminate in specialized nerve and organs. The vascular supply of the hair follicles is provided by a plexus from arterial and venous capillaries as well as from post-capillary venules. These are similar to capillary loops that supply the dermal papillae.

Control over the hair cycle appears to be linked to a complex interaction between the bulge and the papilla of the hair. The 2 primary targets for permanent hair reduction appear to be the region of the bulge that lies near the insertion of the arrector pili muscle and the papilla that extends beyond the dermis, typically 3- to 7-mm deep. Part of the difficulty in eradicating unwanted or excess hair lies in the fact that the follicle has tremendous regenerative capabilities. These capabilities are highly variable among individuals and from one anatomical site to another. The bulge area of the follicle is the chief source of follicular germinal cells. These cells appear to represent a subpopulation of the outer root sheath and possess many features common to stem cells. These are relatively undifferentiated and slow cycling, but can undergo rapid proliferation in response to various signals.

The development of localized or diffuse unwanted hair may occur in association with many inherited syndromes, the use of certain medications, the presence of ovarian or adrenal tumors, and as a normal variant. Hypertrichosis is defined as the presence of increased hair in men or women at any body site, while hirsutism is the term that is typically reserved for the presence of excess hair in women only at androgen-dependent sites.

ELECTROLYSIS AND ELECTROTHERMOLYSIS

The only hair removal technique that can permanently remove hair is electrosurgery. There are two accepted modalities. In "electrolysis," a direct (DC) current is passed into the deep portion of the follicles via electrodes. This results in tissue damage and the destruction of hair follicles by the creation of a chemical reaction occurring at the tip of one of the electrodes. In "electrothermolysis," resistive heating by higher resonant frequency current causes local thermal destruction of the follicles. "Electrothermolysis" is, by far, the more common method, because it can be done quickly. The literature confuses these two terms and typically utilizes the term "electrolysis" to describe any procedure in which electrical current is used for destroying hair.

Both methods are technique dependent and require skill. Each follicle must be entered separately with the electrode. Most needles used in epilation are very finely tapered or are untapered needles with rounded or bulbous tips. An insulated needle for epilation, introduced in 1983, limits heat generation to the base of the follicle only. The insulated probe produces greater damage to the deep peri-bulbar tissue and less necrosis of the upper peri-follicular dermis, thereby reducing the chance of scarring. Correct placement of the insulated needle remains important. The needle is typically inserted into the follicular infundibulum parallel to the hair shaft and advanced slowly until the base of the follicle is reached and resistance is felt. Pain may indicate perforation of the follicular wall or inappropriate placement of the needle tip. Efficacy has not been systematically determined but has been reported to range from 15% to 50% permanent hair loss per treatment. In 1977, when the word "permanent" was approved for electrolysis, the FDA required histologic evidence of damage to the hair follicle before the word could be used. It is unknown what specific conditions affect efficacy, such as age, sex, anatomical site, or depth of hair. Multiple treatments are required with both methods, electrolysis and electrothermolysis, and the process can be painful and tedious, and it is associated with a risk of scarring and infection on the order of 5% to 10%. Electrothermolysis tends to have a higher risk of pain and scarring than galvanic electrolysis. Galvanic electrolysis devices are most often used by lay personnel. They are safer, less painful, and less likely to cause scarring. They are, however, slower than high-frequency electroepilation. With galvanic electrolysis, a bubble of hydrogen gas typically appears at the follicular orifice. This indicates that hydroxides have formed at the base of the follicle causing the desired chemical destruction. The hair papilla has been destroyed when the hair shaft can be removed by gentle traction. A commonly identified problem for both electrolysis and electrothermolysis has been the impracticality of treating large areas of hair growth.

Most aesthetic surgeons work with electrologists to provide permanent hair removal for their patients. For decades, electrolysis has been the only available permanent treatment for unwanted hair. This time-tested modality has been plagued by the problem that very few controlled clinical studies exist, either in the electrologist literature or in the medical literature, specifically highlighting and confirming regrowth rates. Still, most clinicians will routinely inform their patient of the benefits of electrolysis and provide this as one of the treatment options in their armamentarium for the treatment of unwanted hair.

LASERS OR PULSED LIGHT

Lasers and pulsed light sources have recently been introduced as methods of hair modification. These techniques utilize a principle called "selective photothermolysis." Simply stated, a given wavelength of light is absorbed by a specific target. The thermal injury can be restricted to that specific target in a given amount of time, leaving the surrounding tissue unharmed. For there to be an effect on hair growth, damage must be applied to both potential areas of hair follicle germinal cells: the bulge and the papilla. Laser hair modification focuses on laser light being absorbed by melanin in the hair shaft, damaging the follicle epithelium. When an appropriate energy source is directed at the skin, this light is selectively absorbed in the hair shaft melanin and the generated heat diffuses to the surrounding follicular epithelium. Several important parameters for the optimization of laser therapy exist. These include wavelength, fluence, pulse width, number of treatments, and dynamic cooling.

WAVELENGTH

Most laser hair-modification systems are designed to remove unwanted hair through a process coined by Rox Anderson as "selective photothermolysis." Wavelengths between 700 and 1000 nm are selectively absorbed by melanin. Water and oxyhemoglobin are competing chromophores, but between 700 and 1000 nm these competing chromophores absorb less energy than does melanin. Selective photothermolysis involves local selective absorption of the light pulse at wavelengths that are preferentially absorbed by the melanin in hair follicles, but not the surrounding tissue. The wavelength must penetrate adequately into the skin to reach the important targets for inactivation of hair follicles. The laser energy is selectively absorbed by the follicular melanin, which causes thermal damage to the hair shaft and follicle. Sufficient melanin exists in all colors of hair (not in white hair) in the follicular epithelium and matrix to act as the chromophore. Hair growth is subsequently impeded or eliminated, with use of the adequate fluence of the appropriate wavelength, because of the selective damage to the hair follicle.

FLUENCE

Fluence describes energy per unit area. A given amount is necessary to cause follicular damage. While stronger fluences produce better hair-reduction results, the risk of side effects increases as fluence rises.

PULSE WIDTH

The pulse width is one of the most important parameters for achieving effective hair removal. The optimum pulse duration is approximately equal to the thermal relaxation time of the hair follicle. *Thermal relaxation time* is defined as the time required for an object to cool to half the temperature achieved immediately after laser exposure. The thermal relaxation time for follicles of 200 to 300 μm in diameter ranges from 10 to 100 ms. Laser pulses briefer than the thermal relaxation time cause insufficient heating of the target structure (ie, the bulb and papilla). Pulse widths longer than the thermal relaxation time may cause nonselective damage to the surrounding dermis.

NUMBER OF TREATMENTS

The amount of hair reduction per treatment varies among patients, treatment site, and the fluence used per treatment. After each treatment, less hair grows back and the hair that grows back is typically lighter in color and finer in texture.

DYNAMIC COOLING

Because the epidermis also contains melanin, these laser systems can also cause damage to the surrounding epidermis. It has been found that utilizing dynamic cooling allows sufficient laser energy to be delivered to damage hair follicles, while protecting the surrounding epidermis. Since the major targets for hair modification lie at least 1-mm below the skin surface, actively cooling the skin for 0.2 to 1 second allows the epidermal temperature to decrease while the targets remain warm. It has also been found that efficacy increases if the skin can be cooled before, during, and after the laser pulse. Combinations of cooling gels and contact with closed water-loop systems are the most commonly used methods for cooling the skin.

SUMMARY OF SYSTEMS
ND:YAG LASER

The first of the Nd:YAG lasers brought into the market for laser hair modification utilized a photomechanical effect. With poor absorption by melanin at a wavelength of 1064 nm, an oxygenous material placed into the hair follicle was required to absorb the laser energy. This Q-switched Nd:YAG laser employed a topical mineral oil lotion that contained a carbon-based material. This material was applied to the skin surface and massaged into the area to be treated, allowing the lotion to penetrate into the follicle. When the laser energy interacted with the carbon particle, a photomechanical explosion occurred, causing a rapid temperature increase. This thermal energy was thought to cause selective injury to those germinative cells of the follicle in contact with the solution. After the application of the mineral oil/carbon solution, the Nd:YAG laser was utilized with a fluence of 2 to 3 J/cm, a 7-mm spot size, and a pulse duration of 10 ns. Postoperative edema lasted up to 24 hours, with transient erythema being seen for 48 hours. Petechiae were also noted, and these could persist for up to 5 days.

In 1997, Goldberg studied the effect of the topical suspension–assisted Q-switched Nd:YAG laser for hair modification. Thirty-five healthy adult volunteers were treated with a single treatment to selected facial, neck, and axillary sites. Twelve weeks after a single treatment, integrated site scores revealed that the majority of patients had more than 25% fewer hairs. The 12-week mean percentage of hair reduction based on anatomical sites ranged up to 66%.

A newer Nd:YAG laser system with an extended pulse duration operates at a setting between 20 and 100 J/cm with a pulse width ranging from 10 to 50 ms. This laser employs a 5-mm beam diameter with a scanner that covers up to a 25-mm area.

RUBY LASER

The absorption spectrum for melanin is broad; therefore, it overlaps the emission spectrum for a wide variety of lasers. Melanosomes have been targeted by several lasers, including the ruby laser, which delivers light at a wavelength of 695 nm. Melanin is found between matrix cells in the hair bulb and also within the structural elements of the hair shaft, medulla, cortex, and cuticle.

A limiting factor in selecting melanin as the target for hair modification is that it is also found within the epidermis. This can be correlated with the Fitzpatrick classification of skin types, as seen in Table 1. Overzealous therapy can result in epidermal injury, yielding hypopigmentation, hyperpigmentation, or scarring. Epidermal melanin also causes absorptive interference, thereby limiting the amount of light absorbed further down the follicle.

The Epilaser system (Palomar Medical, Lexington, Mass) is a normal mode or non–Q-switched, high-energy pulsed ruby laser. It delivers a 3-ms, 10- to 75-J/cm pulse of red light at a wavelength of 694 nm. A contact cooling handpiece, consisting of a sapphire prism closed-loop system, is used to deliver a convergent beam to the skin with a 20-mm focal length.

The Epitouch laser (Sharplan Lasers [Europe] Ltd, London) is a dual-mode ruby laser designed to operate in a conventional Q-switched mode, as well as in a pulsed mode, for the removal of unwanted hair, similar to the Epilaser system. This system utilizes

TABLE 1.
Fitzpatrick Classification System

Skin Type	Skin Color	Characteristics
I	White	Always burns; never tans
II	White	Usually burns; tans less than average
III	White	Sometimes mild burn; tans about average
IV	White	Rarely burns; tans more than average
V	Brown	Rarely burns; tans profusely
VI	Black	Never burns; deeply pigmented

a cooling device in a transparent gel to minimize reflectants and scattering. The parameters for this system are 0.8-ms pulses with a 4- to 6-mm beam diameter.

In 1998, Dierickx demonstrated hair loss up to 64% ranging from 6 months to 2 years.

Generally speaking, the ruby laser works best on patients with dark hair and light skin such as Fitzpatrick's types I through III. Fitzpatrick's types III through VI, while achieving good hair modification results, are prone to pigmentary changes such as temporary postinflammatory hyperpigmentation and permanent hypopigmentation. Hair color and skin color determine the best fluence to utilize. If tanned patients insist on treatment, 10 to 15 J/cm is typically the maximum fluence used. Fair-skinned types I to III can tolerate the highest fluences; darker skin types should be treated with lower fluences. Treatment should be performed with the highest fluence the skin can tolerate. Studies have shown that the percentage of hair loss depends on the fluence used, with higher percentages of hair loss at higher fluences.

Each skin type has its own threshold fluence at which pigmentation changes occur. To minimize hypopigmentation or hyperpigmentation, one should use, while gaining clinical experience, lower fluences than those suggested. With multiple pulsing, the incidence of pigmentary changes also increases. Therefore, double and triple pulsing is not recommended. An effective fluence is typically one in which the hair carbonizes, followed by very selective follicular swelling and redness. The patient describes a sunburned feeling with mild edema after treatment. This can last anywhere from 2 to 24 hours. If any epidermolysis occurs, the patient should use antibiotic ointment and should be seen daily by the treating physician until it is established that re-epithelialization has occurred satisfactorily.

ALEXANDRITE LASER

Alexandrite systems, such as the Gentle LASE (Candela Corporation) or the Apogee (Cynosure Corporation) system, are cousins to the ruby laser. They utilize wavelengths at 755 nm with pulse durations up to 20 ms. The Candela laser utilizes a cooling device that applies a short burst of cryogen spray to the skin just before the treatment beam.

Generally speaking, the Alexandrite laser yields results similar to that of the ruby laser. Laser hair modification at 1 year is in the 50% to 60% range. Hyperpigmentation and hypopigmentation appear in more than 50% of patients with skin types IV through VI. Erythema is common immediately after treatment and usually resolves in 12 to 48 hours.

LASER DIODE SYSTEM

In 1998, Coherent Medical introduced a new 800-nm high-power, pulsed diode laser system. Laser energy is delivered to the skin surface by means of a water-cooled contact sapphire-chilled tip. The LightSheer diode laser consists of a gallium arsenide diode ray coupled to a novel water-cooled sapphire chilled tip that is placed in contact with the skin during the delivery of the laser energy. A 9-mm imprint can deliver up to 60 J/cm in one of the product's configurations. Select bulb pulse widths range from 5 to 30 ms. Two pulse width selections are available: a fixed 30-ms mode and the Opti Pulse mode, which fixes the pulse duration at one half the delivered fluence. Pulse repetition rate ranges from 1 to 2 Hz.

When compared side by side with the aforementioned systems, the diode system appears to allow for the delivery of higher fluences in darker skin types with improved efficacy of hair modification.

FLASH LAMP

ESC Medical utilizes its flash lamp with a series of filters enabling a wavelength range of 590 to 1200 nanometers. Fluence ranges from 30 to 65 J/cm with a pulse duration of 2.5 to 5 ms. The Epi light utilizes a pulse mode technique which divides the desired fluence into multiple pulses. The subsequent claim was that the Epi light allowed for photo epilation according to hair type being treated and the pigmentation level of the patient's skin. Most scientific studies reveal no greater efficacy than any of the aforementioned systems.

MICROWAVE TECHNOLOGY

Research is ongoing concerning applications of microwave technology. Such a system consists of an electronically controlled unit that simultaneously delivers a pulse of microwave energy and coolant to the surface of the skin through a small-aperture waveguide applicator. Fluences of 9 J delivered for 50 ms have yielded hair modification results comparable with the aforementioned modalities.

PATIENT SELECTION

The great benefit to the patient of the electrologist or the physician is the availability of both electrolysis and laser technology for modifying unwanted hair. Routinely, a combination of electrolysis in facial areas, where permanence is desired, combined with laser hair modification in larger areas, such as the back, legs, arms, and bikini lines, has proved to be a successful combination. The histologic evidence suggests that both systems can successfully damage hair follicles (Figs 1-4). A combination of features contribute to the success of these systems. With each successive treatment, ongoing fibrosis occurs within the hair follicle, leading to a consistent miniaturization of the hair follicle. The hair follicles have a tremendous regenerative potential, yielding smaller follicles near the surface of the skin after treatment. Correlating this clinically, one finds that temporary hair loss occurs in all patients for all hair colors and at all laser fluences. This typically lasts from 1 to 3 months. *Long-term hair reduction* is defined as a

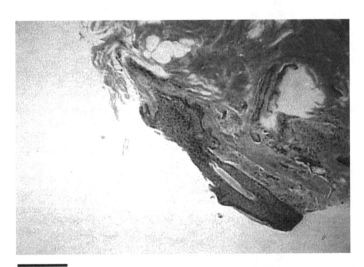

FIGURE 1.
Coherent LightSheer system; 5 treatments 18-30 J/cm² for 30 ms. Note follicular fibrosis, miniaturization with regeneration new follicle.

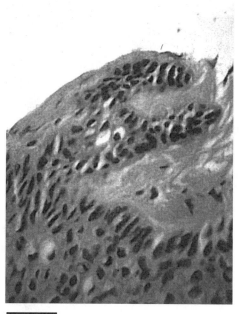

FIGURE 2.
Histology. Coherent LightSheer system; 5 treatments 18-30 J/cm^2 for 30 ms. Follicular regeneration.

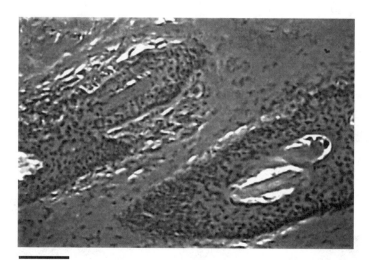

FIGURE 3.
Histology. Laserscope Lyra system; 5 treatments 50 J/cm^2 for 50 ms. Note fibrosis, miniaturization, regeneration new follicle.

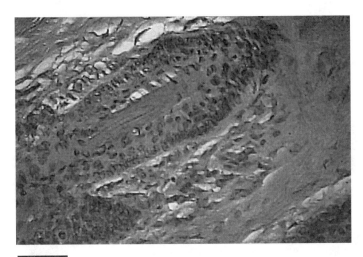

FIGURE 4.
Histology, Laserscope Lyra system; 5 treatments 50 J/cm^2 for 50 ms. Note miniaturization.

significant reduction in the number of terminal hairs at a given body site that is stable for a period of time longer than the follicles' complete growth cycle. Complete hair loss implies that there are no regrowing hairs. This can also be a temporary or a permanent phenomenon. Most laser systems typically produce com-

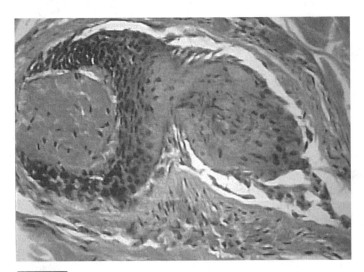

FIGURE 5.
Electrolysis × 4 treatments. Note fibrosis, regeneration new follicle.

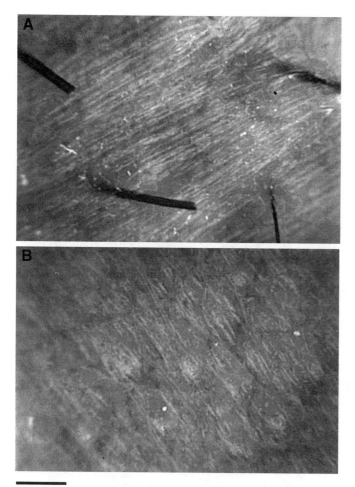

FIGURE 6.
A, Pretreatment. B, Female (45 years old) after 5 treatments at 6 months.

plete, but temporary, hair loss followed by a partial, but long-term, hair reduction.

Those patients who are the happiest with laser hair modification are those with unwanted hair on large areas such as on the legs or back, under arms, and along bikini lines. In most instances, patients with unwanted hair in these regions have stated that they would not undergo electrolysis because of the length of time required per treatment.

By studying hair color and skin type, it is easy to determine which patients will have the best results with laser hair modification. Patients with red, gray, or blond hair can be advised that they should not expect long-term hair reduction. A sun-tanned patient should be instructed to stay out of the sun and to use a bleaching cream and sun block and then to return for treatment when the tan has disappeared.

Since the hair shaft is the chromophore, it is essential that the hair shaft be present in the hair follicle at the time of treatment. Patients are therefore not allowed to pluck, wax, or have electrolysis for a minimum of 6 weeks before undergoing laser therapy. Shaving and depilatory creams are allowed, because they leave the hair shaft in the follicle. It is critical that an adequate patient his-

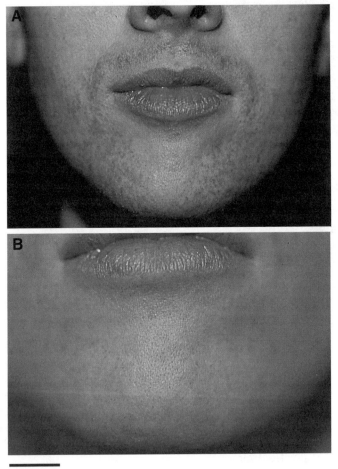

FIGURE 7.
A, Pretreatment. **B,** Female (28 years old) after 6 treatments at 6 months.

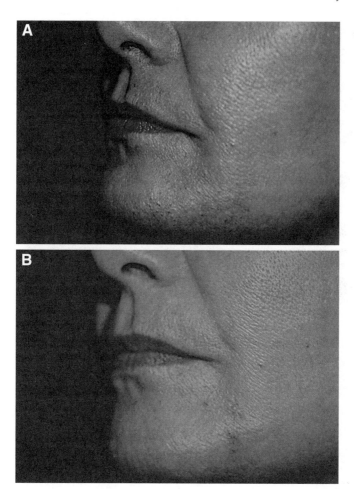

FIGURE 8.
A, Pretreatment. **B,** Female (40 years old) after 6 treatments at 1 year.

tory be taken, with particular attention paid to the endocrine history. Female patients with hirsutism can be treated regardless of the cause. Patients with a history of herpes simplex or genitalis should begin to receive oral antiviral therapy beginning the day before therapy. This is important when treating an upper lip or bikini line because reactivation of herpes simplex and genitalis has been reported after laser therapy. Generally, the drug Acutane should be stopped 6 months to 1 year before laser hair modification. It is critical to match pulse duration and fluence to specific hair color and skin color. This allows for a broad range of thera-

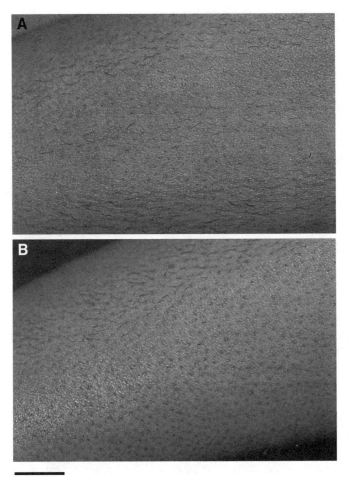

FIGURE 9.
A, Female (25 years old) after 2 treatments. B, Female (25 years old) after 4 treatments.

peutic results. These results can be achieved with few, if any, side effects (Figs 5-9).

SEPARATING FACT FROM FICTION

The great benefit to the patient of the electrologist or the physician is the availability of both electrolysis and lasers for modifying unwanted hair. Within my own office, those who are referring patients for laser hair modification are patients who are also undergoing electrolysis. Routinely, a combination therapy of electrolysis in facial areas where permanence is desired combined with laser hair modification in larger areas, such as the back, legs, arms, and bikini lines, have proved a successful combination to offer patients. The histological evidence suggests that both systems can damage hair follicles. The body's tremendous regenerative capabilities yield sufficient reason why vellous-like hairs regrow in areas of laser hair modification—and electrolysis, in some instances. We are naive to think we can kill something in the body without killing the body. Laser hair modification works tremendously well for some patients, so-so for others, and not well in some instances. The same can be said for electrolysis. Thousands of happy patients have undergone laser hair modification and are shaving areas such as legs, underarms, and bikini lines fewer times during the course of the year than before. These patients openly admit they would not have undergone electrolysis in these areas. Reasons given include perceptions of pain or difficulty in treating larger areas. As mentioned, laser hair modification, in conjunction with electrolysis, is a valuable addition to the armamentarium of therapeutic options available to patients with unwanted hair.

Those instances where honesty and integrity have been compromised through false advertising have tainted the reputations of some physicians involved in the research of these laser systems. "Underselling" the efficacy of these systems has usually yielded the highest degree of satisfaction with patients. After patients are educated on their options of treatment, the ability of providing meticulous care routinely yields very happy patients willing to recommend the treatment modality to others. It behooves physicians and electrologists alike to maintain open doors of communication and common ground in the fields of research, professional practice, and regulation of their respective fields. The future is exciting in the research of laser technology, and further refinements will yield continually improved results. This will benefit patients and therapists alike.

Index

A

Academic performance, and sleep-disordered breathing in children, 5

Accelerators, linear, in frame-based stereotactic surgery, 134-135

Accuracy, in stereotactic surgery, 146, 162

Acoustic neuroma, gamma knife radiosurgery in, 139-141

Adenoidectomy, powered instrumentation for, in children, 33-36
partial, 36

Adenotonsillectomy, for sleep-disordered breathing in children, 6-7

Adolescent
delayed sleep phase syndrome in, 16
thyroid carcinoma in, differentiated, management, 83-84

Aerodigestive tract involvement, in thyroid cancer, management, 81-83

Airway obstruction, and gastroesophageal reflux disease in infants and children, 63

Alexandrite laser systems, hair modification with, 261

Alloderm in chronic facial paralysis, 236-237
for donor site camouflage after temporalis muscle transfer, 234

Alveolar macrophages, lipid-laden, and gastroesophageal reflux disease in infants and children, 58

Amphetamines, for narcolepsy in children, 12-13

Anaerobes in otitis
externa, 169
media, chronic, 168

Anastomosis, twelfth to seventh
end-to-end, for chronic facial paralysis, 231-232
side-to-end, for chronic facial paralysis, 228-229, 230

Anatomy
hair follicle, 254-255
temporomandibular joint, 108-109

Anesthesia, for male rhytidectomy, 243, 245

Angiographic embolization, for epistaxis, 214

Antibiotics, for sinusitis in cystic fibrosis, 45

Antidepressants, for temporomandibular joint syndrome, 118

Anti-inflammatory drugs, nonsteroidal, in temporo-mandibular joint syndrome, 118

Antimicrobial lavage, serial, with endoscopic sinus surgery in cystic fibrosis, 47-48
after lung transplantation, 49

Antrochoanal polyps, powered instrumentation for, in children, 31-32

Antrostomy, large middle meatal, creation during endoscopic sphenopalatine artery ligation for epistaxis, 216

Anxiety, and temporomandibular joint pain, 110

Apnea, and gastroesophageal reflux disease in infants and children, 63-64

Apogee laser system, hair modification with, 261

Appetite, poor, and sleep-disordered breathing in children, 3
Argon plasma coagulation, for epistaxis in hereditary hemorrhagic telangiectasia, 222
Artery
ethmoid, anterior, ligation for epistaxis, 215
maxillary, internal, transantral ligation for epistaxis, 215
sphenopalatine (*see* Sphenopalatine artery)
Arthritis, septic, of temporomandibular joint, 111
Arthrocentesis, in temporomandibular joint syndrome, 120
Arthroplasty, in temporomandibular joint syndrome, 121
Arthroscopy, in temporomandibular joint syndrome, 120
Arthrotomy, in temporomandibular joint syndrome, 120
Aspergillus
fumigatus in otitis externa, 169
niger in otitis externa, 169
Aspiration biopsy, fine-needle
in thyroid cancer, medullary, 92
of thyroid nodule, solitary, 75-76
Aspirin discontinuation, before male rhytidectomy, 242
Asthma
gastroesophageal reflux disease in infants and children and, 64
sinusitis in cystic fibrosis and, 46
Atresia, choanal, repair, powered instrumentation for, in children, 32-33

Attention deficit disorder, and sleep-disordered breathing in children, 4-5
Auditory hallucinations, in narcolepsy in children, 10
Augmentin, for draining ear, 177
Autoregistration headset, with InstaTrak stereotactic system, 148

B

Bacteriology, of draining ear, 168-169
Barium swallow, in diagnosis of gastroesophageal reflux disease in infants and children, 58
Behavior, improvement after treatment for sleep-disordered breathing in children, 5
Behavioral treatment
of narcoleptic children, 12
of temporomandibular joint syndrome, 119
Biofeedback therapy, for temporomandibular joint syndrome, 119
Biopsy
esophageal, in diagnosis of gastroesophageal reflux disease in infants and children, 58
fine-needle aspiration
in thyroid cancer, medullary, 92
of thyroid nodule, solitary, 75-76
Bone scans, in temporomandibular joint syndrome, 117
Botulinum toxin, in chronic facial paralysis, 237
Bragg Peak, 135, 163
Branchio-oto-renal syndrome, molecular genetics of, 205-206

Breathing, sleep-disordered, in children, 3-7
Brow lifting, endoscopic, in chronic facial paralysis, 235
Brown-Roberts-Wells stereotactic frame, 132

C

Calcitonin
  persistently elevated, in medullary thyroid cancer, management, 95-96
  serum, in diagnosis of medullary thyroid cancer, 76, 92
Cancer, thyroid (*see* Thyroid, cancer)
Candida albicans, in otitis externa, 169
Carcinoma, thyroid (*see* Thyroid, cancer)
Cartesian coordinate(s)
  in stereotactic surgery, 130-132
  system, 162
Cartilage, tracheal, invasion by thyroid cancer, management, 82
Cataplexy, in narcolepsy in children, 8-9
Celecoxib, in temporomandibular joint syndrome, 118
Central nervous system
  hypersomnia, idiopathic, in children, 15-16
  stimulants for narcolepsy in children, 12-14
Cervical lymph nodes, in thyroid cancer, management, 80-81
CF protein, 41
Children
  adenoidectomy in, powered instrumentation for, 33-36
    partial, 36
  antrochoanal polyps in, powered instrumentation for, 31-32

breathing in, sleep-disordered, 3-7
choanal atresia repair in, powered instrumentation for, 32-33
cystic fibrosis in (*see* Cystic fibrosis)
delayed sleep phase syndrome in, 16-17
ear in, draining (*see* Draining ear)
gastroesophageal reflux disease in (*see* Gastroesophageal reflux disease in infants and children)
hypersomnia in, idiopathic CNS, 15-16
Lothrop procedure in, modified transnasal endoscopic, 29-30
mucoceles in, powered instrumentation for, 31
narcolepsy in (*see* Narcolepsy in children)
periodic limb movements disorder in, 17-18
respiratory papillomatosis in, powered instrumentation for, 36-37
restless leg syndrome in, 17-18
sinus surgery in, powered instrumentation for
  endoscopic, 26-27
  endoscopic, standard functional, 27-29
  frontal, 29-30
  sphenoid, 30-31
sleep in
  disorders of, management, 1-24
  normal, 2-3
sleepiness in, excessive daytime, causes of, 14-18
thyroid carcinoma in, differentiated, management, 83-84
Choanal atresia repair, powered instrumentation for, in children, 32-33

Chromosome(s)
  genetic diseases and, 184-189
  homologous, in meiosis,
    recombination between, 192
  locations of genes for hereditary
    hearing loss on male
    karyotype, 185
Chronotherapy, for delayed sleep
  phase syndrome in children,
  16
Cimetidine, for gastroesophageal
  reflux disease in infants and
  children, 68
Cisapride, for gastroesophageal
  reflux disease in infants and
  children, 68
Cleaning, of draining ear in office
  treatment, 166-168
Clomipramine, for narcolepsy in
  postpubertal teenagers, 13-14
Coagulation, laser, for epistaxis in
  hereditary hemorrhagic
  telangiectasia, 221-222
Coherent LightSheer laser system
  for hair modification, 261
  posttreatment histology, 262-263
Collimator helmet, in gamma knife
  radiosurgery, 136, 137
Computed tomography (*see* CT)
Computer
  imaging in male rhytidectomy,
    243
  power, Moore's Law graph
    depicting exponential
    growth over past 3 decades,
    130
Congenital abnormalities, of
  temporomandibular joint,
  114
Connective tissue disorders,
  temporomandibular joint in,
  114
Connexin 26 gene, causing hearing
  loss, 195, 198

Corticosteroids (*see* Steroids)
Cough, chronic, and gastroesophageal
  reflux disease in infants and
  children, 61
Cranial
  fossa, middle, frameless stereotactic
    surgery in, 148-151
  nerve, twelfth to seventh
    anastomosis, end-to-end, for
      chronic facial paralysis,
      231-232
    anastomosis, side-to-end, for
      chronic facial paralysis,
      228-229, 230
    graft, interposition, for chronic
      facial paralysis, 229-231, 232
Craniomandibular disorder,
  discussion of term, 108
Croup, recurrent or spasmodic,
  and gastroesophageal reflux
  disease in infants and
  children, 64-65
CT
  scanners in future stereotactic
    surgery, 156-157
  in sinusitis in cystic fibrosis, 41-42
  in temporomandibular joint
    syndrome, 117
  in thyroid cancer long-term
    follow-up, 91
Cx26 gene, causing hearing loss,
  195, 198
Cyclotron generators, 135
Cystic fibrosis
  diagnosis, 43-45
    criteria for, 44
    phenotypic features consistent
      with, 44
  gene therapy in, 50-51
  lung transplantation in, 48-49
  sinonasal symptoms in, 45
  sinus surgery in, powered
    instrumentation for, in
    children, 31

sinusitis in (*see* Sinusitis, in cystic fibrosis)
transmembrane conductance regulator, 41

D

Daytime sleepiness, excessive, causes of, in children, 14-18
Delayed sleep phase syndrome, in children, 16-17
Demineralization, of unicate process in cystic fibrosis, 42
Deoxyribonuclease I, aerosolized recombinant, in cystic fibrosis, 50
Depression
  delayed sleep phase syndrome and, in adolescence, 16
  temporomandibular joint pain and, 110
Desipramine, for cataplexy in children, 14
Development abnormalities, of temporomandibular joint, 114
Diet, mechanical soft, for temporomandibular joint syndrome, 118
Diphosphonates, technetium-99m, bone scans in temporomandibular joint syndrome with, 117
Disk, temporomandibular joint displacement, 110
  repositioning surgery, 120
DNase, aerosolized recombinant, in cystic fibrosis, 50
Dornase alfa, in cystic fibrosis, 50
Draining ear
  bacteriology, 168-169
  office treatment of, 165-181
    cleaning of ear in, 166-168
    examination in, 166-168

ophthalmic preparations for, 172-174
otic preparations for, new, 176
otic preparations for, standard, 170-171
ototopical, 169, 175
patient history in, 166
powder preparations for, 177
systemic, 177-178
Drug(s)
  anti-inflammatory, nonsteroidal, in temporomandibular joint syndrome, 118
  for otomycosis, 178
  therapy (*see* Pharmacotherapy)
Dysphagia, oropharyngeal, and gastroesophageal reflux disease in infants and children, 62

E

Ear, draining (*see* Draining ear)
EDN3 mutations, in Waardenburg syndrome, 205
EDNRB mutations, in Waardenburg syndrome, 205
Ehlers-Danlos syndrome, temporomandibular joint in, 114
Electrolysis, 255-256
  posttreatment histology, 264
Electrothermolysis, 255-256
Embolization, angiographic, for epistaxis, 214
Embryology, temporomandibular joint, 108-109
Emotional
  disturbances in adolescents with narcolepsy, 12
  facial movement, restoration in chronic facial paralysis, 226
Endocrine neoplasia, multiple, type 2, medullary thyroid cancer in, 92-93

Endoscopic
  brow lifting in chronic facial
    paralysis, 235
  ligation of sphenopalatine artery
    for epistaxis (*see*
    Sphenopalatine artery ligation
    for epistaxis, endoscopic)
  Lothrop procedure, modified
    transnasal, in children, 29-30
  sinus surgery
    with antimicrobial lavage, serial,
      for sinusitis in cystic fibrosis,
      47-48
    after lung transplantation in
      cystic fibrosis, 49
    powered instrumentation for, in
      children, 26-27
    for sinusitis in cystic fibrosis,
      46-47
    standard functional, powered
      instrumentation for, in
      children, 27-29
  transsphenoidal surgery, frameless
    stereotactic, 151-155
Enterobacter species, in chronic
  otitis media, 168
Epilaser system, hair modification
  with, 259
Epistaxis
  risk factors, 213-214
  in telangiectasia, hereditary
    hemorrhagic, management,
    221-222
  treatment, 213-223
    nonsurgical, 214
    surgical, 214-215
Epitouch laser, hair modification
  with, 259-260
Escherichia coli, in chronic otitis
  media, 168
Esophageal biopsy, in diagnosis of
  gastroesophageal reflux
  disease in infants and
  children, 58

Ethmoid artery, anterior, ligation
  for epistaxis, 215
Examination
  of draining ear for office treatment,
    166-168
  physical
    before rhytidectomy, male, 242
    in temporomandibular joint
      syndrome evaluation, 116
EYA1 gene, in branchio-oto-renal
  syndrome, 206

F

Facelift, subperiosteal, historical
  review, 241
Facial
  movement
    emotional, restoration in chronic
      facial paralysis, 226
    volitional, restoration in chronic
      facial paralysis, 226
  nerve
    function, preservation in
      gamma knife radiosurgery
      for acoustic neuroma, 145
    grafting in chronic facial
      paralysis, 228
    paralysis (*see* Facial, paralysis
      below)
  paralysis, chronic, 225-238
    anastomosis for, twelfth to
      seventh end-to-end, 231-232
    anastomosis for, twelfth-to-
      seventh side-to-end,
      228-229, 230
    ancillary procedures in,
      235-237
    brow lifting in, endoscopic, 235
    implants in, autologous and
      nonautologous, 236-237
    management, contemporary,
      225-238
    muscle transfers for, temporalis,
      masseter, or free, 232-235

nerve interposition graft for, twelfth to seventh, 229-231, 232
rhytidectomy in, deep-plane or tri-plane, 235-236
Fascia flap, temporoparietal, for donor site camouflage after temporalis muscle transfer, 233, 234
Fat injections, in chronic facial paralysis, 236
Fibrosis, cystic (*see* Cystic fibrosis)
Fiducial, in stereotactic surgery, 133, 162
Fitzpatrick classification, of skin types, 260
Fixation sutures, midface, in male rhytidectomy, 247
Flap
elevation for male deep plane rhytidectomy, 246
temporoparietal fascia, for donor site camouflage after temporalis muscle transfer, 233, 234
Fluoroquinolone agents, otic, 175
Fluoxetine
for cataplexy in children, 14
for narcolepsy, in postpubertal teenagers, 13-14
Follicle, hair, anatomy and physiology, 254-255
Foramen, sphenopalatine, localization for endoscopic sphenopalatine artery ligation for epistaxis, 217
Fossa
middle cranial, frameless stereotactic surgery in, 148-151
pterygopalatine, sphenopalatine artery course after bone removal in, 219

Frame
-based stereotactic surgery, 134-135
stereotactic, Horsley and Clarke's, illustration, 129
Frontal sinus surgery, powered instrumentation for, in children, 29-30
Fundoplication, for gastroesophageal reflux disease in infants and children, 69
Fusobacterium species, in chronic otitis media, 168

G

Gallium citrate scintigraphy, in temporomandibular joint syndrome, 117
Gamma-hydroxybutyrate, for narcolepsy in children, 13
Gamma knife radiosurgery, 135-146, 162
in acoustic neuroma, 139-141
case reports, 139-144
discussion, 144-146
helmet in, collimator, 137
in meningioma, recurrent papillary, 141-144
radiobiology in, 136-137
technique, 137-139
technology, 136-137
Gamma Plan software and workstation, 136
Gamma rays, 162
Gastroesophageal reflux disease in infants and children
airway obstruction and, 63
apnea and, 63-64
asthma and, 64
Children's Hospital of Pittsburgh study, 58-60
cough and, chronic, 61
croup and, recurrent or spasmodic, 64-65

Gastroesophageal reflux disease in
    infants and children *(cont.)*
diagnosis, 57-58
discussion and review of
    literature, 60-68
effects on otolaryngologic
    disorders, 57-73
globus pharyngeus and, 62
hoarseness and, 61-62
laryngitis and, 61-62
laryngomalacia and, 65-66
oropharyngeal dysphagia and, 62
otalgia and, 63
otitis and, 63
pseudolaryngomalacia and, 66-67
rhinopharyngitis and, 60-61
Sandifer's syndrome and, 60
sinusitis and, chronic, 60-61
sore throat and, chronic, 62-63
stridor and, 66-67
subglottic stenosis and, 67-68
throat clearing and, 61-62
treatment, 68-69
vocal cord granulomas and
    ulcers and, 63
vocal cord nodules and, 61-62
Generators, cyclotron, 135
Gene(s)
carriers in medullary thyroid
    cancer, prophylactic surgery
    for, 96-97
Connexin 26, causing hearing
    loss, 195, 198
EDN3, mutations in
    Waardenburg syndrome, 205
EDNRB, mutations in
    Waardenburg syndrome, 205
EYA1, in branchio-oto-renal
    syndrome, 206
hearing impairment, cloned
    syndromic, 202-203
for hearing loss, hereditary, chro-
    mosomal locations of genes
    on male karyotype for, 185

hearing loss, methods of
    identifying, 189-194
KCNE1, mutations in Jervell
    Lange-Nielsen syndrome,
    204
KCNQ1, mutations in Jervell
    Lange-Nielsen syndrome,
    204
KCNQ4, mutations causing hearing
    loss, 198
MITF, mutations in Waardenburg
    syndrome, 205
MYO7A, mutations causing
    hearing loss
    nonsyndromic, 198
    in Usher syndrome, 204
MYO15, mutations causing non-
    syndromic hearing loss, 198
PAX3, mutations in Waardenburg
    syndrome, 205
PDS, mutations causing hearing
    loss, 201
    in Pendred syndrome, 198
single-gene inheritance, basic,
    pedigree patterns of, 187, 188
SOX10, mutations in
    Waardenburg syndrome, 205
TECTA, mutations causing
    hearing loss, 200
therapy in cystic fibrosis, 50-51
Genetic
diseases, and chromosomes,
    184-189
linkage, 190
Genetics
molecular
    of branchio-oto-renal syndrome,
        205-206
    of hearing impairment,
        mitochondrial, 206-207
    of hearing loss, hereditary,
        183-212
    of hearing loss, nonsyndromic,
        194-200

of hearing loss, syndromic, 200-206
of Jervell Lange-Nielsen syndrome, 204
of neurofibromatosis type II, 206
of Pendred syndrome, 201
of Usher syndrome, 204
of Waardenburg syndrome, 205
of narcolepsy in children, 11
Genotype analysis, in cystic fibrosis, 43
Gentle LASE, hair modification with, 261
Globus pharyngeus, and gastroesophageal reflux disease in infants and children, 62
Glucose abnormalities, after prednisone in cystic fibrosis, 50
Gore-Tex implant in chronic facial paralysis, 236-237
for donor site camouflage after temporalis muscle transfer, 233, 234
Gracilis free muscle transfer, for chronic facial paralysis, 234-235
Graft, interposition nerve, twelfth to seventh, for chronic facial paralysis, 229-231, 232
Grafting, facial nerve, in chronic facial paralysis, 228
Granulomas, vocal cord, and gastroesophageal reflux disease in infants and children, 63
Growth retardation, after prednisone in cystic fibrosis, 50

H

H$_2$ blockers, for gastroesophageal reflux disease in infants and children, 68

Haemophilus influenzae, in otorrhea from tympanostomy tubes, 168
Hair
follicle, anatomy and physiology, 254-255
modification
electrolysis for, 255-256
electrothermolysis for, 255-256
laser (*see* Laser, hair modification)
pulsed light, 256-257
reduction, long-term, definition, 262, 264
Hairline alterations, after male rhytidectomy, 249
Hallucinations in narcolepsy in children
auditory, 10
visual hypnagogic, 9-10
Hardware, for future stereotactic systems, 156-157
Head
Mounted Display in future stereotactic surgery, 157-158
and neck surgery, stereotactic advances in, 127-163
Headache in cystic fibrosis, 45
after endoscopic sinus surgery, 46-47
Headset, autoregistration, with InstaTrak stereotactic system, 148
Hearing
impairment
genes, cloned nonsyndromic, 199
genes, cloned syndromic, 202-203
loci, autosomal dominant, nonsyndromic, 196
loci, autosomal recessive, nonsyndromic, 197

Hearing *(cont.)*
  loci, X-linked, nonsyndromic,
    198
  mitochondrial, molecular
    genetics of, 206-207
  loss
  in branchio-oto-renal syndrome,
    molecular genetics of,
    205-206
  genes, methods of identifying,
    189-194
  hereditary, genes for,
    chromosomal locations on
    male karyotype for, 185
  hereditary, molecular genetics
    of, 183-212
  hereditary, nonsyndromic,
    molecular genetics of,
    194-200
  in Jervell Lange-Nielsen
    syndrome, molecular genetics
    of, 204
  in neurofibromatosis type II,
    molecular genetics of, 206
  in Pendred syndrome, molecular
    genetics of, 201
  syndromic, molecular genetics
    of, 200-206
  in Usher syndrome, molecular
    genetics of, 204
  in Waardenburg syndrome,
    molecular genetics of, 205
Helmet, collimator, in gamma
  knife radiosurgery, 136, 137
Hematoma, after male rhytidectomy,
  249
Hemoclips, in endoscopic
  sphenopalatine artery ligation
  for epistaxis, 220
Hemorrhagic telangiectasia,
  hereditary, management of
  epistaxis in, 221-222
Hemostatic effect, of hot water
  irrigation for epistaxis, 214

History
  patient, in office treatment of
    draining ear, 166
  in temporomandibular joint
    syndrome, 115
HLA class II typing, in narcolepsy
  in children, 11
Hoarseness, and gastroesophageal
  reflux disease in infants and
  children, 61-62
Hormone, thyroid, postoperative
  suppression in thyroid
  cancer, 87
  with aerodigestive tract
    involvement, 81
Horsley and Clarke's stereotactic
  frame, illustration, 129
Hot water irrigation, for epistaxis,
  214
y-Hydroxybutyrate, for narcolepsy
  in children, 13
Hypersomnia, idiopathic CNS, in
  children, 15-16
Hypertension, and epistaxis, 214
Hypnagogic hallucinations, visual,
  in narcolepsy in children,
  9-10
Hypocretin levels, in narcoleptic
  children, 11
Hypokalemia, after omeprazole for
  gastroesophageal reflux
  disease in children, 69
Hyponatremia, after omeprazole
  for gastroesophageal reflux
  disease in children, 69

I

Ibuprofen, in cystic fibrosis, 49
Imaging
  (*See also* Scanning)
  computer, in male rhytidectomy,
    243
  magnetic resonance (*see*
    Magnetic resonance imaging)

studies in temporomandibular
joint syndrome, 116-117
Imipramine, for cataplexy in
children, 14
Implants in chronic facial paralysis
autologous and nonautologous,
236-237
Gore-Tex, 236-237
Incisions, in male rhytidectomy,
244, 245
Indium-111 DTPA-Phe-octreotide
scintigraphy, in thyroid cancer
long-term follow-up, 91
Infant
gastroesophageal reflux disease
in (*see* Gastroesophageal
reflux disease in infants and
children)
mucoceles in cystic fibrosis in,
42
Inheritance, basic single-gene,
pedigree patterns of, 187,
188
InstaTrak system, 147-148
Instrumentation, powered (*see*
Powered instrumentation)
Interleukin
-1ß and temporomandibular joint
pain, 109
-6 and temporomandibular joint
pain, 109
Interposition nerve graft, twelfth
to seventh, in chronic facial
paralysis, 229-231, 232
Iodine, radioactive (*see*
Radioiodine)
Iontophoresis sweat test,
pilocarpine, for cystic
fibrosis, 43
Irrigation, hot water, for epistaxis,
214
ISG Viewing Wand, 146
Isocenter, in gamma knife
radiosurgery, 136, 162

Isodose line, in stereotactic
surgery, 162

J

Jervell Lange-Nielsen syndrome,
molecular genetics of, 204
Joint, temporomandibular (*see*
Temporomandibular joint)

K

Karyotype, male, chromosomal
locations of genes for
hereditary hearing loss on,
185
KCNE1 mutations, in Jervell
Lange-Nielsen syndrome,
204
KCNQ1 mutations, in Jervell
Lange-Nielsen syndrome, 204
KCNQ4 mutations, causing hearing loss, 198
Kerrison rongeur, fine-tip, in
endoscopic sphenopalatine
ligation for epistaxis, 217, 218
Knife, gamma knife radiosurgery
(*see* Gamma knife
radiosurgery)

L

Laboratory studies, in
temporomandibular joint
syndrome, 116
Lamina papyracea, and power
instrumentation for
endoscopic sinus surgery in
children, 29
Laryngeal nerve, recurrent, in thyroid
cancer, management, 81
Laryngitis, reflux, in infants and
children, 61-62
Laryngomalacia, and
gastroesophageal reflux
disease in infants and
children, 65-66

Laser
  coagulation for epistaxis in
    hereditary hemorrhagic
    telangiectasia, 221-222
  hair modification, 253-269
    dynamic cooling in, 258
    fluence in, 257
    microwave technology for,
      261-262
    number of treatments, 258
    patient selection for, 262-268
    pulse width in, 257-258
    results, photographs, 265, 266,
      267, 268
    separating fact from fiction,
      268-269
    systems *(see below)*
    wavelength in, 257
  hair modification system(s),
    258-262
    Alexandrite, 261
    diode, 261
    flash lamp, 261
    LightSheer, posttreatment
      histology, 262-263
    Nd:YAG, 258-259
    ruby, 259-260
Laserscope Lyra system, hair
    modification with,
    posttreatment histology,
    263-264
Lavage, serial antimicrobial, with
    endoscopic sinus surgery in
    cystic fibrosis, 47-48
  after lung transplantation, 49
Law, Moore's, 130, 162
Leg, restless leg syndrome, in
    children, 6, 17-18
Leksell stereotactic frame, 132
Lift
  brow, endoscopic, in chronic
    facial paralysis, 235
  face, subperiosteal, historical
    review, 241

Light, pulsed light hair modification,
    256-257
LightSheer laser system for hair
    modification, 261
    posttreatment histology,
    262-263
Limb, periodic limb movements
    disorder, in children, 6,
    17-18
LINAC unit, 134, 135, 162
Linear accelerators, in frame-based
    stereotactic surgery, 134-135
Liothyronine, and radioiodine
    therapy in thyroid cancer, 85
Lipid-laden alveolar macrophages,
    and gastroesophageal reflux
    disease in infants and
    children, 58
Lithium, and radioiodine therapy
    in thyroid cancer, 85-86
Lothrop procedure, modified
    transnasal endoscopic, in
    children, 29-30
Lung transplantation, in cystic
    fibrosis, 48-49
Lymph nodes, cervical, in thyroid
    cancer, management, 80-81

M

Macrophages, lipid-laden alveolar,
    and gastroesophageal reflux
    disease in infants and
    children, 58
Magnetic resonance imaging
  in gamma knife radiosurgery, 138
  of meningioma, recurrent
    papillary, 142
  of pituitary tumor, 152
  in temporomandibular joint
    syndrome, 117
  in thyroid cancer long-term
    follow-up, 91
  units, "open", in future stereotactic
    surgery, 156-157

Masseter muscle transfer, for
chronic facial paralysis,
232-234
Mathematics, of 3-D perception,
exploration by René
Descartes, 131
Matrix metalloproteinases, and
temporomandibular joint
pain, 109
Maxillary
artery, internal, transantral
ligation for epistaxis, 215
sinus volume after endoscopic
sinus surgery in cystic
fibrosis, 47
Mazindol, for narcolepsy in
children, 13
Meatal antrostomy, large middle,
creation in endoscopic
sphenopalatine artery
ligation for epistaxis, 216
Meiosis, 190-191
recombination between
homologous chromosomes
in, 192
Melatonin, for delayed sleep
phase syndrome in children,
16-17
MEN 2, medullary thyroid cancer
in, 92-93
Meningioma, recurrent papillary,
gamma knife radiosurgery
in, 141-144
Metalloproteinases, matrix, and
temporomandibular joint
pain, 109
Metastases, cervical lymph node,
in thyroid cancer,
management, 80-81
Methylphenidate, for narcolepsy
in children, 12
Metoclopramide, for gastroesophageal reflux disease in
infants and children, 68

Microdébrider system, power, in
children, 25-39
Microsurgical ligation, of
sphenopalatine artery for
epistaxis, 215
Microwave technology, for hair
modification, 261-262
MITF mutations, in Waardenburg
syndrome, 205
Mitochondrial hearing impairment,
molecular genetics of,
206-207
Modafinil in children
for hyperinsomnia, idiopathic
CNS, 15-16
for narcolepsy, 13
Molecular genetics (*see* Genetics,
molecular)
Moore's Law, 130, 162
Moraxella catarrhalis, in otorrhea
from tympanostomy tubes,
168
Mouth breathing, and sleep-
disordered breathing in
children, 3
MRI (*see* Magnetic resonance
imaging)
Mucoceles
in cystic fibrosis, 42
powered instrumentation for, in
children, 31
Multiple sleep latency test in
children
in hypersomnia, idiopathic CNS,
15
in narcolepsy, 10-11
in sleep-disordered breathing, 5
Muscle
rectus, medial, and power
instrumentation for
endoscopic sinus surgery in
children, 29
relaxants for temporomandibular
joint syndrome, 118

Muscle *(cont.)*
transfers, temporalis, masseter, or free, for chronic facial paralysis, 232-235
Musculoaponeurotic system, superficial, in midface, description of, 240
MYO7A mutations causing hearing loss
nonsyndromic, 198
in Usher syndrome, 204
MYO15 mutations, causing non-syndromic hearing loss, 198
Myofascial pain and dysfunction, discussion of term, 108

N

Narcolepsy in children, 7-14
clinical presentation, 8-10
diagnosis, 10-11
HLA class II typing and genetics in, 11
treatment
behavioral, 12
pharmacologic, 12-14
strategies, 12-14
Narcotics, for temporomandibular joint syndrome, 118
Nasal
obstruction in cystic fibrosis, 45
potential difference measurements in diagnosis of cystic fibrosis, 43, 45
Nd:YAG laser
coagulation for epistaxis in hereditary hemorrhagic telangiectasia, 221
hair modification with, 258-259
Neck
dissection with thyroidectomy in thyroid cancer, 80-81
surgery, stereotactic advances in, 127-163

Neoplasia *(see* Tumors)
Nerve
cranial *(see* Cranial, nerve)
facial
grafting, in chronic facial paralysis, 228
paralysis *(see* Facial, paralysis)
graft, interposition, twelfth to seventh, for chronic facial paralysis, 229-231, 232
laryngeal, recurrent, in thyroid cancer, management, 81
Nervous system, central
hyperinsomnia, idiopathic, in children, 15-16
stimulants, for narcolepsy in children, 12-14
Neurofibromatosis, type II, molecular genetics of hearing loss in, 206
Neuroma, acoustic, gamma knife radiosurgery in, 139-141
Night terrors, and sleep-disordered breathing in children, 4
Nightmares, and sleep-disordered breathing in children, 4
Nodules
thyroid, solitary, diagnostic evaluation, 75-77
vocal cord, and gastroesophageal reflux disease in infants and children, 61-62
Noise, temporomandibular joint, in TMJ syndrome, 110
NSAIDs, in temporomandibular joint syndrome, 118

O

Octreotide scintigraphy, indium-111, in thyroid cancer long-term follow-up, 91
Office treatment of draining ear *(see* Draining ear, office treatment of)

Ofloxacin, for draining ear, 177
Omeprazole, for gastroesophageal
    reflux disease in infants and
    children, 69
Ophthalmic preparations, for
    office treatment of draining
    ear, 169, 172-174
Oropharyngeal dysphagia, and
    gastroesophageal reflux
    disease in infants and
    children, 62
Osler-Weber-Rendu disease,
    management of epistaxis in,
    221-222
Osteoma, temporomandibular
    joint, 114
Otalgia, and gastroesophageal
    reflux disease in infants and
    children, 63
Otic preparations for office
    treatment of draining ear
    new, 176
    standard, 169, 170-171
Otitis
    externa, bacteriology, 169
    gastroesophageal reflux disease
        in infants and children and, 63
    media, chronic, bacteriology, 168
Otolaryngologic disorders, effects
    of gastroesophageal reflux on,
    in infants and children, 57-73
Otolaryngology
    pediatric, powered instrumentation
        in, 25-39
    stereotactic advances in, 127-163
Otomycosis, agents used in, 178
Otosclerosis, genetics of, 200
Ototopical treatment, of draining
    ear, 169, 175

P

Pain, myofascial pain and
    dysfunction, discussion of
    term, 108

Palate, narrow and high-arched,
    and sleep-disordered breathing
    in children, 4-5
Papillary meningioma, recurrent,
    gamma knife radiosurgery
    in, 141-144
Papillomatosis, recurrent
    respiratory, powered
    instrumentation for, in
    children, 36-37
Paralysis
    facial (*see* Facial, paralysis)
    sleep, in narcolepsy, in children,
        9
Paranasal sinus infection, after
    lung transplantation for
    cystic fibrosis, 49
PAX3 mutations, in Waardenburg
    syndrome, 205
PDS mutations causing hearing
    loss, 201
    in Pendred syndrome, 198
Pedigree patterns, of basic single-
    gene inheritance, 187, 188
Pemoline, for narcolepsy in
    children, 12-13
Pendred syndrome, molecular
    genetics of, 201
Penicillin, for draining ear, 177
Peptostreptococcus species, in
    chronic otitis media, 168
Pergolide, for periodic limb move-
    ments disorder and restless
    leg syndrome in children, 17
Periodic limb movements disorder,
    in children, 6, 17-18
PET
    scanner, 162
    in future stereotactic surgery, 156
    in thyroid cancer long-term
        follow-up, 91
pH probe, 24-hour, in diagnosis of
    gastroesophageal reflux disease
    in infants and children, 58

Pharmacologic therapy (*see* Pharmacotherapy)

Pharmacotherapy
  for gastroesophageal reflux disease in infants and children, 68-69
  for narcolepsy in children, 12-14
  for temporomandibular joint syndrome, 118, 119

Phenotypic features, consistent with diagnosis of cystic fibrosis, 44

Photographs, in male rhytidectomy, 243

Phototherapy, for delayed sleep phase syndrome in children, 16

Physical
  examination
    before rhytidectomy, male, 242
    in temporomandibular joint syndrome evaluation, 116
  therapy for temporomandibular joint syndrome, 118-119

Physiology, hair follicle, 254-255

Pilocarpine iontophoresis sweat test, for cystic fibrosis, 43

Piperacillin, for sinusitis in cystic fibrosis, 48

Pituitary tumor, MRI of, 152

Pixel, in stereotactic surgery, 131, 162

Polar coordinate systems, in stereotactic surgery, 132, 163

Polygraphic monitoring, in diagnosis of idiopathic CNS hypersomnia, in children, 15

Polypectomy, for sinusitis in cystic fibrosis, 46

Polyps, antrochoanal, powered instrumentation for, in children, 31-32

Polysomnogram in children
  in narcolepsy, 10
  in sleep-disordered breathing, 5

Porphyromonas species, in chronic otitis media, 168

Positron emission tomography (*see* PET)

POU4F3 mutations, causing hearing loss, 200

Powder preparations, for office treatment of draining ear, 177

Powered instrumentation in children, 25-39
  for adenoidectomy, 33-36
    partial, 36
  for antrochoanal polyps, 31-32
  for choanal atresia repair, 32-33
  for mucoceles, 31
  for respiratory papillomatosis, recurrent, 36-37
  for sinus surgery
    in cystic fibrosis, 31
    endoscopic, 26-27
    endoscopic, standard functional, 27-29
    frontal, 29-30
    sphenoid, 30-31

Pramipexole, for periodic limb movements disorder and restless leg syndrome in children, 17

Precision, in stereotactic surgery, 146, 163

Prednisone, alternate-day, in cystic fibrosis, 49-50

Pregnancy, thyroid cancer during, 84

Prevotella species, in chronic otitis media, 168

Prokinetic agents, for gastroesophageal reflux disease in infants and children, 68

Protein, CF, 41

Proteus mirabilis, in chronic otitis media, 168

Proton, in stereotactic surgery, 135, 163

Proto-oncogene mutations, *ret,* in hereditary medullary thyroid cancer, 93-94

Pseudolaryngomalacia, and gastroesophageal reflux disease in infants and children, 66-67

Pseudomonas aeruginosa
  in otitis externa, 169
  in otitis media, chronic, 168
  in otorrhea from tympanostomy tubes, 168
  infection after lung transplantation for cystic fibrosis, 49

Psychological therapies, for temporomandibular joint syndrome, 119

Psychosocial etiologies, of temporomandibular joint syndrome, 114-115

Pterygopalatine fossa, sphenopalatine artery course after bone removal in, 219

Pulmozyme, in cystic fibrosis, 50

Pulsed light hair modification, 256-257

R

Radiobiology, in gamma knife radiosurgery, 136-137

Radiography, in temporomandibular joint syndrome, 117

Radioiodine
  scanning in long-term follow-up of thyroid cancer, 89
  therapy, postoperative, in thyroid cancer, 85-86
  for aerodigestive involvement, 81

Radionuclide scanning, of solitary thyroid nodule, 76

Radiosurgery
  gamma knife (*see* Gamma knife radiosurgery)
  stereotactic, 163

Radiotherapy
  external beam postoperative, in thyroid cancer, 87-88
  with aerodigestive tract involvement, 81
  medullary, 95
  stereotactic, 134, 163

Ranitidine, for gastroesophageal reflux disease in infants and children, 68

Recombination, 191
  between homologous chromosomes in meiosis, 192

Rectus muscle, medial, and power instrumentation for endoscopic sinus surgery in children, 29

Reflux, gastroesophageal (*see* Gastroesophageal reflux)

Registration, in stereotactic surgery, 132-133, 163

REM sleep onset, early, in narcolepsy in children, 8

Respiratory papillomatosis, recurrent, powered instrumentation for, in children, 36-37

Restless legs syndrome, in children, 6, 17-18

ret proto-oncogene mutations, in hereditary medullary thyroid cancer, 93-94

Retinoic acid, and radioiodine therapy in thyroid cancer, 86

Rhinopharyngitis, and gastroesophageal reflux disease in infants and children, 60-61

Rhytidectomy
  composite, historical review, 240

Rhytidectomy *(cont.)*
  deep-plane
    in facial paralysis, chronic,
      235-236
    historical review, 240
    in men, 245
    in men, flap elevation for, 246
  historical review, 240-241
  male, 239-251
    incisions in, 244
    intraoperative considerations,
      244-248
    postoperative considerations,
      248-249
    preoperative considerations,
      241-243
    sutures in, midface fixation,
      247
  triplane, in chronic facial paralysis,
    235-236
Robotics, active stereotactic, 157
Rofecoxib, in temporomandibular
  joint syndrome, 118
Rongeur, fine-tip, in endoscopic
  sphenopalatine ligation for
  epistaxis, 217, 218
Ruby laser, hair modification with,
  259-260

S

Sandifer's syndrome, and
  gastroesophageal reflux
  disease in infants and
  children, 60
Scanners
  CT, in future stereotactic surgery,
    156-157
  PET, 162
    in future stereotactic systems,
      156
Scanning
  (See also Imaging)
  bone, in temporomandibular
    joint syndrome, 117

octreotide, indium-111, in thyroid
  cancer long-term follow-up,
  91
radioiodine, in long-term follow-
  up of thyroid cancer, 89
radionuclide, of solitary thyroid
  nodule, 76
tetrofosmin, technetium-99m, in
  thyroid cancer long-term
  follow-up, 91
thallium-201, in thyroid cancer
  long-term follow-up, 91
Scintigraphy *(see* Scanning)
Scintiscans, in diagnosis of
  gastroesophageal reflux
  disease in infants and
  children, 58
Septic arthritis, of
  temporomandibular joint,
  111
Sinonasal symptoms, in cystic
  fibrosis, 45
Sinus
  frontal, surgery, powered
    instrumentation for, in
    children, 29-30
  maxillary, volume after endoscopic
    sinus surgery in cystic fibrosis,
    47
  paranasal, infection after lung
    transplantation for cystic
    fibrosis, 49
  sphenoid, surgery, powered
    instrumentation for, in
    children, 30-31
  surgery, endoscopic, powered
    instrumentation for, in
    children, 26-27
    standard functional, 27-29
Sinusitis
  chronic, and gastroesophageal
    reflux disease in infants and
    children, 60-61
  in cystic fibrosis, 41-55

endoscopic sinus surgery with
serial antimicrobial lavage
for, 47-48
management, 41-55
management, medical, 45
management, surgical, 45-47
treatment, new, 49-50
Skin types, Fitzpatrick classification
of, 260
Sleep
delayed sleep phase syndrome in
children, 16-17
-disordered breathing in children,
3-7
disorders in children,
management, 1-24
latency test, multiple (*see*
Multiple sleep latency test)
normal childhood, 2-3
paralysis in narcolepsy in
children, 9
position, and sleep-disordered
breathing in children, 4
REM, early onset, in narcolepsy
in children, 8
Sleepiness, excessive daytime,
causes of, in children, 14-18
SMAS, in midface, description of,
240
Smoking discontinuation, before
male rhytidectomy, 242
Snoring, and sleep-disordered
breathing in children, 4
Software
future, for stereotactic systems, 157
Gamma Plan, 136
Sore throat, chronic, and gastroesophageal reflux disease in
infants and children, 62-63
SOX10 mutations, in Waardenburg
syndrome, 205
Speech defects, and sleep-
disordered breathing in
children, 3

Sphenoid sinus surgery, powered
instrumentation in, in
children, 30-31
Sphenopalatine artery ligation for
epistaxis, 215
endoscopic
clinical experience, 221
hemoclips in, 220
meatal antrostomy creation in,
large middle, 216
sphenopalatine artery course in
pterygopalatine fossa after
bone removal in, 219
sphenopalatine foramen
localization in, 217
technique, 215-220
microsurgical, 215
sphenopalatine foramen
localization in, 217
Splint therapy, for temporomandibular joint syndrome,
118
Staphylococcus aureus
in otitis
externa, 169
media, chronic, 168
in otorrhea from tympanostomy
tubes, 169
Stenosis, subglottic, and gastroesophageal reflux disease in
infants and children, 67-68
Stereoendoscope, Vista, 159
Stereotactic
advances in otolaryngology—
head and neck surgery,
127-163
developments, future, 156-158
accessories for, 157-158
hardware for, 156-157
software for, 157
frame, Horsley and Clarke's,
illustration, 129
principles, 129-133
radiosurgery, 163

Stereotactic *(cont.)*
  radiotherapy, 134, 163
  robotics, active, 157
  surgery
    Cartesian coordinates in,
      130-132
    discussion of term, 127
    frame-based, 134-135
    frameless *(see below)*
    functional, 128, 162
    historical developments,
      128-129
    registration in, 132-133
  surgery, frameless, 146-155,
    162
    case reports, 148-155
    in cranial fossa, middle, 148-151
    discussion, 155
    endoscopic transsphenoidal,
      151-155
    systems, 147
    technique, 147-148
    technology, 146-147
  technology, 129-130
Steroids in cystic fibrosis
  inhaled, 50
  oral, 49-50
  topical nasal, 45
Streptococcus
  pneumoniae in otorrhea from
    tympanostomy tubes, 168
  in otorrhea from tympanostomy
    tubes, 168
Stridor, and gastroesophageal
  reflux disease in infants and
  children, 66-67
Subglottic stenosis, and
  gastroesophageal reflux
  disease in infants and
  children, 67-68
Submalar implants, in chronic
  facial paralysis, 236
Subperiosteal facelift, historical
  review, 241

Superficial musculoaponeurotic
  system, in midface,
  description of, 240
Sutures, midface fixation, in male
  rhytidectomy, 247
Swallowing difficulties, and sleep-
  disordered breathing in
  children, 3
  for cystic fibrosis, 43
Sweating, nocturnal, and sleep-
  disordered breathing in
  children, 4

T

Technetium-99m
  diphosphonates, bone scans in
    temporomandibular joint
    syndrome with, 117
  tetrofosmin scintigraphy in
    thyroid cancer long-term
    follow-up, 91
Technology
  gamma knife radiosurgery,
    136-137
  stereotactic, 129-130
  stereotactic surgery, frameless,
    146-147
TECTA mutations, causing hearing
  loss, 200
Telangiectasia, hereditary
  hemorrhagic, management
  of epistaxis in, 221-222
Temporalis muscle transfer, for
  chronic facial paralysis,
  232-234
Temporomandibular joint
  anatomy, 108-109
  arthritis, septic, 111
  embryology, 108-109
  noise in TMJ syndrome, 110
  replacement, artificial, for TMJ
    syndrome, 121
  syndrome, 107-125
  diagnosis, 107-125

diagnosis, differential, 115-117
etiologies, intracapsular and
extracapsular, 112-113
evaluation, 115-117
history in, 115
imaging studies in, 116-117
laboratory studies in, 116
management, 107-125
medications for, 118
pathogenesis, 109-115
physical examination in, 116
signs, 109-115
symptoms, 109-115
syndrome, treatment, 117-121
medical, 118-119
nonsurgical, 118-119
surgical, 119-121
Temporoparietal fascia flap, for
donor site camouflage after
temporalis muscle transfer,
233, 234
Tetrofosmin scintigraphy,
technetium-99m, in thyroid
cancer long-term follow-up, 91
Thallium-201 scintigraphy, in
thyroid cancer long-term
follow-up, 91
Therabite, for temporomandibular
joint syndrome, 119
Thermal relaxation time, in laser
hair modification, 258
3-D perception, mathematics of,
exploration by René
Descartes, 131
Throat
clearing and gastroesophageal
reflux disease in infants and
children, 61-62
sore, chronic, and gastroesophageal
reflux disease in infants and
children, 62-63
Thyroglobulin, serum, in long-
term follow-up of thyroid
cancer, 89-90

Thyroid
cancer, 75-106
aerodigestive tract involvement
in, management, 81-83
differentiated, in children and
adolescents, management,
83-84
follow-up, long-term, 88-91
follow-up, long-term, other
diagnostic modalities in,
90-91
follow-up, long-term, radioiodine
scanning in, 89
follow-up, long-term, serum
thyroglobulin in, 89-90
laryngeal nerve in, recurrent,
management, 81
lymph nodes in, cervical,
management, 80-81
management, 75-106
management, surgical, 78-84
medullary (*see below*)
in pregnancy, 84
radioiodine therapy in, adjuvant,
85-86
radiotherapy for, external beam
postoperative, 87-88
staging, 77-78
thyroid hormone suppression
in, adjuvant, 87
thyroidectomy for, outpatient,
83
treatment, adjuvant, 84-88
cancer, medullary, 91-97
calcitonin in, persistently
elevated, management, 95-96
gene carriers in, prophylactic
surgery for, 96-97
radiotherapy in, adjuvant, 95
ret proto-oncogene mutations
in, 93-94
surgical management, initial, 95
carcinoma (*see* Thyroid, cancer
above)

Thyroid *(cont.)*
  hormone suppression,
    postoperative, in thyroid
    cancer, 87
  for aerodigestive tract
    involvement, 81
  nodule, solitary, diagnostic
    evaluation, 75-77
Thyroidectomy in thyroid cancer,
    78-80
  medullary, 95
  as prophylactic surgery in gene
    carriers, 96-97
  outpatient, 83
Tissue, connective tissue disorders,
    temporomandibular joint in,
    114
Tobramycin, for sinusitis in cystic
    fibrosis, 47-48
Tomography
  computed *(see* CT)
  positron emission *(see* PET)
Toxin, botulinum, in chronic
    facial paralysis, 237
Tracheal cartilage invasion by
    thyroid cancer, management,
    82
Transcription factor *POU4F3*
    mutations, causing hearing
    loss, 200
Transplantation, lung, in cystic
    fibrosis, 48-49
Transsphenoidal surgery, frameless
    stereotactic endoscopic,
    151-155
Tubes, tympanostomy, bacteriology
    of otorrhea from, 168-169
Tumor(s)
  endocrine, multiple, type 2,
    medullary thyroid cancer in,
    92-93
  necrosis factor and temporo-
    mandibular joint pain, 109
  pituitary, MRI of, 152

temporomandibular joint, 114
Tympanostomy tubes,
  bacteriology of otorrhea
  from, 168-169

U

Ulcers, vocal cord, and gastroesophageal reflux disease in
  infants and children, 63
Ultrasound
  -guided fine-needle aspiration
    biopsy of solitary thyroid
    nodule, 76
  intraoperative, in future
    stereotactic surgery, 156
  in thyroid cancer follow-up,
    long-term, 90
  of thyroid nodule, solitary, 77
Unicate process demineralization,
  in cystic fibrosis, 42
Usher syndrome, molecular genetics
  of, 204

V

Vista head-mounted display, in
  future stereotactic systems,
  157-158
Vista stereoendoscope, 159
Visual hypnagogic hallucinations,
  in narcolepsy in children,
  9-10
Vocal cord
  granulomas and gastroesophageal
    reflux disease in infants and
    children, 63
  nodules and gastroesophageal
    reflux disease in infants and
    children, 61-62
  ulcers and gastroesophageal
    reflux disease in infants and
    children, 63
Voice recognition software, in
  future stereotactic systems,
  158

Volitional facial movement, restoration in chronic facial paralysis, 226

Voxel, in stereotactic surgery, 131, 163

W

Waardenburg syndrome, molecular genetics of, 205

Water, hot water irrigation for epistaxis, 214

X

X-linked hearing-impairment loci, nonsyndromic, 198

Y

YAG laser
Nd:
coagulation for epistaxis in hereditary hemorrhagic telangiectasia with, 221
hair modification with, 258-259